On-Call Geriatric Psychiatry

Ana Hategan • James A. Bourgeois
Calvin H. Hirsch
Editors

On-Call Geriatric Psychiatry

Handbook of Principles and Practice

Springer

Editors

Ana Hategan
Department of Psychiatry and
Behavioural Neurosciences
Division of Geriatric Psychiatry
McMaster University
Hamilton, Ontario
Canada

Calvin H. Hirsch
Department of Internal Medicine
Division of General Medicine
University of California Davis
Sacramento, California
USA

James A. Bourgeois
Department of Psychiatry/Langley Porter
Psychiatric Institute
University of California San Francisco
San Francisco, California
USA

ISBN 978-3-319-30344-4 ISBN 978-3-319-30346-8 (eBook)
DOI 10.1007/978-3-319-30346-8

Library of Congress Control Number: 2016938224

Printed on acid-free paper

This Springer imprint is published by Springer Nature
The registered company is Springer International Publishing AG Switzerland

We dedicate this book to the aging adults around the world who grow old along with us.

Foreword

An older man sits in the waiting room of a busy emergency department. He has refused to eat for 3 days, hardly speaks to family, and fainted at his home, prompting his family to bring him in for an evaluation. He saw his primary care physician 1 month prior who diagnosed "depression." She prescribed sertraline for him and scheduled an appointment to see him at 6 weeks for follow-up. "It will take that long to determine if the medication is working." The man took the medicine for a week then stopped because he did not think it was working. Therefore, in the ED sits this older man with his daughter for 3 h waiting to be seen. The daughter had no idea of where else she can turn.

When the on-call psychiatrist arrives, what does she do? Does the patient need hospitalization? Is another prescription in order? Are beds available if admission is required? Will the patient and family agree for him to be admitted? If not, is commitment appropriate? If outpatient treatment is the best next step, to whom does the on-call psychiatrist refer the patient? Where does the responsibility of the on-call psychiatrist end and another provider's begin, that is, how does the provider assure a safe clinical handover? If, as is often the case, a geriatric psychiatrist or even a psychiatrist is not available, who will make the diagnosis and provide the care needed? What must these providers know in order to provide adequate care? These questions must be answered and care provided within the context of the busy, fast-paced environment of an emergency department. The same issues arise for on-call psychiatry in a general hospital, on an inpatient psychiatric unit, not to mention in the outpatient setting.

The historical practice of psychiatry, at its best, was slow medicine, practiced by a physician who works in a setting that encourages time to listen and follow a patient closely.[1] On-call psychiatry is embedded in fast medicine, and our practice must be embedded within this context. Practitioners therefore can be thankful for this excellent book edited by Ana Hategan, James Bourgeois, and Calvin Hirsch which calls out this unique yet critical slice of psychiatric practice so often neglected. I am not aware of a book which addresses the specific needs of on-call psychiatry (though there are a number of books on emergency psychiatry – not quite the same). The

[1]Victoria Sweet. God's Hotel: A Doctor, a Hospital, and a Pilgrimage To the Heart of Medicine. New York, Riverhead Books, 2012

book is a hefty one, yet the authors and editors have provided many aids to permit the practitioner to find essential information quickly.

The first such aid is a series of clinical pearls. These highlighted paragraphs provide the reader the type of insights that a seasoned practitioner conveys to a student on rounds, historically one of the foundations for the training of physicians. At the end of each chapter, a list of key points can be found which provide a quick summary of the main points of the chapter. Clinical vignettes are sprinkled throughout the book, and these bring the real world of on-call psychiatry continually to the attention of the reader. We have neglected the value of the "case report" in our journals and textbooks in recent years in favor of empirical data. These case reports bring to life the world of the psychiatrist and other practitioners who finds themselves on call at night or over a weekend or during the midst of a busy clinical day.

Among the aids available, however, I would especially call to the reader's attention the tables and figures. For example, the tables in Chap. 12 provide a primer for much of what is needed when evaluating the side effects of psychotropic drugs and the ever central issue of drug-drug interactions that are so critical given the polypharmacy experienced by older adults. The reader could gain much by simply looking through these tables periodically as a method of keeping critical information necessary for competent practice ever before him.

No foreword can do justice to the wealth of useful and practical guidance in this book. Yet I want to focus on a few critical issues which I believe to be especially relevant yet undervalued by those who provide mental health care in on-call situations. The first, which is sprinkled throughout the book, is the importance of teamwork. Those who write texts can easily emphasize teamwork in theory, yet these writers provide numerous examples of how teamwork can be practiced in the service of patients during emergent situations.

In Chap. 2, the authors emphasize the importance of the physical exam. No on-call psychiatrist can assume that a thorough physical exam has been performed, especially in an emergency department or in an outpatient clinic. If the patient is agitated, unruly, or abusive, the physical is easily neglected. Not only must the on-call practitioner have the skills to perform the physical (and obtain necessary lab work), that practitioner must also have the skill to calm the patient so that a physical exam can be performed with consent. The need to approach the patient with dignity and a plea for cooperation is emphasized in Chap. 5. The authors call practitioners to an anti-oppressive approach (respect of the patient). In a fast-moving on-call situation where time is of the essence, it is so easy to be authoritative (and some emphatic decision-making is necessary). Yet an autocratic approach may not only undermine the immediate attempts to intervene, it may also reduce the chances that a patient and family will seek emergency help in the future, perhaps leading to tragic consequences because of delay in obtaining adequate care. First impressions are critical impressions, and the on-call psychiatrist is an exemplar of first impressions. In addition, such an approach is just the right thing to do.

Emergency departments are locations of risk for older adults. In Chap. 16, the major issue of boarding in the ED (keeping patients on hold for days and perhaps even weeks) is highlighted, and the risk for adverse consequences is clearly noted.

To the medical community at large, not to mention the public, this inhumane and ineffective way to manage psychiatric patients is a major public health challenge. Emergency departments are dangerous places for older adults with psychiatric disorders when patients are boarded, even though they may be lifesaving in an acute situation.

In Chap. 25, the authors focus upon suicide and violence. Though any practitioner working with older adults should be acutely aware of the high rates of suicides among white males, we tend to forget the possibility of violence in elders. Just recently I read of a person murdered in a long-term care facility by a roommate, probably due to agitation resulting from cognitive impairment. The authors are to be commended in recognizing this potential critical problem and providing guidance, a public health approach to guidance, that can be implemented. Though we cannot predict accurately when a violent act will occur any more than we can predict a heart attack, we can take steps to reduce the risk.

The psychiatric community should be thankful that this resource is now available and thankful that these thoughtful clinicians have devoted their time to providing guidance for practitioners who are "on call."

Durham, NC, USA Dan Blazer, MD, MPH, PhD

Preface

With the worldwide graying of the population, owing to lower birth rates (in many countries) combined with longer lifespan due to management of infectious diseases, diabetes mellitus, stroke, and heart and renal diseases, clinicians urgently need to enhance their skills in managing older, sicker patients, in whom complex age-related physiology and psychosocial needs interact with multiple comorbidities and their treatment. Added to this is the longer life expectancy of patients diagnosed with schizophrenia and bipolar disorder with modern psychiatric treatment, plus greater surveillance and interventions for neurocognitive disorders. Despite these trends, access to inpatient geriatric psychiatric beds remains tragically limited. All of this conspires to increase the likelihood that clinicians will encounter (while on call to cover various healthcare institutions) geriatric psychiatric urgencies and emergencies. Drawing on the current clinical literature in geriatric psychiatry and psychosomatic medicine, the chapter authors have endeavored to provide a current, pragmatic, and concise guide to the expedient clinical assessment and management of the various clinical problems encountered in on-call geriatric psychiatry.

The after-hours setting offers specific challenges, as consultants are expected to exhibit a high degree of competence and confidence in approaching complex clinical situations. In particular, medical trainees (resident physicians and medical students alike) and other mental health professionals may have limited experience in geriatric psychiatry. Due to the shortage of psychiatrists available to provide on-call consultation in many care delivery systems, on-call clinical urgencies in the management of psychiatric illness in geriatric patients are the province of many medical specialists, nurse practitioners, physician assistants, and other health professionals. As such, the editors hope that many clinicians will (we hope) find this volume useful. Similarly, we hope that this volume serves as a concise refresher for other psychiatrists (e.g., general adult psychiatrists, child and adolescent psychiatrists), who may primarily be office- or clinic-based, but may occasionally see geriatric patients in an on-call circumstance. All this is to make the geriatric psychiatry subspecialty more accessible and less daunting to clinicians who do not see geriatric and/or consultation-liaison cases that often but need to be able to function capably "when the time comes."

This handbook refers to the care provided to an older adult, or geriatric patient, and to evidence-based contemporary care strategies. It covers basic principles and practice tips for on-call psychiatric and general medical care of the geriatric psychiatric patient in various institutional settings, where an on-call clinician may be required to provide care for conditions and in circumstances that differ from accustomed daily practice, approach the boundaries of clinical expertise, or invade the clinician's comfort zone. In particular, crisis and on-call interventions in care settings may require the psychiatry resident physician or the psychiatric consultant:

(i) To evaluate the psychiatric patients in the emergency department and if needed admit them to the inpatient psychiatric units
(ii) To respond to any urgent psychiatric consults called in by another inpatient medical service
(iii) To respond to any medical or psychiatric urgencies on the inpatient psychiatric units
(iv) To manage on-call psychiatric consultation requests at other care institutions, e.g., nursing facilities, rehabilitation units

An older adult is not just a person who is age 65 years or older. Socioeconomically challenged adults (including homeless and incarcerated persons), as well as those with chronic substance abuse, may physiologically age more rapidly than their age-matched, less disadvantaged counterparts in the community. An adult who is younger than age 65 can be a victim of elder mistreatment if the circumstances of abuse relate to dependence on others due to developmental or acquired physical or mental disability. This book also covers the utility of contemporary technology, such as telepsychiatry/telemedicine, which can overcome geographic and transportation barriers by making state-of-the-art geriatric psychiatric consultation available to clinicians and their patients at clinics remote from consulting psychiatrist. The medicolegal context for the practice of medicine is also ever changing. Decisions such as to allow natural death and advance directives, the use of restraint, and seclusion, among others, are complex and strictly regulated.

The editors were motivated to mobilize our many chapter authors to compose this concise on-call geriatric psychiatry handbook based on years of experience in geriatric psychiatry (AH), medical center-based psychosomatic medicine and emergency psychiatry (JAB), and geriatric internal medicine (CHH). *On-Call Geriatric Psychiatry*: *Handbook of Principles and Practice* compiles resources to help clinicians respond effectively to the types of calls they are likely to encounter regarding geriatric patients, details a pragmatic approach to diagnosing and managing psychiatric illness in these often patients, facilitates communicating with colleagues and patients' families, and helps clinicians avoid common pitfalls that arise from these calls. Finally, we are deeply grateful to our many chapter authors from various professional disciplines, who care for geriatric patients in a variety of institutional settings, and to our patients, who are our ultimate teachers and without whom this volume would not be possible.

Hamilton, ON, Canada — Ana Hategan, MD
San Francisco, CA, USA — James A. Bourgeois, OD, MD
Sacramento, CA, USA — Calvin H. Hirsch, MD

Contents

Contributors

Mariam Abdurrahman, MD, MSc, Dip (GHEI) Department of Psychiatry, St. Joseph's Health Centre, Toronto, ON, Canada

Daniel L. Ambrosini, LLB/BCL, MSc, PhD Legal Counsel, St. Joseph's Healthcare Hamilton, Hamilton, ON, Canada

Department of Psychiatry and Behavioural Neurosciences, Forensic Psychiatry Program, McMaster University, Hamilton, ON, Canada

Rebecca Anglin, MD, PhD Department of Psychiatry and Behavioural Neurosciences, McMaster University, Hamilton, ON, Canada

Division of Gastroenterology, Department of Medicine, McMaster University, Hamilton, ON, Canada

Debra Bakerjian, PhD, APRN, FAAN, FAANP NP/PA Clinical, Education and Practice, Betty Irene Moore School of Nursing, University of California, Davis, Sacramento, CA, USA

Lauren S. Barney, BA, JD St. Joseph's Healthcare Hamilton, Hamilton, ON, Canada

Julia Baxter, BSc. HK, MHS Department of Psychiatry and Behavioural Neurosciences, McMaster University, Hamilton, ON, Canada

James A. Bourgeois, OD, MD Department of Psychiatry/Langley Porter Psychiatric Institute, University of California San Francisco, San Francisco, CA, USA

Consultation-Liaison Service, University of California San Francisco Medical Center, San Francisco, CA, USA

Gary Chaimowitz, MD Department of Psychiatry and Behavioural Neurosciences, Division of Forensic Psychiatry, McMaster University, Hamilton, ON, Canada

Simon Chiu, MD, PhD Department of Psychiatry, Lawson Health Research Institute, University of Western Ontario, London, ON, Canada

James M. Ellison, MD, MPH Swank Foundation Endowed Chair in Memory Care and Geriatrics, Christiana Care Health System, Wilmington, MA 19801, USA

Research Associate, McLean Hospital, Belmont, MA 02478, USA

Howard H. Fenn, MD Department of Psychiatry and Behavioral Sciences, Stanford University, Stanford, CA, USA

Deborah C. Francis, RN, MSN, GCNS-BC Geriatric Clinical Nurse Specialist Co-Chair Bioethics Committee, Kaiser Permanente South Sacramento Medical Center, Sacramento, USA

Claudia Garcia, MD Post-graduate Medical Education, Department of Psychiatry, University of Toronto, Toronto, ON, Canada

Lisebeth Gatkowski, RN, BScN St. Joseph' Healthcare Hamilton, Faculty Mohawk College of Applied Arts & Technology, Institute for Applied Health Sciences at McMaster, Hamilton, ON, Canada

Caroline Giroux, MD Department of Psychiatry and Behavioral Sciences, APSS Stockton Clinic, University of California, Davis Health System, Sacramento, CA, USA

Psychiatry and Behavioral Sciences, UC Davis Medical Center, University of California, Davis Health System, Sacramento, CA, USA

Jeremy Goldberg, MD Department of Psychiatry and Behavioural Neurosciences, McMaster University, Hamilton, ON, Canada

Randi Hagerman, MD Department of Pediatrics, University of California Davis Medical Center, Sacramento, CA, USA

University of California MIND Institute, Sacramento, CA, USA

Sheila Harms, MD Department of Psychiatry and Behavioural Neurosciences, Faculty of Health Sciences, Michael G. Degroote School of Medicine, McMaster University, McMaster University Medical Centre, Hamilton Health Sciences Corporation, Hamilton, ON, Canada

Ana Hategan, MD Department of Psychiatry and Behavioural Neurosciences, Division of Geriatric Psychiatry, Michael G. DeGroote School of Medicine, Faculty of Health Sciences, McMaster University, Hamilton, ON, Canada

Donald M. Hilty, MD Department of Psychiatry and Addiction Medicine, Kaweah Delta Medical Center and Keck School of Medicine at USC, Visalia, CA, USA

Calvin H. Hirsch, MD Department of Internal Medicine, Division of General Medicine, University of California Davis Medical Center, Sacramento, CA, USA

Ashkan Javaheri, MD, CMD Mercy Medical Group, Geriatric Division, University of California at Davis School of Medicine, Sacramento, CA, USA

Tara La Rose, MSW, PhD Social Work Program, Trent University, Oshawa, ON, Canada

Margaret W. Leung, MD, MPH Department of Palliative Care Services, Kaiser Permanente, Roseville, CA, USA

Andrew Ligsay, MD University of California, Davis School of Medicine and MIND Institute, Sacramento, CA, USA

Emily MacKillop, PhD, ABPP Department of Psychiatry and Behavioural Neurosciences, McMaster University, Hamilton, ON, Canada

Shyam Maharaj, BSc. Pharm, PhD Department of Psychiatry and Behavioural Neurosciences, McMaster University, Hamilton, ON, Canada

Kolja Paech, MD Kaiser Permanente, Roseville, CA, USA

Usha Parthasarathi, MBBS Department of Psychiatry and Behavioural Neurosciences, McMaster University, St. Joseph's Healthcare, Hamilton, ON, Canada

Sebastien Prat, MD Department of Psychiatry and Behavioural Neurosciences, McMaster University, Hamilton, ON, Canada

Terry Rabinowitz, MD, DDS Division of Consultation Psychiatry and Psychosomatic Medicine, Psychiatry and Family Medicine, Telemedicine, University of Vermont College of Medicine, University of Vermont Medical Center, Burlington, VT, USA

Jason G. Roof, MD Division of Psychiatry and the Law, Department of Psychiatry and Behavioral Sciences, University of California, Davis Medical Center, Sacramento, CA, USA

Karen Saperson, MBChB Department of Psychiatry and Behavioural Neurosciences, Division of Geriatric Psychiatry, Faculty of Health Sciences, Michael G. Degroote School of Medicine, McMaster University, St. Joseph's Healthcare, Hamilton, ON, Canada

Lorin M. Scher, MD Department of Psychiatry, University of California Davis, Davis, CA, USA

W. Edwin Smith, MD Department of Psychiatry, Saint John Regional Hospital, Dalhousie and Memorial Universities, Saint John, NB, Canada

Sidney R. Stacey, MHSc, FCCHL, FACHE Department of Psychiatry and Behavioural Neurosciences, Faculty of Health Sciences, McMaster University, St. Joseph's Healthcare, Hamilton, ON, Canada

Dane E. Stevenson, MD, MS Department of Emergency Medicine, University of California Davis, Davis, CA, USA

Katren Tyler, MD Geriatric Emergency Medicine Fellowship Director, Department of Emergency Medicine, University of California, Davis, Sacramento, CA, USA

Albina Veltman, MD Department of Psychiatry and Behavioural Neurosciences, McMaster University, Hamilton, ON, Canada

Ilse R. Wiechers, MD, MPP, MHS Psychotropic Drug Safety Initiative, Office of Mental Health Operations, Department of Veterans Affairs, Northeast Program Evaluation Center, West Haven, CT, USA

Department of Psychiatry, Yale University School of Medicine, West Haven, CT, USA

Tricia Woo, MD Division of Geriatric Internal Medicine, McMaster University, Hamilton, ON, Canada

Glen L. Xiong, MD, CMD Department of Psychiatry and Behavioral Sciences, University of California at Davis, Sacramento, CA, USA

Department of Psychiatry and Behavioral Sciences, University of California, Davis Medical Center, Sacramento, CA, USA

Elmira Yessengaliyeva, MD Department of Psychiatry and Behavioral Sciences, Stanford University, Stanford, CA, USA

Part I

On-Call Geriatric Psychiatry: General Principles and Clinical Practice

Psychiatric Examination 1

Ana Hategan and James A. Bourgeois

1.1 Background

The psychiatric examination is a process of gathering information about a patient with the purpose of making a diagnosis, which is a prerequisite for any treatment process. This can be performed in an institutional (emergency department, inpatient unit, or skilled nursing home) setting, ambulatory (outpatient) setting, or community (as a home-based assessment performed by a mobile crisis team) setting. A description of these settings with the common on-call or crisis chief complaints for a clinician to encounter is detailed elsewhere in this book (see Part III).

The on-call psychiatric examination of the geriatric patient, particularly in hospital settings, is typically a multidisciplinary process, with contributions from various clinicians (e.g., nurses, social workers, crisis counselors). An on-call nursing assessment includes (1) a risk assessment (e.g., risk of suicide and self-harm, aggression, elopement from hospital, sexual safety in hospital, medication adherence) and (2) obtaining background personal and health information from geriatric patients being evaluated and/or their caregivers. The immediate purpose of the nursing assessment is to determine the required level of care and supervision and to determine an immediate plan to manage disturbed behavior until the patient is being

A. Hategan, MD (✉)
Department of Psychiatry and Behavioural Neurosciences, Division of Geriatric Psychiatry, Michael G. DeGroote School of Medicine, Faculty of Health Sciences, McMaster University, Hamilton, ON, Canada
e-mail: ahategan@stjosham.on.ca

J.A. Bourgeois, OD, MD
Department of Psychiatry/Langley Porter Psychiatric Institute, University of California San Francisco, San Francisco, CA, USA

Consultation-Liaison Service, University of California San Francisco Medical Center, San Francisco, CA, USA

A. Hategan et al. (eds.), *On-Call Geriatric Psychiatry: Handbook of Principles and Practice*, DOI 10.1007/978-3-319-30346-8_1

assessed by the on-call physician. The on-call psychiatric consultant takes a history and performs a mental status examination and physical examination as described below. Most on-call psychiatric examinations, which are performed under the constraints of time, tend to be more directed than the routine, more comprehensive psychiatric examinations. Although on-call clinicians resort to traditional patient interview techniques, they often solicit input from family members, home caregivers, nursing staff, and other clinicians.

1.2 The On-Call Psychiatric Examination and General Principles

The on-call psychiatric examination of the geriatric patient incorporates all aspects of a routine psychiatric assessment including demographic data, chief complaint, history of present illness, past and current psychiatric and medical illnesses, family and social history, mental status examination, and physical and laboratory examination. On-call clinicians can find it challenging to obtain objective historical information, especially when it is subject to geriatric patients with impaired cognition and the lack of reliable informants. It is prudent to note your assessment of the historian's objectivity and reliability. The clinician must determine whether the patient responds to initial questions and can provide a coherent history. Otherwise, information is sought from family members, community caregivers and caseworkers, or other collateral sources (e.g., nursing staff and other clinicians). Even when a patient is communicative, caseworkers, family members, and friends may provide additional information that the patient has omitted. With limited exceptions (such as duty to warn/protect), the clinician cannot disclose patient information to collateral sources without the patient's or (in the case of an incompetent patient) substitute decision-maker's permission. Receiving information from collateral sources does not violate patient confidentiality. However, clinicians should follow the usual caution of not "keeping secrets" from competent patients. Therefore, the clinician reserves the right to tell the competent patient all information *with attribution of source(s)*, the principle being "clinicians do not keep secrets from patients." Previous psychiatric assessments, treatments, and degree of adherence to past treatments are reviewed, and relevant medical records are obtained as soon as possible.

Clinical Pearl

Conducting an interview with closed-ended questions (following a more rigid system review) often precludes patients from revealing relevant information. It is advisable to begin the interview with a relatively open-ended question to elicit the patient's chief complaint or primary concern.

The principal tasks for on-call clinicians in conducting a psychiatric examination in geriatric patients are summarized in Fig. 1.1.

Tasks for the on-call clinician

- Establish rapport
- Communicate emphatically
- Maintain appropriate boundaries
- Adjust the interview style according to patient's situation; optimize sensory function
- Shorten the interview for acutely agitated, aggressive patients
- Use open-ended questions to increase depth of understanding
- Use close-ended questions to increase breadth of understanding
- Assess patient's education, language, and cultural needs; use a translator if necessary
- Verify that patient understands and hears you
- Assess patient and informant reliability
- Assess patient safety (suicide risk, dangerousness); develop a safety plan
- Cover all key elements of the psychiatric examination
- Review advance directives and end-of-life care
- Review available medical records/test results before assessment is completed
- Formulate the data gathered and develop a biopsychosocial formulation
- Formulate a differential diagnosis
- Develop a treatment plan
- Verify that the patient understands the plan and affords treatment
- Document if patient refuses treatment
- Assess capacity to make treatment decisions
- Establish follow-up plans
- Document accurately

Fig. 1.1 Main tasks for on-call clinicians conducting a psychiatric examination in geriatric patients

1.3 Biographical and Demographic Data

A standard part of any psychiatric examination is obtaining of biographical and demographic data. This includes the patient's name, age, address, first language, education achievement, housing and financial status, marital status, and family contact details.

1.4 Chief Complaint and Present Illness

The on-call clinician should first explore (1) what prompted the need for psychiatric examination of a patient (e.g., unwanted or unpleasant emotions or thoughts, undesirable or unsafe behavior), (2) the extent to which the presenting symptoms affect the patient or interfere with the patient's social and interpersonal functioning, and (3) the required legal hospitalization status of the patient. The account of present illness describes the onset, nature, and development of the patient's current symptoms. The clinician further attempts to gain a broader perspective on the patient's personality by reviewing significant life events (current and past) and the patient's responses to them. This may reveal personality traits that may "get better," or adaptive, with time (e.g., emotional stability, agreeableness, conscientiousness), or maladaptive (e.g., decreased openness to experience, dependency), which may explain the current coping mechanisms employed [1, 2]. Focusing only on the presenting symptoms may result in omitting psychiatric comorbidities. Therefore, a review of systems (ROS) to check for concurrent psychiatric syndromes is essential and helps with the differential diagnosis. In addition, the general medical ROS provides important information about the physical symptoms of psychiatric disorders (e.g., changes in appetite, weight, energy, sleep) and somatic expressions of psychiatric disorders (e.g., pain complaints, physical symptoms without clear physiological explanation).

It is important to remember that, unlike their younger counterparts, geriatric patients rarely present with a clearly identifiable diagnosis. Geriatric patients may seek medical attention complaining of unspecific physical symptoms (e.g., vague, unspecific abdominal pain or discomfort) or no complaints at all (due to fear or denial). They may not seek medical attention for perceived "trivial" complaints, such as insomnia. This is for several reasons, including (1) interpretation of their emotional, memory, or sleep dysfunction as "normal" signs of aging, (2) predilection for complex pathophysiology presenting in clinically complex ways in geriatric age, (3) communication barriers or hearing impairment, or (4) cultural incompatibilities, which may contribute to an inadequate description of the chief complaint and present illness. Being familiar with common screening tools used specifically in the geriatric population for identifying various psychiatric syndromes is essential for the on-call practice (see Chap. 10 for details on the screening tools and their utility).

1.5 Past Psychiatric History

This includes an exploration of the patient's past diagnoses, including substance use, previously prescribed treatments (e.g., pharmacotherapy, somatic treatments, psychotherapies), and hospitalizations. The patient should also be asked about attitudes regarding pharmacotherapy and psychotherapy, so that this information can be incorporated into the management plan.

1.6 Past Medical History and Medications

This section of the geriatric psychiatric examination is similar to the information obtained from other patient populations. However, patients and their caregivers may not recall important details from medical or surgical events taking place several decades ago. It is essential for the on-call clinician to readily have access to electronic medical records from multiple sources. Polypharmacy is common in geriatric patients (see Chap. 3). Careful documentation of all current medications (prescription and over the counter), doses, indications, and side effects is greatly recommended.

1.7 Family History

Family history provides useful information about known diagnoses and familial predisposition to diseases that are virtually always late in onset (e.g., major neurocognitive disorder (NCD) due to Alzheimer's disease – formerly dementia).

1.8 Social History

The social evaluation comprises information ranging from a patient's developmental, educational, and employment history to advance directives and views on end-of-life care. For most on-call clinical settings, this is a complex area to cover. One or several members of the medical team (e.g., nurses, social workers, counselors) will often collect socially relevant information during the encounter with the patient before being seen by the psychiatric consultant. The on-call psychiatric examination must explicitly incorporate some critical points of a social evaluation, which will be enlisted below.

1.8.1 Employment History

It is important to remember that enjoying retirement is a legitimate "vocation." Many older adults who have retired from their careers continue to work part time or volunteer. This facilitates personal accomplishment, community connections, and financial independence, all of which are potential determinants of health [3].

1.8.2 Living Arrangements and Social Supports

One of the on-call assessment's roles is the determination of appropriate living arrangements. There are three basic types of living arrangements for geriatric patients, such as (1) private homes in the community, (2) assisted living residences, and (3) skilled nursing facilities and nursing homes. Some geriatric patients may have no fixed address, such is the case of homelessness, which requires immediate social work intervention (see Chap. 27). Respite stay is a short-term (usually about 2 weeks) type of admission in which patients living at home occupy a nursing home bed. It is important to ask about the extent and quality of social networks, including cohabitants, number of children and the frequency of their visits, and involvement of close relatives, friends, and reliable neighbors, both to determine the level of interpersonal support and to evaluate for the possibility of caregiver stress. Ask about abusive behavior directed at the patient. Elder mistreatment (or elder abuse) may take the form of physical, psychological, financial, and sexual abuse and neglect (see Chaps. 13 and 14). The patient is also often a caregiver to a disabled family member. Ask whether the caregiver's responsibilities cause stress or unacceptable loss of independence.

1.8.3 Sexual History

Older adults maintain a sexual life, and, thus, sexually transmitted infections, including human immunodeficiency virus (HIV), are relevant to explore in those at increased risk [4]. Sexual dysfunction, diminished libido, and dyspareunia are common with age, despite geriatric patients' own reservations to raise the subject. A nonjudgmental, open-ended question inviting the geriatric patient to share information may be best [4] (e.g., "Part of my interview is to ask the patient about all important areas of function, including sexual function. What would you like to tell me about your sexual life?"). More detailed questions can follow once a dialogue has been initiated.

1.8.4 Lifestyle Choices

Patients are routinely asked about lifestyle choices and behaviors (e.g., regular exercise, alcohol drinking, sleep habits) that may place them at risk of harm. If specific behaviors have distinct relevance to the chief complaint, the clinicians include it in the present illness section.

1.8.5 Response to Life Adversities

Recent psychosocial stressors such as the death of a spouse, friend, or family member, retirement, or extrication from a community can be factors associated with increased rates of depression and mortality in the geriatric population and warrant full exploration [3].

1.8.6 Access to Community Services

Clinicians should inquire about the patient's access to community services. In-home support includes physician house calls, visiting nurses, home health aides, meals on wheels, and paid homemakers. Out-of-home support comprises adult day centers and group counseling services. Community-based healthcare services involve primary care physicians, ambulatory care centers, and rehabilitation facilities.

1.8.7 Functional Performance

Functional performance is assessed at two levels: (a) instrumental activities of daily living (IADLs) (e.g., driving or ability to use public transportation, shopping, meal preparation, telephone skills, housework, laundry, medication administration, handling finances) and (b) basic activities of daily living (ADLs) (e.g., bathing, dressing, transferring, feeding, toileting, continence). Ask who helps patients perform each specific task.

Clinical Pearl
Performance-based screens can be readily available to the on-call clinician to incorporate into their on-call medical practice. An occupational therapy and/or social work assessment, either in hospital or in-home environment, can help reveal patient's level of functioning, support at home, or eligibility for assistance programs.

Physicians frequently find themselves in the position of determining whether the patients are fit to drive due to medical conditions (e.g., NCDs, vision impairment, or treatment-related adverse effects). Inquire whether the patient has a valid driver's license, how many traffic violations, accidents, and related injuries there have been in the past year.

1.8.8 Advance Directives

Clinicians must have an open discussion with patients and their family about their views on therapeutic interventions and end-of-life care. Review of advance directives (such as identification of a healthcare proxy) to guide the future decisions of physicians and family members is essential.

1.9 Mental Status Examination

The mental status examination (MSE) represents a cross-sectional description of a patient's current state of mind. The data are collected through a combination of direct and indirect methods of observation and questions to evaluate several domains of mental function, including appearance, behavior, speech, mood and affect, thought process, thought content, perception, cognition, insight, and judgment. Brief standardized screening questionnaires are available for assessing certain components of the MSE (see Fig. 10.2). Standardized assessments can help identify the chief symptoms and provide a baseline for measuring response to treatment, but such tools cannot take the place of a detailed MSE. Since time constraints can preclude a detailed evaluation of the on-call psychiatric examination, a thorough MSE is, however, essential to obtain.

1.9.1 General Appearance and Behavior

Observation of the general appearance can provide evidence of underlying psychiatric disorders ("Is the patient malnourished, unkempt, disheveled, or dressed inappropriately for the weather?"). The behavior may reveal evidence of attitudes and feelings denied by the patient ("Does the patient pace back and forth despite denying anxiety, worry, concern, or "nervousness"?"; "Does the patient seem sad, "down," or "blue" despite denying feelings of depression?"; "Has the patient engaged in substance abuse and/or attempted self-harm?," when they have an odor of alcohol and/or self-inflicted injury, respectively). Patients can appear (1) actively violent (assaulting staff members, throwing or breaking things), (2) belligerent and hostile (e.g., potentially violent), or (3) not threatening to the clinicians but express intent to harm another person (which should trigger an assessment of homicidal ideation).

1.9.2 Speech

Clinicians should note the patient's rate, volume, and prosody of speech (i.e., variation in intonation, melody, accents, and vocal quality). A patient with depression may speak softly and slowly, whereas a patient with mania may speak loudly and rapidly. However, older patients may also speak loudly because of hearing impairment. Abnormalities such as dysarthria and aphasia may indicate a physical cause (e.g., stroke, neurodegenerative disorders, traumatic brain injury).

1.9.3 Emotional Expression

The clinician asks patients to describe their feelings. Mood (i.e., emotions reported by the patient) and affect (i.e., emotional states observed by the clinician) should be assessed. The patient's posture, hand gestures, tone of voice, eye contact, and facial expressions are all carefully examined. Incongruities between mood and affect should be noted.

1.9.4 Thoughts

Clinicians should assess *how* (process) and *what* (content) is communicated by the patient. The clinician should assess whether ideas appear coherent and goal directed and whether transition from one thought to the next is logical. Patients with psychotic or manic symptoms may have disorganized thoughts or flight of ideas. The symptoms of formal thought disorder (e.g., tangentially, digression, circumstantiality, illogicality, incoherence, perseveration, thought blocking) attributable to new-onset schizophrenia spectrum illness are rare after age 60 [5]. However, some/all of these symptoms can be seen in delirium and major

NCDs, which are common in older patients. Abnormal content may take the form of obsessions (i.e., unwanted and distressing thoughts, urges, or images), compulsions (i.e., excessive, repetitive behaviors or mental acts), overvalued ideas (i.e., unreasonable, strongly held beliefs, but with less than delusional intensity), and delusions (i.e., fixed, false beliefs). Persecutory and partition delusions are more common in patients with late-onset psychotic disorders than their earlier-onset counterparts [5]. The assessment can determine whether psychological distress is expressed as excessive preoccupations with physical symptoms (e.g., headache or abdominal pain).

Clinical Pearl
Clinicians should *always* assess for self-harm, suicidal, or homicidal ideation and behavior. The threat to self also includes inability to care for self, leading to self-neglect in geriatric patients.

1.9.5 Perception

Screening for perceptual disturbances is critical for detecting dissociative symptoms (e.g., derealization, depersonalization), illusions (i.e., things are perceived differently by the patient, but distinguishes they are not real), and hallucinations (i.e., things are perceived differently by the patient, but does not distinguish they are not real). Hallucinations can affect all sensory modalities, although visual, tactile, olfactory, and auditory types are more common in late-onset psychotic disorders [5] (see Sect. 10.2.3). Command hallucinations to harm (i.e., voices instructing the patient to harm self and/or others) should be thoroughly investigated as these can range from innocuous to life threatening [6].

1.9.6 Cognition

Cognitive functions include the patient's level of alertness; orientation to time, place, and person; attentiveness and concentration; memory; abstract reasoning; problem solving; and decision-making. When these processes are disrupted, the consequences for the patient can be considerable (e.g., unintentional medication overdose, mismanaged life savings, motor vehicle accidents). Before testing cognition, it is important to know that the patient's sensory abilities (vision and hearing) are intact, since attribution of sensory impairment could well be misconstrued as cognitive impairment. For example, visually impaired patients may experience "empty sensory field" hallucinations (the sensory system with functional impairment produces hallucinatory experiences in the sensory deficit state, such as the Charles Bonnet syndrome); these same patients may score poorly on the first 5 items of the Montreal Cognitive Assessment (MoCA), which require intact visual processing of test items. There are many ways to assess cognition.

Clinical Pearl
An impression for the cognitive abilities of a patient by way of the psychiatric interview is not recommended, since many cognitively impaired patients may be able to compensate for deficits and appear to be intact unless explicit capacities are tested (see Chap. 10 for the brief cognitive screening tools).

In particular, memory testing involves remote memory (e.g., ask basic knowledge questions such as who the first president or the first prime minister of a respective country was), recent memory (e.g., ask questions about current events or news stories), and immediate memory (e.g., test if the patient can accurately repeat a short list of words several minutes later; no multiple choice or other cues are required in a normal situation). Attention can be tested with serial subtractions of the same number from a starting point or naming the days of the week or the months of the year, backward.

1.9.7 Insight and Judgment

Insight and judgment are particularly important in making decisions about safety. Insight refers to the ability to identify pathological events (e.g., hallucinations, delusions), understand possible treatment options, and adhere to these. Insight can be rated as poor, limited, fair, or good. Judgment refers to a patient's problem-solving ability in general. Judgment can be assessed by exploring recent decision-making process or by posing a practical dilemma (e.g., "What should you do if you see smoke coming out of the house?").

1.10 Physical and Laboratory Examination

A thorough physical examination is regarded as an integral part of a comprehensive psychiatric examination. During on-call practice, a more directed physical examination is determined based on the chief medical complaint. See Chap. 2 for further details on the on-call physical examination. Laboratory tests may be performed to exclude any co-occurring medical disorder and treatment-related adverse effects that could induce or worsen a preexisting psychiatric disorder.

Table 1.1 summarizes the main domains and some key elements of the on-call psychiatric examination of a geriatric patient [7–9].

Table 1.1 Main domains and key elements of the on-call psychiatric examination of the geriatric patient [7–9]

Domain	Key elements
Biographical and demographic data	Name, age, address, first language, education achievement, financial status, marital status and family contact details, housing status
Chief complaint and present illness	Account of onset and development of current symptoms, legal hospitalization status
	Potential for harm to self or others (e.g., suicidal thoughts, plans, and intent, prior suicide attempts and means used)
	Review of systems
	Psychiatric screening instrument results
Psychiatric history	Known current and past psychiatric illness
	Substance use (e.g., use or abuse of alcohol, tobacco, illicit drugs)
	List of prescribed treatments (e.g., medications, somatic treatments such as ECT or rTMS, psychotherapy)
	Hospitalizations
Medical history and medications	Known disorders and chronic conditions
	New-onset physical symptoms
	Current treatments
Family history	Known neuropsychiatric diagnoses, including major NCDs
Social history	Developmental history (e.g., developmental milestones, family composition, childhood experience)
	Educational history (e.g., schooling experience, educational level)
	Employment history (including retirement, volunteering)
	Legal history (e.g., arrests, incarcerations)
	Relational/marital history (e.g., marital status, quality and stability of marriage(s)/other significant relationships)
	Living arrangements (e.g., alone, cohabitants, supervised setting, homeless)
	Sexual history (e.g., identity, orientation, adaptation, experiences, function)
	Lifestyle choices (e.g., exercise, alcohol/drug use pattern, sleep habits)
	Social supports (e.g., friends, family members, social groups, quality of relationships, abuse)
	Response to life adversities (e.g., divorce, illness, losses)
	Access to community services
	Functional performance (e.g., IADLs and ADLs)
	Advance directives (e.g., power of attorney, conservatorships, code status)

(continued)

Table 1.1 (continued)

Domain	Key elements
Mental status examination	Appearance (e.g., distinctive features, clothing, hygiene, grooming)
	Behavior (e.g., posture, facial expression, eye contact, body language, gestures)
	Speech (e.g., rate, volume, tonality)
	Mood (e.g., happy, depressed, irritable, anxious) and affect (e.g., range, appropriateness, stability, congruity)
	Thoughts
	Process (e.g., loose associations, flight of ideas, circumstantial or tangential thinking)
	Content (e.g., delusions, overvalued ideas, preoccupations, obsessions, suicidal and/or homicidal ideation)
	Perception (e.g., dissociative features, illusions, hallucinations)
	Cognition (e.g., orientation, concentration, memory, abstract reasoning, MoCA result)
	Insight (i.e., acknowledgment of a possible psychiatric problem)
	Judgment (i.e., problem-solving ability)
Physical and laboratory examination	Determine appropriate timing, scope, and intensity of the on-call physical exam. Determine who the most appropriate examiner is (psychiatrist vs. other clinician)
	Detect abnormalities in general appearance, vital signs, organ systems
	Determine if more detailed physical exam is necessary for specific diseases
	Laboratory tests for systemic medical causes of neuropsychiatric presentation: TSH (for hypo- or hyperthyroidism); CBC, electrolytes, serum calcium, fasting glucose, B_{12}, TSH, liver enzymes (for major/mild NCDs and metabolic disturbance); CBC (for systemic infection or chronic disease); rheumatological markers; additional tests depending on presentation; liquid biomarkers for Alzheimer's disease (e.g., CSF Aβ1-42 and tau): used in research protocols and have no clinical utility as of now [7]
	Structural neuroimaging for major/mild NCDs (MRI or CT): indicated in most, but not required in all [7]
	Laboratory tests for serum drug levels (e.g., lithium, valproic acid, carbamazepine)
	Laboratory tests for antipsychotic monitoring: serum glucose and lipids for metabolic syndrome, electrocardiogram for iatrogenic cardiac arrhythmias, WBC and ANC for neutropenia with clozapine or carbamazepine use [8, 9]

Note: ADLs activities of daily living, *ANC* absolute neutrophil count, *CBC* complete blood count, *CSF* cerebrospinal fluid, *CT* computed tomography, *ECT* electroconvulsive therapy, *IADLs* instrumental activities of daily living, *MRI* magnetic resonance imaging, *NCDs* neurocognitive disorders, *rTMS* repetitive transcranial magnetic stimulation, *TSH* thyroid-stimulating hormone, *WBC* while blood cell count

Key Points

- On-call or crisis psychiatric examination is commonly performed in various settings such as institutional, ambulatory, and community environments.
- The psychiatric examination is a process of gathering information about a patient with the purpose of making a diagnosis, which is a prerequisite for any treatment process.
- Performing an on-call psychiatric examination of the geriatric patient, particularly in hospital settings, is typically a multidisciplinary process, with contributions from various clinicians.
- Most on-call psychiatric examinations, which are performed under the constraints of time, tend to be more directed than the routine psychiatric examination.
- Formal cognitive assessment (e.g., by using MoCA, available freely on the Internet at http://www.mocatest.org) should always be done in patients with cognitive impairment.
- Although on-call clinicians resort to traditional patient interview techniques, they often solicit input from family members, home caregivers, nursing staff, and other clinicians.

References

1. Caspi A, Roberts BW, Shiner RL. Personality development: stability and change. Annu Rev Psychol. 2005;56:453–84.
2. Cooper LD, Balsis S, Oltmanns TF. Aging: empirical contribution. A longitudinal analysis of personality disorder dimensions and personality traits in a community sample of older adults: perspectives from selves and informants. J Pers Disord. 2014;28(1):151–65.
3. The chief public health officer's report on the state of public health in Canada 2010. Chapter 3: The health and well-being of Canadian seniors. http://www.phac-aspc.gc.ca/cphorsphc-respcacsp/2010/fr-rc/cphorsphc-respcacsp-06-eng.php. Accessed 28 Oct 2015.
4. Chow ES, Hategan A, Bourgeois JA. When it's time for 'the talk': sexuality and your geriatric patient. Current Psychiatry 2015;14(5):13–14, 16–19, 29–30.
5. Howard R, Rabins PV, Seeman MV, Jeste DV. Late-onset schizophrenia and very-late-onset schizophrenia-like psychosis: an international consensus. The international Late-Onset Schizophrenia Group. Am J Psychiatry. 2000;157(2):172–8.
6. Braham LG, Trower P, Birchwood M. Acting on command hallucinations and dangerous behavior: a critique of the major findings in the last decade. Clin Psychol Rev. 2004;24(5):513–28.
7. Gauthier S, Patterson C, Chertkow H, Gordon M, Hermann N, Rockwodd K, et al. Recommendations of the 4th Canadian Consensus Conference on the Diagnosis and Treatment of Dementia (CCCDTD4). Can Geriatr J. 2012;15(4):120–6.
8. U.S. Food and Drug Administration. FDA Drug Safety Communication: FDA modifies monitoring for neutropenia associated with schizophrenia medicine clozapine; approves new shared REMS program for all clozapine medicines. 9-15-2015. http://www.fda.gov/Drugs/DrugSafety/ucm461853.htm. Accessed 1 Nov 2015.
9. Health Canada: Clozapine. http://webprod5.hc-sc.gc.ca/dpd-bdpp/dispatch-repartition.do?lang=eng. Accessed 1 Nov 2015.

Physical Examination

2

Tricia Woo and Calvin H. Hirsch

2.1 Background

The physical examination remains an essential part of the psychiatrist's tool kit, especially when called to medically evaluate a patient on the psychiatric unit or to assess a psychiatric inpatient because of neuropsychiatric manifestations of new-onset delirium. The examination may provide clues to the etiology of the psychiatric illness, such as finding an enlarged thyroid in a patient presenting with psychotic features or a smooth tongue and impaired proprioception in a patient with a progressive neurocognitive disorder (formerly dementia). Although it is impossible to review the entire physical examination in a brief chapter, important clinical findings more commonly encountered in geriatric patients are herein emphasized. Their recognition and interpretation can guide diagnosis, management, and the assessment of a psychiatric patient's medical acuity.

2.2 The On-Call Physical Examination and General Principles

The physical examination should begin with assessing the clinical stability of the patient. Unstable vital signs, visible distress, and labored breathing would be indicative of the need of more immediate medical consultation. Can he/she talk in full sentences or have to stop frequently to catch his/her breath? If the patient has limited ability to articulate symptoms, facial expression, and posture, as well as any

T. Woo, MD (✉)
Division of Geriatric Internal Medicine, McMaster University, Hamilton, ON, Canada
e-mail: twoo@HHSC.CA

C.H. Hirsch, MD
Department of Internal Medicine, Division of General Medicine, University of California
Davis Medical Center, Sacramento, CA, USA

A. Hategan et al. (eds.), *On-Call Geriatric Psychiatry: Handbook of Principles and Practice*, DOI 10.1007/978-3-319-30346-8_2

part of their body that they may be clutching, provide clues to acuity and where the exam should be targeted. Distress with diaphoresis represents a red flag for a potentially serious condition, and if the patient has a history of diabetes mellitus should prompt an immediate point-of-care finger-stick blood glucose. Leaning forward with hands on the knees ("tripoding") may be an indicator of respiratory distress or chest pain. Lying with knees bent may be a clue for an intra-abdominal process or nausea.

Clinical Pearl
Limit the time the patient is in the supine position as this may cause back pain for patients with osteoarthritis or kyphoscoliosis and shortness of breath for those with cardiopulmonary disease – consider having extra pillows on hand.

2.3 Vital Signs

In healthy older adults, the mean oral temperature is 97.2 °F (36.2 °C) and lower than in other age groups. Absence of fever does not exclude infection in older adults. Hypothermia (<36 °C) is often considered the clinical equivalent of fever in this population [1] and is a systemic inflammatory response syndrome (SIRS) criteria.

It is advisable to check blood pressure and pulses in both arms. The pulse should be taken for at least 30 seconds, and any irregularity is noted. Blood pressure may be overestimated in geriatric patients due to calcification in their blood vessels which cannot be compressed. This is known as "pseudohypertension" and should be suspected if dizziness develops after antihypertensives are begun or doses are increased to treat elevated systolic BP [2]. All geriatric patients should be evaluated for orthostatic hypotension, as it occurs frequently in the frail patient and may be associated with falls and symptoms of pre-syncope. Blood pressure is measured with patients in the supine position and then after they have been standing for 3–5 min. If systolic BP falls ≥20 mmHg after patients stand, orthostatic hypotension is diagnosed [3]. Measuring the patient's current weight and comparing to baseline values may be useful in assessing cardiac volume status. A respiratory rate greater than 20 bpm indicates tachypnea and should prompt measuring oxygen saturation, even if dyspnea has not been reported.

Clinical Pearl
Premature beats may not generate a sufficient pulse pressure to be palpated in the wrist or carotid artery. The most reliable way to evaluate the pulse is by auscultation of the heart. This should always be done to determine heart rate in patients with atrial fibrillation.

2.4 Head and Neck Exam

The dentition of older patients should be inspected. Missing, broken, or carious teeth may reflect self-neglect or neglect by others and can adversely affect nutrition and self-image. If the patient is missing teeth or is edentulous, check if there is a well-fitting dental appliance or dentures. Inspect the tongue if normally papillated. A red, smooth, beefy-looking tongue suggests B_{12} or folate deficiency. The temporal arteries should be palpated for tenderness or nodularity which may indicate temporal arteritis in a patient complaining of headache. Although a fundoscopic examination may not be necessary, inspect the corneas for opacities and evaluate vision with a wall-mounted Snellen chart or handheld card in both eyes with corrective lenses in place. If visual acuity is <20/100 corrected in either eye, the patient's vision is severely impaired, which can impact gait safety and increase fall risk. Check for presbyopia with corrective lenses in place. If the patient cannot read standard printed text with corrective lenses, they may not be able to read instructions or the labels of prescriptions. (Assessing visual acuity also can be used to discretely test literacy.)

2.5 Cardiopulmonary Exam

2.5.1 Lungs

Except when performed in conjunction with a complete admission history and physical, the lungs will be examined when there is suspicion of a pulmonary process because of a cough, elevated respiratory rate, shortness of breath, and/or a fever. Ideally, examination of the lung should begin with inspection, followed by percussion and auscultation. Inspection compliments the general impression of the patient's medical status and should focus on whether intercostal and neck strap muscles are being used to increase ventilation. In patients with shortness of breath (SOB), the use of these accessory muscles and worse SOB when lying indicates higher medical acuity and needs for urgent medical evaluation. Pursed lip breathing, resembling lips configured for whistling, also is a sign of medical acuity when the patient is at rest. Percussion is helpful when looking for signs of a pleural effusion or pneumonia, but from a practical standpoint can be omitted in most cases when chest radiography is readily available [4].

Clinical Pearl

Percussion requires that the fingers of the nondominant hand be laid flat against the skin to create a seal and then struck forcefully with the index and middle fingers. The utility of this technique is compromised when the patient is obese or when a forceful strike is difficult. In such circumstances, a standard triangular rubber reflex hammer can be used to strike the fingers, generating a more forceful percussion and facilitating the distinction between resonance (normal) and dullness (consolidation, effusion, or lung collapse).

Auscultation is a skill that requires practice and is affected by the quality of the stethoscope. The purpose of auscultating the lung is to identify concerning adventitious sounds, such as wheezing, rhonchi, crackles (rales), inspiratory stridor, and an asymmetric decrease in breath sounds. Wheezing is high pitched and indicates airway obstruction, but their loudness and duration during exhalation are important. Generally, the longer the wheezes last during exhalation, the more severe the bronchial obstruction. The loudness of the wheeze also reflects severity, but the clinician should be aware that when the bronchi are severely narrowed, loudness declines. Rhonchi are low-pitched sounds that generally reflect mucus within the large airways that the patient is having trouble clearing. Crackles suggest alveolar fluid from pneumonia or heart failure, but can be heard in localized atelectasis. They almost always merit chest radiography. Stridor is an *inspiratory* wheeze-like sound that reflects focal narrowing of an airway. If loudest over the trachea, it can represent a medical emergency (e.g., adult croup). An asymmetric decrease in breath sounds generally should also prompt chest radiography.

Clinical Pearl
Do not forget to auscultate the anterior chest and the sides of the thorax. Auscultation of the anterior chest is required to assess the upper lobes. The sides of the thorax overlie the middle lobe (right) and lingula (left).

2.5.2 Heart

Auscultation of the heart permits more accurate assessment of an irregular pulse (see Sect. 2.3, above) as well as detection of murmurs, rubs, and gallops. Accurate auscultatory assessment of heart murmurs in the stable patient has become less important with the increased availability of echocardiography, but auscultation for new or worse murmurs plays an essential role in patients presenting with a suspected myocardial infarction or experiencing new or acutely worse heart failure. The most common cardiac murmurs that the on-call psychiatrist will encounter in geriatric patients result from mitral regurgitation and/or aortic stenosis/sclerosis. The on-call psychiatrist should be able to differentiate potentially serious murmurs from stable, chronic ones. Fortunately, most murmurs that can be easily auscultated will have been documented previously, so review of the medical record often can provide a frame of reference. Mitral murmurs usually are heard best at the lower left sternal border or the apex and may radiate toward the axilla. A new loud or worse mitral murmur ($\geq$ grade 3; see Table 2.1) may suggest serious underlying cardiac decompensation and requires urgent medical/cardiologic consultation or transfer to the emergency department. Aortic outflow tract murmurs can be heard best at the right upper sternal border, but in older patients may be prominent at the apex. Early-peaking aortic valvular murmurs are associated with a brisk carotid upstroke that barely follows S1 and usually do not require urgent evaluation with echocardiography. The later in systole the aortic murmur occurs, the more severe the stenosis, and

Table 2.1 Guide to describing and rating cardiac murmurs

Descriptors	Grade and definition	
Early, middle, or late in systole	1	A very soft, easily missed murmur that is usually not clinically significant
Crescendo-decrescendo vs. constant loudness: S1 and S2 can be distinctly heard	2	A soft murmur that can be readily heard over a localized area
Holosystolic: Murmur begins at the end of S1 and continuous to the beginning of S2; both S1 and S2 distinctly heard	3	A moderately loud murmur
Pansystolic: Murmur heard from the beginning of S1 to the end of S2; S1 and S2 indistinct	4	A loud murmur that can be heard over a wide area but unaccompanied by a thrill (vibration felt over the precordium)
	5	A loud murmur over a wide area of the precordium accompanied by a thrill
	6	A very loud murmur that can be appreciated with the stethoscope raised just above the precordium; a thrill also should be present

the longer the delay in the carotid upstroke. Of note, the loudness of the murmur may *soften* in very advanced, clinically significant aortic stenosis. Geriatric patients with dyspnea on exertion, exertional chest pain, or syncope should be evaluated for clinically significant aortic stenosis.

Physical findings associated with myocardial infarction may be nonspecific but may include signs of acute heart failure including a new S3 or new mitral regurgitation murmur. A pericardial rub is a grating or rubbing sound that is loudest near the left sternal border and most apparent when the patient is sitting upright. A rub may be a sign of pericarditis which can be caused by a variety of disorders including infection, myocardial infarction, and trauma. Palpation for the point of maximal impulse (PMI) may not be as reliable in geriatric patients due to displacement of the PMI with significant kyphosis, as well medial placement in severe obstructive lung disease or lateral displacement in obesity. Measurement of the jugular venous pressure may be very useful in determining volume status. To measure the patient's venous pressure, the clinician should examine the veins on the right side of the heart as they have the most direct route to the heart. An elevated jugular venous pressure is defined as the top of the neck veins more than 3 cm above the sternal angle. Chest pain which is reproducible by tenderness to palpation may suggest costochondritis, which is the most common musculoskeletal cause of chest pain [5].

2.6 Abdominal Exam

Patients who are unable to assume and maintain the supine position (e.g., kyphoscoliosis, cardiopulmonary disease) may give the appearance of distension. The abdomen is palpated to check for weak abdominal muscles, which is common among older adults and which may result in hernias. In some thin older adults, a normal aorta is palpable, but the vessel and pulsations do not extend laterally. Most abdominal aortic aneurysms are palpable as a pulsatile mass and their lateral width can be measured on physical examination. Geriatric patients with peritonitis may lack classic peritoneal signs of rebound and guarding. For patients with symptoms of constipation, palpation may reveal hard, palpable stool in the ascending, descending, and sigmoid segments of the colon [6].

2.7 Lower Extremity Exam

On general observation, look for swelling at the ankles, feet, and legs. Gently compress the patient's soft tissue with your thumb on the shin for several minutes and then observe for indentation. In patients that are unable to arise out of bed, edema may also be present in the sacral and coccygeal areas. Lower limb edema that is acute and symmetric in both limbs may be suggestive of right heart failure. Unilateral swelling may suggest venous thromboembolism, and if the patient also has concurrent complaints of chest pain or dyspnea, then consider evaluation for pulmonary thromboembolism. Signs of arterial insufficiency (e.g., hair loss, decreased peripheral pulses) may be seen in patients with known peripheral vascular disease [7].

2.8 Neurological Exam

A *directed* neurological exam can be indispensable for on-call situations and can guide the triaging of the patient to the most appropriate consulting service. The neurological examination is based on the principles of anatomical localization that aim to identify lateralized neurological findings suggestive of local pathology or multifocal disease. The examination consists of the following: mental status examination, cranial nerves, motor, sensory, coordination, gait, and reflexes. Knowledge of the normal neurological examination in the healthy older patient is essential for proper interpretation of the neurological exam.

2.8.1 Level of Consciousness

The neurological examination of the unconscious patient is by necessity brief and focused and the goal is to determine underlying etiology. The Glasgow Coma Scale (GCS) is commonly utilized to assess the severity of impaired consciousness both on initial and subsequent assessments. Mild brain injury is classified as GCS >13, moderate injury GCS 9–12, and severe with GCS <8–9 which may require intubation [8] (see Table 2.2). Note that a depressed GCS can reflect excessive sedation as well as brain injury.

Table 2.2 Glasgow Coma Scale

Eye opening (E)	Verbal response (V)	Motor response (M)
4 – spontaneous	5 – normal conversation	6 – normal
3 – to voice	4 – disoriented	5 – localizes pain
2 – to pain	3 – incoherent words	4 – withdrawal from pain
1 – none	2 – incompressible sounds	3 – decorticate posture
	1 – none	2 – decerebrate posture
		1 – none

Assessment of spontaneous and elicited movements and reflexes will be important. Lack of spontaneous movement and reduced muscle tone may indicate acute structural disease. Tremor, asterixis, and myoclonic jerks suggest metabolic or toxic etiology. Pupillary light reflexes should be examined for both direct and consensual response. Eye position should be examined as cerebral lesions can produce a persistent deviation toward the side of the lesion. If there has been head trauma, the cervical spine will need to be immobilized.

2.8.2 Cranial Nerves (CN)

On routine examination, testing olfaction (CN I) is often omitted but diminished sense of smell occurs in half of those aged 65–80 [9]. It is very important to screen for visual problems (CN II) in older patients as impairment may not be reported accurately by patients and may represent a potentially correctable problem. Bedside assessment of visual fields is performed by confrontation testing (finger counting) in the four quadrants of each eye separately.

Clinical Pearl
Older patients may have smaller pupils and their pupillary reflexes may be sluggish. Pupillary abnormalities such as Horner's syndrome (small pupil and ptosis) can suggest prior brain stem stroke.

Fundoscopy can reveal causes of visual loss such as cataracts, optic atrophy, as well as optic disk edema. Abnormalities of eye movements can be helpful in diagnosis of stroke syndromes and neurodegenerative disorders.

The on-call psychiatrist may be asked to evaluate a patient with the rapid onset, over several hours, of unilateral facial paralysis, which includes inability to close the eye, drooping of the corner of the mouth, and loss of the nasolabial fold. In the absence of any other acute neurological abnormality, the facial paralysis most likely represents Bell's palsy, due to idiopathic injury of the ipsilateral seventh cranial nerve. Other symptoms may include loss of taste on the anterior two thirds of the tongue as well as either decreased hearing or hyperacusis in the ipsilateral ear. In geriatric patients, contrasted head computed tomography or magnetic resonance imaging should be performed to rule out stroke, and a formal neurological consultation is recommended.

Facial motor function and sensation can be assessed by examining the facial (CN VII) and trigeminal (CN V) nerves. Inspect the fact for symmetry and test the ability to close the eyelids against resistance. Then ask the patient to purse their lips, blow out their cheeks, and show their teeth.

Clinical Pearl
A unilateral upper motor neuron facial palsy suggests a stroke or other lesion in the contralateral hemisphere. In lower motor neuron lesions of the facial nerve (e.g., Bell's palsy), the entire face on one side is weak with both voluntary and involuntary movements affected (see above).

To test hearing (CN VIII), whisper in each ear while causing an occlusion in the other ear. CN IX and X are tested in tandem and manage the gag reflex and palatal movement, respectively. Ask the patient to say "ahh" and look for smooth upward palatal movement. CN XI is tested by asking the patient to shrug their shoulders (trapezius muscles) and turn their head (sternocleidomastoid muscles) against resistance. To test CN XII, ask the patient to stick out their tongue and observe for fasciculation and tongue deviation. If there is unilateral weakness, the tongue will deviate toward the weaker side [10].

2.8.3 Motor

The motor examination is comprised of inspection for fasciculation, muscle bulk, and testing for tone and power. With normal aging, there is some mild decline in motor function, reduced strength, and speed of movements. *Fasciculation* is defined as fine, fast intermittent contraction of muscle fibers that are visible below the dermis. Benign causes of fasciculation include medications such as caffeine, salbutamol, and anticholinergic medications used over a long period of time. *Tone* is defined as the resistance of a muscle to passive movement and can be rated as increased, normal, or decreased. Testing for tone in the upper extremities can be performed by brisk supination of the relaxed forearm. Increased tone can be described as spastic or rigid. Spasticity is a velocity-dependent resistance to movement (described as a "clasp-knife" response) which primarily affects the flexors in the arm and suggests an upper motor pathology (e.g., stroke). Rigidity is a velocity-independent "lead pipe" response that affects the flexor and extensor muscles equally and is associated with parkinsonism. The examiner grasps the hand in a handshake, and after asking the patient to let his muscle go limp, supinates and pronates the wrist. Above the elbow, the examiner places a thumb on the biceps tendon while flexing and contracting the arm. A ratcheting or stuttering sensation instead of smooth movement ("cogwheel" rigidity) can often be seen as well as felt. Muscle *strength* testing identifies patterns of weakness between upper and lower extremities and right and left sides. The six-point Medical Research Council grading scale is commonly used to describe strength [11]:

0 – no contraction
1 – muscle contraction but no movement
2 – can move but not against gravity
3 – can move against gravity but not resistance
4 – weak movement against resistance
5 – normal power

Clinical Pearl
Inquire about other neurological symptoms such as difficulty with fine motor skills (e.g., buttoning clothes) and drooling or changes in handwriting; all of these features would be consistent with Parkinson's disease. Multiple extrapyramidal signs (muscle rigidity, tremor) may indicate either adverse effects of antipsychotic medication or parkinsonism.

Tremor is an important and frequent clinical sign among older patients and requires a logical approach to diagnosis. The underlying etiology may be physiologic or suggestive of a pathological condition such as Parkinson's disease (PD), essential tremor (ET), cerebellar disease, or alcohol withdrawal (see Table 2.3). A tremor is defined as a rhythmic oscillatory type of involuntary movement produced by contractions of reciprocally opposed muscles and is classified on the basis of when it occurs: at rest, during an action, or while holding a specific posture (e.g., when holding the arms outstretched). Constant, rhythmic tremors can be seen in

Table 2.3 Differential diagnosis of tremor

Tremor	Description
Physiologic tremor	Fine, high frequency (>7 Hz) tremor noted in hands. It is exacerbated by anxiety, caffeine, and medications[a]
Parkinsonian tremor	Resting tremor (3–6 Hz) often with a "pill-rolling" quality. May occur asymmetrically in one hand or leg
Essential tremor	Bilateral postural tremor in the hands, larynx, or head. Often has a positive family history and absence of other neurological findings
Alcohol withdrawal tremor	Similar to ET and often occurs 8–12 h after alcohol cessation
Cerebellar tremor	May be postural or action. Often associated with dysmetria (lack of coordinated movement with undershoot or overshoot of intended target) and gait ataxia

[a]See text for list of medications

both PD and ET and sometimes are difficult to differentiate. Past-pointing during rapid movement of the patient's index finger between his nose and the examiner's finger suggests ET.

ET is the most common movement disorder in older adults and has a prevalence of 4–6 % in the community. This tremor is typically a symmetrical postural tremor frequently affecting the hands and larynx (producing wobbling of the voice) and less commonly the head, tongue, and legs. The head can rhythmically and rapidly bob up and down (titubation) or sway left and right. In PD, the tremor usually – but not always – dampens as the finger approaches its target. In ET, muscle tone is normal and there is no evidence of the bradykinesia, stooped posture, and shuffling gait of PD. Severe ET and cerebellar dysfunction may be hard to distinguish.

Physiologic tremor is a normal variant and generally occurs during maintenance of a posture and has a high frequency of >7 Hz. Medications such as fluoxetine, methylphenidate, haloperidol, lithium, salbutamol, and valproic acid may also exacerbate a physiological tremor. Individuals with physiologic tremor should be encouraged to reduce their caffeine intake and their medication list should be reviewed, and offending medications should either have their dose reduced or discontinued altogether [12].

Clinical Pearl

Take a *handwriting sample*; patients with Parkinson's disease will have micrographia and those with essential tremor will have normal-sized script. Considered features are consistent with *psychogenic tremor* if there is abrupt onset, spontaneous remission, equivocating tremor characteristics, and extinction with distraction. In new-onset tremor, a comprehensive *review of medications* (e.g., antipsychotics, antidepressants, lithium) including over-the-counter medications (e.g., pseudoephedrine, caffeine), with specific attention to newly started medications, is cardinal. A fine motor tremor frequently may result from frequent treatments with a beta-agonist bronchodilator or the use of theophylline (chemically similar to caffeine). A trial off of the implicated medication should be accomplished.

2.8.4 Coordination and Gait

Cerebellar function does not change in normal aging. Ischemic stroke syndromes and alcoholic degeneration are the dominant causes of cerebellar dysfunction in older patients. In psychiatric patients, irreversible cerebellar dysfunction can occur from lithium toxicity; in the geriatric patient, lithium levels in the therapeutic range have been associated with cerebellar dysfunction. Anticonvulsants used for bipolar disorder also may lead to cerebellar dysfunction. Pan-cerebellar dysfunction may result from a form of multisystem atrophy. Examination of the cerebellum involves testing the trunk for balance and the limbs for coordination. Limb ataxia is assessed by the finger-to-nose test in the upper extremities and the heel-to-skin test in the lower extremities. For patients with cerebellar ataxia, there may be dysmetria (overshooting or undershooting of the intended target). The truncal imbalance gives the patient a wide-based stance and a gait ataxia and inability to perform tandem gait. Alcohol-related cerebellar degeneration presents with truncal imbalance and a wide-based gait without a tremor of dysmetria. Gait and mobility problems are common in the geriatric population and increase with age. For patients with falls risk, consider performing the get up and go test, e.g., instruct the patient to start from sitting in chair, get up, walk 10 feet, turn around, and walk back. This test should be performed rapidly and smoothly. Timed values >20 s are associated with functional impairment and increased risk of falls [13].

2.8.5 Reflexes

Deep tendon reflexes (DTR) are routinely tested and the results are described based on their presence or absence and whether or not they are symmetrical. These reflexes tend to diminish with aging, and it is often necessary to use reinforcement techniques (e.g., teeth clenching) to bring out reflexes that appear absent or diminished. The National Institute of Neurological Disorders myotatic reflex scale grades reflexes as follows [14]:

0 – Absent
1 – Trace response or reinforcement required
2 – Reflex in lower half of normal range
3 – Reflex in upper half of normal range
4 – Reflex greater than normal, including clonus

Reflexes that are significantly diminished or absent suggest disease in the peripheral nervous system. Hyperreflexia is abnormal in older patients and suggests a central nervous system (pyramidal tract) lesion. Although hyperreflexia can be associated with hyperthyroidism, this association is seen less in the older compared to younger patients. Unilateral hyperreflexia may be a residual finding from hemiparesis due to stroke. Sustained rhythmic beating at a joint during forceful flexion (e.g., the ankle) indicates clonus. Up to 3–4 beats can be within normal limits. Nonsustained clonus will extinguish after 5–10 beats and sustained clonus lasts >10 beats; both are pathologic.

Babinski Reflex The extensor plantar response is not part of normal aging, and its presence suggests an interruption in the corticospinal tract (e.g., stroke, mass lesion, spinal cord compression). To test the reflex, the patient should first be placed in the supine position. Use a thumbnail or thin stick, gently stroke along the lateral aspect of the sole of the foot toward the base of the toes and across the balls of the foot. Be careful to avoid producing pain or tickling the patient. The normal response is a downward flexion of the toes. The classic abnormal response is the up-going great toe [15].

Clinical Pearl
Upper motor neuron signs indicate that the lesion is above the anterior horn cell (brain stem, motor cortex, and spinal cord); these signs are characterized by spasticity, weakness, increased reflexes and positive Babinski reflex. Lower motor neuron signs indicate the lesion is either in or anterior to the horn cell (root, plexus, and peripheral nerve); these signs are characterized by reduced muscle tone, muscle wasting, fasciculation, and areflexia.

Primitive Reflexes Primitive reflexes (frontal release signs) are present in infancy and disappear with the development of the central nervous system. The seven reflexes include the snout, palmo-mental, glabellar, sucking, rooting, corneo-mandibular, and grasp. Reappearance of these reflexes may occur in late life both in normal older adults and in certain disease conditions. For example, an abnormal glabellar tap may be relevant in a diagnosis of PD. To perform this reflex, tap the area above the nose on the forehead (glabella) at 1 second intervals. A normal response would be to initially blink and then this response will extinguish. In a patient with frontal lobe injury or PD, this blinking does not extinguish.

2.8.6 Sensory

Spinothalamic (pain, temperature, and light touch), dorsal column (vibration, proprioception, and touch localization), and hemispheric (graphesthesia) sensory functions should be screened. The stimulation should be applied lightly and should be compared bilaterally as well as distal versus proximally. Vibration sensation is reduced in the lower limbs of normal older adults and may not be attributable to disease. Loss of proprioceptive position sense in the great toes is pathologic and can occur in B_{12} deficiency or after peripheral nerve injury. With the patient's eyes closed and the patient instructed not to move the toe, the examiner grasps the great toe on the sides and moves it up and down several times before asking the patient if the toe is "up or down." The test should be repeated several times to ensure consistency of response (correct or incorrect localization). There are age-related increases in sensory thresholds for sensory modalities, but these changes are not clinically apparent on bedside testing [16].

Romberg's Sign Romberg's sign is a useful test of sensory (proprioceptive) function of the feet which requires healthy dorsal columns of the spinal cord. To perform this test, have the patient stand with feet together and eyes closed. Stand close by in case the patient becomes off balance. The test is positive if the patient sways or falls while their eyes are closed. These patients may also have an abnormal gait due to sensory ataxia.

Clinical Pearl
In patients with major neurocognitive disorder (dementia), sensory examination may be unreliable and difficult. Patients with cerebellar ataxia will have difficulty standing with feet together with eyes open or closed. This is a useful test to distinguish cerebellar and sensory ataxia.

Key Points

- The on-call physical examination can be judiciously guided by the patient's history in order to assist the on-call psychiatrist with the differential diagnosis in geriatric psychiatric patients.
- Physical examination is important in the geriatric population where an accurate history may be difficult to obtain, and atypical presentations of disease are common.
- Unstable vital signs or signs of distress will signify higher level of acuity and need for immediate medical consultation.
- Although indispensable for on-call situations, a directed neurological exam can guide the triaging of the patient to the most appropriate consulting service.
- Utilize the Glasgow Coma Scale (GCS) as part of the initial assessment of the patient with an altered level of consciousness.
- Auscultation of a new or worsening cardiac murmur is very helpful in the assessment of a patient with suspected myocardial infarction or heart failure.

References

1. Lu SH, Leasure AR, Dai YT. A systematic review of body temperature variations in older persons. J Clin Nurs. 2010;36:234–5.
2. Messerl FH. Osler's maneuver, pseudohypertension and true hypertension in the elderly. Am J Med. 1986;80(5):906–10.
3. Ooi WL, Barret S, Hossain M, Kelley-Gagnon M, Lipsitz LA. Patterns of orthostatic blood pressure change and their clinical correlates in a frail, elderly population. JAMA. 1997;277:1299–304.
4. Mahler DA, Fierro-Carrion G, Baird JC. Evaluation of dyspnea in the elderly. Clin Geriatr Med. 2003;19:19–33.
5. Chun AA, McGee SR. Bedside diagnosis of coronary artery disease: a systematic review. Am J Med. 2004;117(5):335–43.
6. Yen EL, McNamara RM. Abdominal pain. Clin Geriatr Med. 2007;23(2):255–70.

7. Blankfield RP, Finkelhor RS, Alexander JJ, Flocke SA, Maiocco J, Goodwin M, et al. Etiology and diagnosis of bilateral leg edema in primary care. Am J Med. 1998;105:192–7.
8. Teasdale G, Jennett B. Assessment of coma and impaired consciousness. A practical scale. Lancet. 1974;2(7872):81–4.
9. Doti RL, Shannon P, Applebaum SL, Giberson R, Siksorsia L, Rosenberg L. Smell identification ability: changes with age. Science. 1984;226:1491–3.
10. Gladstone DJ, Black SE. The neurological exam in aging, dementia and cerebrovascular disease – Part 1: introduction, head and neck and cranial nerves. Geriatr Aging. 2002; 5(7):36–43.
11. Medical Research Council. Aids to examination of the peripheral nervous system. Memorandum no. 45. London: Her Majesty's Stationary Office; 1976.
12. Jankovic J, Fahn S. Physiologic and pathogenic tremor. Diagnosis, mechanism and management. Ann Intern Med. 1980;93:460–5.
13. Podsiadlo D, Richardson S. The timed up and go: a test of basic functional mobility for frail elderly persons. J Am Geriatr Soc. 1991;39:142–8.
14. Litvan I, Mangone CA, Werden W, Bueri JA, Estol CJ, Garcea DO, et al. Reliability of the NINDS Myotatic reflex scale. Neurology. 1996;47:969–72.
15. van Gijin J. The Babinski sign. Pract Neurol. 2002;2:42–4.
16. Gladstone DJ, Black SE. The neurological exam in aging, dementia and cerebrovascular disease – Part 4 – reflexes and sensory examination. Geriatr Aging. 2002;5(10):51–7.

Psychopharmacology Principles

3

Glen L. Xiong, Ashkan Javaheri, and Ilse R. Wiechers

3.1 Background

This chapter aims to cover general principles of geriatric psychopharmacology as they may apply to the on-call primary care clinician or psychiatrist. This chapter limits the "clinical encounter" to telephone calls where a face-to-face mental status examination of the patient and access to complete medical records is not possible. Please refer to Chap. 10 for medication treatment of specific psychiatric complaints and Chap. 12 for detailed coverage of chief adverse side effects of psychotropic medications.

3.2 Basic Principles of On-Call Geriatric Psychopharmacology

Table 3.1 summarizes some basic principles of using psychiatric medications in the on-call setting. While this is not comprehensive, the authors distilled some of the basic rules and mental shortcuts based on their collective clinical experience, citing

G.L. Xiong, MD, CMD (✉)
Department of Psychiatry and Behavioral Sciences, University of California, Davis, 2230 Stockton Blvd., Sacramento, CA 95817, USA
e-mail: gxiong@ucdavis.edu

A. Javaheri, MD, CMD
Mercy Medical Group, Geriatric Division, University of California, Davis, School of Medicine, 3000 Q Street, Sacramento, CA 95816, USA

I.R. Wiechers, MD, MPP, MHS
Psychotropic Drug Safety Initiative, Office of Mental Health Operations, Department of Veterans Affairs, Northeast Program Evaluation Center, West Haven, CT, USA

Department of Psychiatry, Yale University School of Medicine, 950 Campbell Ave, NEPEC/182, West Haven, CT 06516, USA

A. Hategan et al. (eds.), *On-Call Geriatric Psychiatry: Handbook of Principles and Practice*, DOI 10.1007/978-3-319-30346-8_3

Table 3.1 Basic principles of on-call geriatric psychopharmacology (AVOID)

*A*void prescribing medications when possible	Time limit the on-call physician order for a medication, especially for high-risk medications such as benzodiazepines and hypnotics Avoid drug-drug interactions when starting a new medication
*V*erify medications actually taken	Adjust timing or the dosing of current medications before adding new medications
*O*ptimize current medications and medication dosages	Avoid treating the side effects of one medication with another agent Adjust timing or the dosing of current medications before adding new medications Ensure medications are given a good trial – "start low, go slow, but go all the way" Take advantage of desired side effects such as sedation and weight gain
*I*dentify the most effective mode of medication delivery	In acute agitation, consider appropriate modes of drug administration When indicated, consider checking serum levels of medications for clinical efficacy and medication adherence
*D*iagnose correctly and determine the target symptoms	Use the diagnosis to guide medication selection and titrate to target dose Determine the underlying etiology of symptoms before starting medications Many symptoms and behaviors can be reversible without required medication

relevant empirical evidence as much as possible. We proposed the following five clinical pearls with the acronym AVOID.

3.2.1 *Avoid* Prescribing a Psychiatric Medication Without Clear Indication Whenever Possible

Pharmacotherapy can be challenging in geriatric patients due to age-related changes in pharmacokinetics and pharmacodynamics and high rates of medical comorbidities, all of which lead to increased risks of polypharmacy, drug-drug interactions, and adverse drug events [1]. Nearly every psychotropic medication is listed in the American Geriatrics Society Beers Criteria, as each class of psychotropic medication has substantial risks of harm in geriatric patients [2]. Coupled with the limitations of the on-call clinical encounter mentioned above and the tenet of the Hippocratic Oath to "first do no harm," on-call clinicians should avoid prescribing new medications for geriatric patients as much as possible. Since the clinical diagnosis becomes ever more elusive without a clinical examination and complete access to medical records, medication indication is more likely to be based on second-hand reports of symptoms rather than on a clear clinical diagnosis. Should a medication be prescribed, it should be initiated for a time-limited course and with a clear monitoring plan to assess for drug-drug interactions, medication adverse events, and effectiveness. This monitoring plan should also ensure reevaluation of the patient before continuing medication for a longer trial, ideally with an inpatient follow-up the following day or a follow-up outpatient visit within 1–2 weeks.

3.2.2 Verify Medications Actually Taken

A complete medication review with information about medications that have actually been taken in the last 24–72 h is imperative. Regardless of setting, patients often do not take all their medications exactly as they have been prescribed and instructed. Missed doses can results from patients with cognitive impairment forgetting to take their medications, hospitalized patients being too busy getting a medical procedure at the time medications are due, or nursing home patients being already drowsy at the time of medication administration. Before adding a new medication, first review with the nursing staff, caregivers, and patients the current medication administration. Consider adjusting the timing or the dosing of the current medications to help address reported symptoms.

3.2.3 Optimize Current Medications and Dosages

3.2.3.1 Reduce Medications Before Adding a Medication

In the USA, 50 % of Medicare beneficiaries take five or more medications and polypharmacy is a well-known problem in geriatric patients [3]. It is especially important to review recently added medications to determine if any new symptoms are due to a medication adverse event. Avoid treating the side effects of one medication with another medication. Instead, consider decreasing dose to reduce side effects or find a better-tolerated alternative.

3.2.3.2 Ensure Medications Are Given a Good Trial

While the adage of "start low and go slow" is time tested and wise guidance, clinicians must also avoid starting too low and going too slow and ensure they "go all the way." Medications such as benzodiazepines can exhibit a J-curve phenomenon where low doses can be associated with a paradoxical disinhibition or agitation, and higher doses can produce the necessary sedation to manage acute agitation and physical aggression [4]. While risk factors for benzodiazepines-related paradoxical reaction remain poorly understood [5], we know from clinical experience that patients with occult alcohol use disorder are at high risk since they have developed tolerance for alcohol (through activity on the GABA receptors), and therefore smaller doses of benzodiazepines are more likely to cause disinhibition (similar to having an "alcohol buzz").

Another common geriatric psychiatry prescribing adage is to utilize the potential benefit of medication side effects. For example, the sedation and weight gain side effects of mirtazapine are frequently used to treat insomnia and weight loss.

Nevertheless, low doses of multiple concomitant medications without achieving target dose range contribute to problematic polypharmacy. Similarly, "slow" titration of some medications that are needed to produce the clinical effects during the on-call settings will lead to undertreatment. The consequence of undertreatment of acute agitation and physical aggression could potentially result in physical injury to the patient, staff, and caregivers.

3.2.4 *I*dentify the Most Effective Mode of Medication Delivery

Once a medication is prescribed, it is important to ensure that the patient receives the desired dose. Often there can be delays in the drug actually being delivered to the patient due to insurance coverage, drug availability, or delay in drug administration (which can be common in long-term care settings). In truly emergent situations, such as acute agitation, it is rare that oral pill or tablet administration will be accepted by the patient; thus, alternative modes of delivery should be considered. Medication injection, liquid, orally dissolving tablets, crushed medications with food or beverage, and topical formulations are potential alternatives. When in doubt, consider checking serum levels of antidepressants or antipsychotics, and when indicated, check serum levels of valproic acid, lithium, or carbamazepine [6]. Although drug levels may not necessarily correlate with clinical efficacy, getting the serum drug level can be helpful in monitoring medication adherence.

3.2.5 *D*iagnose Correctly and Determine the Target Symptoms

Use the diagnosis to guide medication selection and titrate to target dose. Many geriatric patients have cognitive impairment and are unable to fully express their needs or feelings. Various "unmet" needs such as environmental changes, unfamiliar caregiver, sitting in a soiled diaper, or uncontrolled pain can cause agitation. It is important to ask about these factors and determine the underlying etiology of symptoms before starting psychopharmacotherapy. Many of these symptoms and behaviors can be reversed without requiring medication [7].

3.3 Age-Related Changes in Pharmacokinetics and Pharmacodynamics

3.3.1 Pharmacokinetics

In general terms, pharmacokinetics refers to "effects of the body on drugs." This includes medication *absorption, metabolism, distribution, and excretion.* With aging comes reduced medication absorption due to reduced gastric emptying and intestinal

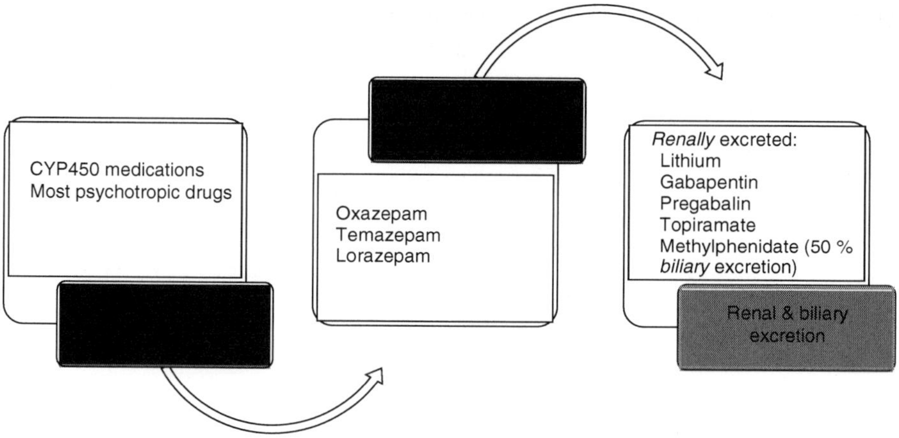

Fig. 3.1 Pathways of drug metabolism and excretion [8–11]

motility and reduced gastric acidity (especially for those taking proton pump inhibitors). Inhibitors of P-glycoprotein in the intestinal wall (e.g., garlic and grapefruit juice and common psychiatric medications such as amitriptyline, fluoxetine, paroxetine, haloperidol, and risperidone) can lead to increased absorption and high serum levels for P-glycoprotein substrates (e.g., amitriptyline, citalopram, paroxetine, venlafaxine, quetiapine) [8]. Overall, reduced absorption due to aging is thought to reduce the time to achieve serum drug levels but not necessarily the magnitude of the levels [9].

Most psychotropic drugs are metabolized by the liver (via phase 1 oxidation and phase 2 glucuronidation) and excreted through the bile or unchanged through the kidney. Other drugs are converted to active metabolites that pass through the kidney (e.g., metabolites of risperidone, bupropion, venlafaxine) [8–11] (see Fig. 3.1). Choosing a psychotropic drug that does not require phase 1 biotransformation or only requires glucuronidation (e.g., lorazepam, oxazepam, temazepam) may be considered in patients with liver disease.

While drug metabolism may be reduced in geriatric patients, genetic polymorphism (especially for various cytochrome P450 enzymes) tends to account for more individual differences than aging. Approximately 8 % of Caucasians lack the capacity to metabolize CYP2D6 substrates and are classified as poor metabolizers, whereas the rest are extensive metabolizers (the majority of individuals). CYP2D6 metabolizing capacity should be considered when psychotropics are coadministered with drugs that inhibit CYP2D6 [12, 13].

The volume of drug distribution is increased for lipophilic drugs (e.g., diazepam) since body fat composition may increase by more than 30 % in geriatric patients leading to increased half-life for lipophilic drugs [8]. However, geriatric patients with malnutrition may in fact have reduced body fat composition [9] so that lipophilic drugs may have lower than anticipated half-lives. Lithium and other water-soluble drugs distributed in total body water can be especially difficult to manage in renal disease or other medical conditions, which can result in rapid hemodynamic changes (e.g., aggressive diuresis, excessive diarrhea, or vomiting) and which could further result in severe drug toxicity. As the total body water volume decreases, a previously therapeutic drug level can become acutely toxic.

Drug excretion is most significantly affected by reduced glomerular filtration rate (GFR), which can progressively decline by nearly 50 % starting from age 30 to 80 years. Medical comorbidities, such as congestive heart failure and chronic renal disease, are more common in the geriatric patients and further contribute to the effect of an already reduced GFR, which influence the excretion of water-soluble drugs and the metabolites of certain drugs [8, 9].

3.3.2 Pharmacodynamics

Pharmacodynamics refers to "effects of the drug on the body." In general, aging leads to reduced neurotransmitter receptor activity in the brain, and this necessitates lowering of the target doses for most medications. Some important age-related changes include decreased baroreceptor responsivity (leading to increased risk of orthostatic hypotension from alpha antagonists), decreased D_2 receptor density (leading to increased sensitivity to parkinsonism), decreased cholinergic activity (resulting in increased response to anticholinergic agents), increased sensitivity of GABA-aminergic system (leading to increased sensitivity to benzodiazepines), and decreased serotonin reuptake receptor binding and attenuated concentrations in 5-HT_1A and 5-HT_2A receptor density (leading to mood dysregulation and anxiety). Geriatric patients may only need 30–50 % of the serum concentration of benzodiazepines to achieve the same effect compared to younger patients [14]. As for antipsychotics, a recent positron emission tomography study in geriatric patients with schizophrenia confirms previous clinical adage that the dopamine D_2 and D_3 receptor occupancy for optimum antipsychotic effect should be lowered to 50–60 % rather than 65–80 % for younger patients [15]. While less is known about antidepressant receptor physiology, lower target doses are recommended as higher doses are more likely to cause adverse events such as altered heart rate, increased risk of bleeding, and cardiovascular risks such as QT_C prolongation (e.g., citalopram and TCAs). Figure 3.2 summarizes the common age-related and non-age-related pharmacokinetics and pharmacodynamics in the geriatric population [13–15].

3.4 Common On-Call Medications

On-call clinicians will often receive calls about depression, anxiety, agitation, confusion, or insomnia. Table 3.2 lists the most commonly prescribed medications in geriatric patients by drug class for the most common psychiatric presentations that

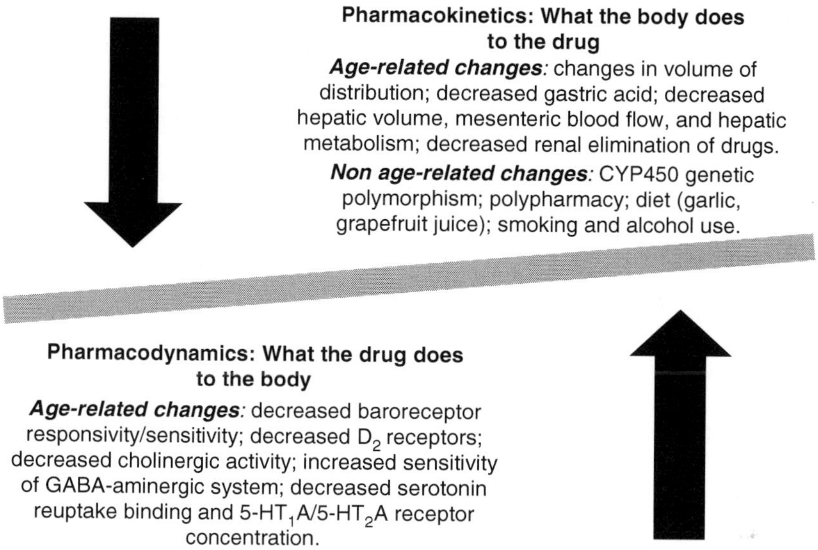

Fig. 3.2 Pharmacokinetics and pharmacodynamics in geriatric patients [13–15]

clinicians are likely to be addressing in the on-call setting [10, 11]. We also list other medications that clinicians may encounter. Although clinicians may not start all these medications while on call, they should be mindful of the adverse effects and possible need to reduce the dosage or discontinue some of these medications. We present below some strategies and interventions for common on-call psychiatric presentations.

3.4.1 Depression and Anxiety

Depression and anxiety should rarely be treated by starting a new medication without an initial face-to-face diagnostic assessment. However, since patients may develop side effects, it is not uncommon to make dose adjustments or switch to a different antidepressant over the phone with proper informed consent. As for anxiety disorders, the most common call is for acute anxiety or panic attack where the caregiver or nursing staff requests a benzodiazepine (such as lorazepam). Most of these calls should be managed by giving specific instructions to the caller to use behavioral interventions (e.g., deep breathing techniques). The use of benzodiazepines in the geriatric patients should be limited due to the many risks (e.g., falls, hip fracture, motor vehicle accidents, cognitive impairment) [16–19], but when absolutely necessary, the preference should be for short-acting agents and agents that avoid first-pass metabolism in the liver and thus have no active metabolites, e.g., oxazepam, temazepam, and lorazepam (also known as OTL for "outside the liver") (see Fig. 3.1).

Table 3.2 Common on-call medications in geriatric psychiatry [10, 11]

Medication (starting dose/day)[a]	Dose adjustments	Side effects and other considerations
Antidepressants		
Citalopram (10 mg) [escitalopram (5 mg)]	Renal impairment: no adjustment necessary Hepatic impairment: citalopram max dose 20 mg/day	SIADH/hyponatremia, risk of bleeding, risk of falls, anorexia Akathisia, headache, agitation, GI complaints, diarrhea, constipation, sexual side effects QTc prolongation warning by the US FDA and Health Canada: risk at dose >40 mg/day, max 20 mg/day in patients over 60 Escitalopram is an enantiomer of citalopram and is twice as potent as citalopram
Sertraline (25 mg)	Renal impairment: no adjustment necessary Hepatic impairment: lower or less frequent dosing	SIADH/hyponatremia, risk of bleeding, risk of falls, anorexia Akathisia, headache, agitation, GI complaints, diarrhea, constipation, sexual side effects
Venlafaxine (37.5 mg XR)	Mild to moderate renal impairment: 25–50 % dose reduction Hemodialysis: 50 % dose reduction Hepatic impairment: 50 % dose reduction	Dose-related increase in BP, nausea, constipation, sexual side effects Useful for pain May need to start at 12.5–25 mg IR for frail elderly SIADH/hyponatremia, risk of bleeding, risk of falls
Duloxetine (30 mg)	Renal impairment: avoid use Hepatic impairment: avoid use	Dry mouth, nausea, constipation, sexual side effects, diarrhea Useful for neuropathic pain, fibromyalgia SIADH/hyponatremia, risk of bleeding
Mirtazapine (7.5–15 mg) [ODT]	Renal impairment: clearance reduced, increase dose slowly Hepatic impairment: clearance reduced, increase dose slowly	Sedation, weight gain, constipation, mild anticholinergic effects Decreased WBC More sedating when used at lowest doses (<15 mg)
Bupropion (37.5–50 mg)	Renal impairment: consider reducing frequency and/or dose Hepatic impairment: consider reducing frequency and/or dose	Dry mouth, agitation, constipation Can lower seizure threshold No data to support use in anxiety disorders

Mood stabilizers		
Lithium (150–300 mg qhs) [liquid]	Severe renal impairment: relative contraindication	Tremor, benign leukocytosis, hypothyroidism, hyperparathyroidism, interstitial nephropathy, diabetes insipidus, neurotoxicity (with overdose/toxicity), cardiac conduction abnormalities, GI upset, acne Pretreatment and monitoring studies: Ca, renal panel, CBC, TSH, eGFR, serum lithium level, ECG
Valproate (125–250 mg qd-bid-tid) [IV, liquid, sprinkles]	Hepatic impairment: use lower dose, contraindicated in severe liver disease Avoid in hyperammonemia, pancreatitis, thrombocytopenia/leukopenia, pregnancy	Headache, tremor, dizziness, ataxia, nausea, vomiting, diarrhea, constipation, reduced appetite, weight gain, somnolence, thrombocytopenia, hepatotoxicity, pancreatitis, hyponatremia, suicidal behavior and ideation, hyperammonemia Pretreatment and monitoring studies: CBC, liver enzymes, serum valproate level Check for serum hyperammonemia if altered mental status (and consider urea cycle enzyme deficiency as cause of hyperammonemia)
Lamotrigine (12.5–25 mg qd-bid)	Hepatic impairment: reduce target dose	Dizziness, sedation, ataxia, confusion, headaches, nausea, vomiting, diarrhea, blurred vision, Stevens-Johnson syndrome Increased risk of suicidal ideation and behavior Start at 12.5 mg when used with valproate to avoid increased risk of skin rash
Antipsychotics	Class-wide side effects: sedation, anticholinergic symptoms, orthostatic hypotension, extrapyramidal symptoms (EPS), akathisia, QTc prolongation, metabolic side effects, acute kidney injury, cognitive decline, cerebrovascular adverse events, and death in patients with neurocognitive disorders. Prominent side effects for specific medications noted below	

(continued)

Table 3.2 (continued)

Medication (starting dose/day)[a]	Dose adjustments	Side effects and other considerations
Haloperidol (0.25–0.5 mg bid) [IM, LAI, liquid]	Renal impairment: no adjustment necessary Hepatic impairment: mild to moderate, no adjustment necessary; severe, use is contraindicated Avoid if QTc >500 ms	EPS: rigidity/parkinsonism, akathisia, dyskinesia Increased mortality
Olanzapine (2.5–5 mg) [IM, LAI, ODT]	No adjustment necessary Avoid in diabetes	Anticholinergic, weight gain, hyperglycemia, hypertriglyceridemia
Risperidone (0.25–0.5 mg qd-bid) [IM, LAI, ODT, liquid]	Renal impairment: reduce dose Hepatic impairment: reduce dose	EPS, hyperprolactinemia
Quetiapine (12.5–25 mg)	Hepatic impairment: reduce dose	QTc prolongation, orthostatic hypotension, anticholinergic, weight gain, hyperglycemia, hypertriglyceridemia
Sedatives/hypnotics		
Lorazepam (0.25–0.5 mg qd-bid) [IM, IV, topical gel, liquid]	Renal impairment: mild to moderate, no adjustment necessary; renal failure, use not recommended Hepatic impairment: mild to moderate, no adjustment necessary; hepatic failure, use not recommended	Elderly are prone to CNS depression even after low doses; start very low initial doses, depending on the response of the patient, to avoid oversedation or neurological impairment Paradoxical reactions (including anxiety, agitation, and excitation) can occur
Trazodone (12.5–50 mg qhs)	Hepatic impairment: caution	Orthostasis, QTc prolongation, priapism
Doxepin (3–6 mg qhs)	Hepatic impairment: 3 mg max dose Renal impairment: 3 mg max dose; contraindicated in patients with urinary retention	Anticholinergic side effects in doses >6 mg/day
Melatonin (1–3 mg qhs)	No adjustment necessary	Drowsiness, headache, dizziness, nausea Indicated for use in jet lag, circadian rhythm sleep disorders, delayed phase sleep disorder

Note: [a]Use lower dose for patients aged >75 or those >60 with frailty and multiple medication comorbidities. *IM* (available as intramuscular formulation for acute treatment; dose often needs reduction as intramuscular is more bioavailable than oral), *LAI* (available as long-acting injectable formulation, check prescriber guide for dose conversion), *ODT* (available as oral dissolving/disintegrating tablet)

3.4.2 Acute Agitation and Physical Aggression

The first-line treatment for behavioral disturbance in patients with major neurocognitive disorders (NCDs) (formerly dementia) is non-pharmacological interventions for the unmet needs [7]. However, medication may be required, especially if the agitated or aggressive behavior is escalating, has not responded to non-pharmacological approaches, and may cause physical injury to or put the patient and/or caregivers at risk of imminent harm. Often a medical work-up is limited as the patient will not provide urine or blood samples nor permit physical examination during an acute episode. In such instances a one-time low dose of antipsychotic, preferably second-generation atypical, is usually a reasonable choice. Careful evaluation of the underlying etiology of the agitation, such as unmet needs, should be conducted once the acute crisis has passed and prior to establishing regular use of an antipsychotic. The use of antipsychotics in patients with major NCDs has been associated with increased risk of cerebrovascular adverse events and death [20–22], which led many regulatory agencies to issue black box warnings. Thus, the use of antipsychotics in patients with major NCDs requires close monitoring for adverse events and a time-limited course with attempts at gradual dose reduction when clinically appropriate. It is important to note that risperidone is approved in Canada for "short-term symptomatic management of aggression or psychotic symptoms in patients with severe dementia of the Alzheimer's type unresponsive to non-pharmacological approaches and when there is a risk of harm to self or others" [23] and in the UK for up to 6 weeks for the treatment of "persistent aggression due to moderate to severe" major NCD [24]. Antipsychotics do not have such specific approval for the treatment of NCD-related psychosis or aggression in the USA by the Food and Drug Administration.

3.4.3 Delirium

Delirium management starts with a strategy that attempts discontinuation of new medications (e.g., anticholinergic medication) that could contribute to delirium and identifies and treats the underlying medical condition (e.g., acute infection). Non-pharmacological interventions are of the utmost importance and are addressed elsewhere. The treatment of delirium with short-term (<1 week) use of antipsychotic medications is recommended for patients in acute distress and who may pose danger to themselves or others [25]. Patients with history of Parkinson's disease and major NCD with Lewy bodies may be particularly sensitive to high-potency antipsychotics, which often cause worsening of movement disorder and agitation in these patients. Although the strongest evidence supports the use of clozapine for Parkinson's-related psychosis, quetiapine is often the first-line antipsychotic in patients with Parkinson's disease and major NCD with Lewy bodies for psychosis and for delirium due to ease of administration [26]. Clozapine is almost never used in delirium for various reasons including its anticholinergic effects. Finally, delirium and delirium tremens related to benzodiazepine and alcohol withdrawal necessitate primary treatment with benzodiazepines and adjunctively with antipsychotics and anticonvulsants when needed [27].

3.4.4 Insomnia

Sleep disturbances are common in geriatric patients, especially with Parkinson's disease and NCDs. Benzodiazepines and hypnotics should be avoided for long-term use given all the risks discussed above. Nonetheless, the inability of the patient to sleep can be very stressful for caregivers to patients with major NCDs who may stay awake with the patient at night and thus precipitate a crisis phone call request to their primary care physician for management of insomnia. It is important to encourage patients to stay active during the daytime, decrease or eliminate naps, get adequate sunlight exposure, limit or eliminate alcohol or caffeine, and improve sleep hygiene. (See Sect. 10.2.8.2, *Management* of the patient with insomnia.) For cognitively intact geriatric patients, referral for cognitive behavioral therapy for insomnia should be a first-line treatment option and a long-term solution to the problem of insomnia [28, 29]. When non-pharmacological efforts have failed, medication choices should include the use of sedating antidepressants (e.g., low-dose doxepin, mirtazapine, trazodone), ramelteon, melatonin, or prazosin (specifically for the treatment of posttraumatic stress disorder-associated sleep disturbance). Avoid antihistamines to treat insomnia in the geriatric patients due to their high anticholinergic burden and risk for side effects. Consider treating underlying anxiety when ruminations and worries appear to be causing sleep-onset insomnia.

Case Vignette Mrs. A was an 82-year-old female with history of ischemic stroke, hypertension, depression, anxiety, and major NCD due to Alzheimer's disease, who had become more restless over the previous 2 days. The patient's daughter called the community mobile crisis team at 1:00 AM complaining that Mrs. A had been talking to her deceased parents, was calling out and appeared distraught, and attempted to leave the house. Her regular medications included citalopram 10 mg daily, lorazepam 0.5 mg at noon, atenolol 25 mg daily, aspirin 81 mg daily, and acetaminophen 500 mg as needed for pain. She moved to her daughter's house 3 days previously, after her husband (her primary caregiver) was hospitalized. The daughter suspected that Mrs. A might not have taken her medications that day while the daughter was away at work. You were the on-call clinician and responded to the daughter's call. The daughter was asking for a medication to calm Mrs. A down because she was getting "out of control." Based on the information presented, you concluded that Mrs. A was in a new environment, most likely she was not taking her medications properly and that the daughter (or other caretaker) needed to supervise her. You advised the daughter to try to redirect Mrs. A. You explained to the daughter that giving Mrs. A a dose of the prescribed lorazepam 0.5 mg (already available to the daughter) could help her to relax, but the daughter should watch her closely for falls and other adverse events. You advised the daughter to schedule a visit with

Mrs. A's primary care physician to be seen shortly (within 1 week) for full assessment and medication reconciliation.

Key Points

- The acronym AVOID may be used as a set of clinical pearls to approach geriatric psychopharmacology: *A*void medication when possible; *V*erify medications actually taken; *O*ptimize timing and dosing of active medications; *I*dentify the most optimal delivery method; and *D*iagnose correctly.
- Genetic polymorphism may account more for individual medication metabolism than aging. More specifically, CYP2D6 metabolizing capacity should be considered when psychotropic medications are coadministered with drugs that inhibit CYP2D6.
- In general, aging leads to reduced neurotransmitter receptor activity in the brain, and this leads to lowering of the target doses for most medications.
- The first-line treatment for behavioral disturbance in patients with major NCDs is non-pharmacological interventions. Medication may be required, especially if the aggressive behavior is escalating, has not responded to non-pharmacological interventions, and may cause physical injury to patient and/or caregivers.

References

1. Steinman MA, Hanlon JT. Managing medications in clinically complex elders: "There's got to be a happy medium". JAMA. 2010;304(14):1592–601.
2. American Geriatrics Society 2015 Beers Criteria Update Expert Panel. American Geriatrics Society 2015 Updated Beers Criteria for potentially inappropriate medication use in geriatric adults. J Am Geriatr Soc. 2015. doi:10.1111/jgs.13702.
3. Kaufman DW, Kelly JP, Rosenberg L, Anderson TE, Mitchell AA. Recent patterns of medication use in the ambulatory adult population of the United States: the Slone survey. JAMA. 2002;287(3):337–44.
4. Zimmerman K, Rudolph J, Salow M, Skarf LM. Delirium in palliative care patients: focus on pharmacotherapy. Am J Hosp Palliat Care. 2011;28(7):501–10.
5. Mancuso CE, Tanzi MG, Gabay M. Paradoxical reactions to benzodiazepines: literature review and treatment options. Pharmacotherapy. 2004;24(9):1177–85.
6. Lonergan E, Luxenberg J. Valproate preparations for agitation in dementia. Cochrane Database Syst Rev. 2009;(3):CD003945.
7. Kales HC, Gitlin LN. Lyketsos CG; Detroit Expert Panel on assessment and management of neuropsychiatric symptoms of dementia. Management of neuropsychiatric symptoms of dementia in clinical settings: recommendations from a multidisciplinary expert panel. J Am Geriatr Soc. 2014;62(4):762–9.
8. Oesterheld JR. Transports. In: Wynn GH, Oesterheld JR, Cozza KL, Armstrong SC, editors. Clinical manual of drug interaction: principles for medical practice. Washington, DC: American Psychiatric Publishing; 2009. p. 43–60.
9. Carlo AD, Alpert JE. Geriatric psychopharmacology: pharmacokinetic and pharmacodynamic considerations. Psychiatr Ann. 2015;45(7):336–41.

10. Crone CC, Gabriel GM, DiMartini A. An overview of psychiatric issues in liver disease for the consultation-liaison psychiatrist. Psychosomatics. 2006;47(3):188–205.
11. McIntyre RS, Baghdady NT, Banik S, Swartz SA. The use of psychotropic drugs in patients with impaired renal function. Prim Psychiatry. 2008;15(1):73–88.
12. Wilkinson GR. Drug metabolism and variability among patients in drug response. N Engl J Med. 2005;352(21):2211–21.
13. Pollock B, Forsyth C, Bies R. The critical role of clinical pharmacology in geriatric psychopharmacology. Clin Pharmacol Ther. 2009;85(1):89–93. 14.
14. Stegemann S, Ecker F, Maio M, Kraahs P, Wohlfart R, Breitkreutz J, et al. Geriatric drug therapy: neglecting the inevitable majority. Ageing Res Rev. 2010;9(4):384–98.
15. Graff-Guerrero A, Rajji TK, Mulsant BH, Nakajima S, Caravaggio F, Suzuki T, et al. Evaluation of antipsychotic dose reduction in late-life schizophrenia: a prospective dopamine D2/3 receptor occupancy study. JAMA Psychiatry. 2015;72(9):927–34.
16. Woolcott JC, Richardson KJ, Wiens MO, Patel B, Marin J, Khan KM, et al. Meta-analysis of the impact of 9 medication classes on falls in elderly persons. Arch Intern Med. 2009;169(21):1952–60.
17. Dassanayake T, Michie P, Carter G, Jones A. Effects of benzodiazepines, antidepressants and opioids on driving: a systematic review and meta-analysis of epidemiological and experimental evidence. Drug Saf. 2011;34(2):125–56.
18. Wang PS, Bohn RL, Glynn RJ, Mogun H, Avorn J. Hazardous benzodiazepine regimens in the elderly: effects of half-life, dosage, and duration on risk of hip fracture. Am J Psychiatry. 2001;158(6):892–8.
19. Billioti de Gage S, Moride Y, Ducruet T, Kurth T, Verdoux H, Tournier M, et al. Benzodiazepine use and risk of Alzheimer's disease: case–control study. BMJ. 2014;349:g5205.
20. Schneider LS, Dagerman KS, Insel P. Risk of death with atypical antipsychotic drug treatment for dementia: meta-analysis of randomized placebo-controlled trials. JAMA. 2005;294(15):1934–43.
21. Kales HC, Valenstein M, Kim HM, McCarthy JF, Ganoczy D, Cunningham F, et al. Mortality risk in patients with dementia treated with antipsychotics versus other psychiatric medications. Am J Psychiatry. 2007;164(10):1568–76. quiz 1623.
22. Schneeweiss S, Setoguchi S, Brookhart A, Dormuth C, Wang PS. Risk of death associated with the use of conventional versus atypical antipsychotic drugs among elderly patients. CMAJ. 2007;176(5):627–32.
23. Health Canada. Risperidone product monograph. http://webprod5.hc-sc.gc.ca/dpd-bdpp/dispatch-repartition.do?lang=eng. Accessed 16 Oct 2015.
24. Public Assessment Report of the Medicine Evaluation Board in the Netherlands. 2008. http://db.cbg-meb.nl/mri/par/nlh-1078-001-002-003-004-005-006.pdf. Accessed 9 Oct 2015.
25. National Institute for Health and Clinical Excellence (NICE). 2010. Delirium: diagnosis, prevention and treatment. https://www.nice.org.uk/Guidance/CG103. Accessed 13 Oct 2015.
26. Weintraub D, Hurtig HI. Presentation and management of psychosis in Parkinson's disease and Dementia with Lewy bodies. Am J Psychiatry. 2007;164(10):1491–8.
27. Amato L, Minozzi S, Davoli M. Efficacy and safety of pharmacological interventions for the treatment of the Alcohol Withdrawal Syndrome. Cochrane Database Syst Rev. 2011;(6):CD008537.
28. Trauer JM, Qian MY, Doyle JS, Rajaratnam SM, Cunnington D. Cognitive behavioral therapy for chronic insomnia: a systematic review and meta-analysis. Ann Intern Med. 2015;163(3):191–204.
29. Baillargeon L, Landreville P, Verreault R, Beauchemin J-P, Grégoire J-P, Morin CM. Discontinuation of benzodiazepines among geriatric insomniac adults treated with cognitive-behavioural therapy combined with gradual tapering: a randomized trial. CMAJ. 2003;169(10):1015–20.

Psychotherapy Principles

4

Caroline Giroux and W. Edwin Smith

4.1 Background

Let's reach out and smile at each other
For we can march together
We have to knock on all the doors, at least try
Until the day we die.
(Quoted from *The Revolutionaries*, by Caroline Giroux, MD [1])

As we age, losses of all kinds accumulate. Depending on how we negotiate these inevitable life challenges, a crisis with various manifestations (e.g., sadness, panic, somatization, substance misuse) can ensue and may benefit from a specific psychotherapeutic approach. During brief on-call encounters, the assessment can be therapeutic and fruitful as long as the clinician is able to be fully present and interested. During the intervention, evaluation and therapy intermingle to set the foundations for more prolonged growth later.

The following is a description of general principles of implementing psychotherapy approaches and types of brief psychotherapy techniques which can be used with patients regardless of psychiatric diagnosis. Excessive emphasis on psychiatric diagnoses may lead to less appreciation of the patient's specific psychology and thus is often *counterproductive* in the everyday psychotherapy of less severely impaired patients and is incompatible with the therapeutic venture that Yalom described as "spontaneous, creative, and uncertain" [2]. Instead, with a technique that digs through all the symptomatic layers, it is possible to envision that more than

C. Giroux, MD (✉)
Department of Psychiatry and Behavioral Sciences, APSS Stockton Clinic, Davis Health System, University of California, Sacramento, CA, USA
e-mail: cgiroux@ucdavis.edu

W.E. Smith, MD
Department of Psychiatry, Saint John Regional Hospital, Dalhousie and Memorial Universities, Saint John, NB, Canada

A. Hategan et al. (eds.), *On-Call Geriatric Psychiatry: Handbook of Principles and Practice*, DOI 10.1007/978-3-319-30346-8_4

one approach will be used for the same patient. As a general rule, any of these approaches could be combined in various ways, depending on the patient's specific situation and needs.

Case Vignette Mrs. R was a 73-year-old woman living in a semi-independent apartment complex for seniors. She was found on the floor by the housekeeper. She was semiconscious, whimpering, and had soiled her underwear. Empty vodka bottles were lying around the floor. She was brought to the emergency department (ED) and was diagnosed with worsening knee osteoarthritis, mild renal failure, and alcohol intoxication. Shortly before her discharge, she started crying and screaming and threatened to hang herself because she did not want to suffer a slow death like her husband. You were the on-call psychiatrist. The ED nurse who called you mentioned that Mrs. R's second husband had passed away from heart failure a few days earlier. Upon assessing Mrs. R, you found out that she used to drink heavily after her menopause and then became fully abstinent on her own, but she returned to drinking alcohol a few weeks prior to her husband's deteriorating condition. Around that time, her only daughter stopped calling her after an argument.

4.2 General Principles

4.2.1 Frame

This initial consultation (which in most cases remains the only encounter due to the on-call structure) is of crucial importance. Ideally, the patient should be evaluated in his/her living environment, because it decreases the patient's anxiety, helps confiding about inner life, and facilitates the working relationship [3]. Flexibility in general is an important parameter to optimize the meaning of each clinical encounter.

4.2.2 Time Allocation

If feasible, allow as much time as necessary (sometimes up to 2 h) to follow the patient's pace, deal with physical limitations (e.g., decreased audition, cognitive impairment), and implement adequate crisis intervention. Avoiding a hospital admission is usually more fruitful and less traumatic.

4.2.3 The Therapist's Role and Attitudes: Being Curious and Interested

For a therapist to "be curious and interested" in all he/she does with the patient is the foundation of working alliance because it helps in engaging the patient. The concept *curious and interested* is the mentalizing mindset which, according to Fonagy, refers to the ability to understand people in terms of their feelings, desires, beliefs, and expectations [4]. It is likely one of the most powerful connection tools available to humans. It takes work and time to develop, but when practiced, it improves the value of every interaction between people. It makes even brief emergency assessments meaningful and productive. Most importantly, it helps in establishing safety and trust. It is a prerequisite to a clear understanding of the patient's reality and has special value for the older adults who seek to be heard and accepted. Being curious and interested starts with deepening awareness of one's self, one's thoughts, feelings, and blind spots, and their possible origins ("Know thyself"). Deepening awareness means that we never cease working on it ourselves and that we work similarly to know our patients' experiences and their origins. *Who are they really?*

Much of what happens in psychotherapy depends on the clinician's ability to understand the mind of another. Mentalizing expands the relaxation response (self in the moment) to past, future, and others. We all have a native mentalizing ability that can be put at the service of psychotherapy.

Being curious and interested regardless of the psychotherapeutic school (e.g., behavioral, psychodynamic, motivational) leads to interactions at greater depth than usual because it rapidly establishes connection, does not make premature assumptions, and keeps the mind open to the unexpected. After all, the patient is the expert on his/her own life. It finds relevant topics as choices that both patient and therapist suggest. It seeks compromise between the solutions that the psychotherapist believes are relevant and practical and what the patient really wants.

Concluding an interview where we genuinely became "Mr. Curious" or "Ms. Interested" is usually associated with greater understanding of issues and possible options as well as a sense of how another human being responds to one's own experience of reality. The improvement in outlook following a real connection with another real person is one of the big gains. Patients often seek a similar experience with future psychotherapists and with others in their lives.

4.3 Brief Psychotherapy Approaches

We all can practice new skills that we have not yet had the opportunity to develop in our lives. Specific psychotherapies allow specific learning to occur. In order to identify which ones will be most appropriate, one uses intuition (sometimes called "right cerebral functions") and active listening. In any psychotherapeutic journey, the clinician must follow the patient. It is even more accurate for geriatric patients, whose limitations might require extra flexibility.

4.3.1 Supportive Therapy

Warmth and empathy are key components of this approach, like the oxygen of the therapeutic dyad. Use positive supportive statements (such as genuinely felt compliments when appropriate) [2]. A handshake at the beginning and/or at the end of the session as well as physical assistance when the patient is frail can represent a nice reassuring gesture, a gentle emotional holding to facilitate the connection if there is some sensory impairment. Grief support counseling should be done early on. Recovery from grief means "discovering and completing" the unfinished emotions or elements regarding the unique lost relationship [5]. Contradictory emotions will be looked at and eventually integrated, in a whole perspective of what has been.

Case Analysis Again, continuous interest in Mrs. R's story will facilitate the process. Here are some ways of achieving the connection:

- Offer condolences.
- Ask if she would like to talk about the deceased (late husband but also other significant losses) and give her opportunity to do so.
- Allow for tears to flow and emotions to be spoken; grieving people need to be heard, not fixed [5].
- Try not to touch during the emotionally intense part of narration as it usually stops feelings [5].
- Be interested in the rituals and ask if she has assistance from family.
- Suggest that she tries journaling, drawing, painting, or other artistic modalities to process and maintain good memories of this relationship alive.
- Normalize grief as a validation approach.

4.3.2 Ongoing Interventions While Assessing for Suicidal Risk

While managing one's own anxiety, validation of the patient's feelings should take place. At the same time, you can remind him/her of your role to ensure safety and support alternatives that would allow self-growth. Remaining interested will help the life story to unfold.

Case Analysis Since Mrs. R could be experiencing an acute grief reaction with depressive manifestations, one should assess at various stages of the interview where does she situate herself in terms of desires for life versus death. Working to establish a more accurate perspective is an intervention, at the end of which, suicidal ideation may be much lower. Explaining current medical conditions and prognoses after reviewing the charts and discussing with primary care clinician if possible can help address hopelessness by dissipating misunderstandings and anxiety. Giving the patient a different outlook on his/her future and orienting him/her to possible goals during the subsequent phase of the therapeutic work is often lifesaving. Following with questions about what Mrs. R needs to know and which problems she needs to solve provides a good indication of lowered suicide risk.

4.3.3 Cognitive Behavioral Therapy (CBT)

(a) Cognitive Part An increasing amount of data suggests that the salient mechanism of change in cognitive therapy is the development of metacognition (e.g., responding to negative thoughts as transitory events rather than as an inherent aspect of self) [6].

(b) Behavioral Strategies They include exercise and socialization. Explain that the studies have shown that these lifestyle elements enhance brain health (mood and cognition). For example, brief alcohol interventions (such as *brief alcohol counseling*) are time-limited counseling strategies that focus on changing behavior and increasing treatment compliance. As your active listening (of both the narrative and the nonverbal cues) establishes a good therapeutic rapport, alcohol use disorder should be ruled out. If the patient screened positive on the CAGE, for instance, you can inquire about the impact of the alcohol drinking on the patient's life and proceed with psychoeducation about its effects on health. Two randomized trials studying brief interventions (consisting of two 15 min counseling sessions and two follow-up phone calls) for patients who screened positive for alcohol misuse showed there was a 50–75 % reduction in drinking to moderate levels [7].

Case Analysis Exploring Mrs. R's views on her current drinking pattern and then sharing your concerns about the effects of alcohol on her health and the interference with the grief process are important components.

4.3.4 Trauma-Informed Care

Trauma is common and is often at the root of psychiatric symptoms. Since it is overwhelming and can result in fear, shame, or helplessness, most individuals will try everything to avoid experiencing such feelings again. In times of high stress and crises, individuals are at risk of developing trauma-based reactions. It is essential to detect potential triggers for maladaptive behaviors. In order to do so, it is important to keep in mind the likelihood that any individual has experienced trauma in some form or another; therefore, one should conduct a brief trauma history screen (see Chap. 14).

Case Analysis In Mrs. R's case, the on-call psychiatrist found out that losing her husband was reminding her of her father's death and her former husband's suicide. Some comforting statements such as "I'm sorry this happened to you" followed by questions asked while remaining curious and interested like "How did you cope with that?" can facilitate the processing of past and current events. Reminding the person that she is more than the sum of events in her life can give rise to personal growth and self-empowerment goals.

Finally, concrete tools geared toward stress/trigger management and self-care (e.g., healthy diet, restorative sleep, self-soothing strategies) should be given. Psychoeducation about the manifestations of trauma response (including suicidal ideation) should be provided.

4.3.5 Corporal Mediation

To deal with anxiety, some mindfulness techniques can be demonstrated to induce relaxation by focusing on the body and can be used later by the patient. The patient is instructed to "experience" exactly what is happening at the moment [4]. The six core skills are (i) observing, (ii) describing, (iii) participating, (iv) taking a nonjudgmental stance, (v) focusing on one thing at the moment, and (vi) being effective. Moreover, the attention to the body sensations can later be generalized to an awareness of behaviors or thought patterns. These techniques can be necessary prior to more in-depth therapeutic work. Deep breathing is easy to use at the bedside. Other approaches are progressive relaxation of Jacobson, Schultz' training, yoga, and meditation [8].

Case Analysis Ask Mrs. R about her emotional experiences: e.g., "What is going on now inside?"or "Where in your body are you experiencing the sadness/fear/anger?" Show her to inhale by counting to three, then exhale by counting to three. Repeat the cycle. Examples of situations and settings for the patient to continue practicing mindfulness exercises include:

- Focusing on breathing
- Eating an apple
- Preparing tea or coffee
- Cleaning the dishes
- Folding laundry
- Walking
- Paying attention to an object's physical characteristics
- Wrapping/unwrapping a present
- Smelling lavender

4.3.6 Other Approaches

The following are useful tools that can be incorporated easily during the on-call assessment (by asking questions that the patient can continue to reflect on after the session or by using immediate occurrences of the encounter, the "here and now," to reflect on current difficulties) or at the end, as an encouragement to engage in a specific psychotherapeutic journey.

4.3.6.1 Psychodynamic/Existential

Through the personal narrative, Mrs. R can make some correlations between the past and the present and be assisted in finding a meaning of her difficulties in her life as a whole. Therefore, active listening of her own story will likely be therapeutic, and questions should be asked for the purposes of clarifying, reformulating (a way to mirror, validate), and manifesting a genuine interest in the patient's life trajectory.

4.3.6.2 Motivational Interviewing

The patient is assisted in making an exhaustive list of the pros of drinking and then the cons of an unhealthy behavior (such as excessive use of alcohol) versus abstinence.

4.3.6.3 Interpersonal

It addresses four components that are hypothesized to lead or maintain depression [6]:

- Grief (e.g., death of spouse, loss of faith)
- Interpersonal disputes (e.g., conflicts with adult children)
- Role transitions (e.g., retirement, move)
- Interpersonal deficits (e.g., isolation, acting-outs, suicidal threats)

Case Analysis The on-call psychiatrist learned that Mrs. R's first baby (a daughter) died shortly after birth and she was not allowed to hold her and say goodbye. She suddenly remained silent and seemed angry. Upon asking her what was happening, she admitted that you looked like her former husband who at the time silenced her tears, told her she had to be strong in order to conceive a "boy." Stay present and validate her uncompleted emotions. You can coach her in writing a "loss graph" [6].

4.3.6.4 Dialectical Behavioral Therapy (DBT) and Acceptance Commitment Therapy (ACT)

For older patients, by targeting cognitive/behavioral rigidity and emotional constriction, they help the patient in finding healthier coping skills.

Case Analysis Mrs. R developed the assumption that "everything I love leaves me." You can help her question this belief by looking for evidence supporting a less "black-and-white" thinking. She should be assisted in making a plan or schedule for the next day, with a concrete step-by-step approach, such as eating breakfast, taking a shower, cleaning up the apartment, calling Alcoholics Anonymous, or scheduling an appointment with a counselor for grief support. In preparation of future crises, putting together an individualized "soothing kit" (e.g., backpack with enjoyable music, positive mementos, aromatherapy, modeling clay, pictures of loved ones, diary, books) can be fun and increases self-efficacy and empowerment. Concluding the session when she is comfortable with the plan will provide a form of corrective emotional experience. Hence, she will have prepared herself for what is natural termination of the process (as opposed to death or abandonment) when she feels ready.

4.3.6.5 Bibliotherapy (e.g., Book, Electronic Audio Formats)

This can be used as an adjunct to other forms of therapy. Among its advantages, the material is processed at the patient's pace, self-administered (which can decrease fear of stigmatization), and a good option for those with decreased mobility. Check that the patient is comfortable with reading. Table 4.1 enlists a few self-help book materials that an on-call clinician can recommend to a patient in crisis [5, 10–17].

Table 4.1 Self-help bibliotherapy in counseling [5, 10–17]

Title	Author
The Grief Recovery Handbook	John W. James and Russell Friedman
The Necessary Losses	Judith Viorst
The Courage to Grieve	Judy Tatelbaum
Looking at Mindfulness[a]	Christophe André
Peace is Every Step	Thich Nhat Hanh
The Mindful Way through Depression[a]	Mark Williams et al.
Feeling Good	David Burns
The Places that Scare You	Pema Chödrön
Inventing the Rest of Our Lives	Suzanne Braun Levine

[a]CD included

4.4 Age-Specific Considerations

Highly effective treatments originally developed in younger adult populations (like CBT or DBT) have been successfully modified to meet the specific needs of older adults [6]. Here are some examples of procedural adaptations to consider when implementing brief techniques during the on-call practice [9]:

- Find a room that is quiet, well ventilated, and well lit.
- Give written materials to the patient; fonts for written material should be larger; memory aids (handouts) can be very helpful.
- Psychoeducation is an integral part of almost all psychotherapy modalities and should be reiterated as needed.
- Ask the patient to repeat the recommendations and invite questions.

Key Points

- Total attention in the form of *active listening* (as opposed to a checklist diagnosing approach) is the main modality during on-call crisis interventions using brief psychotherapy. The clinician should remember that diagnoses are made of words that communicate with other professionals but do not capture the human being's essence.
- During an encounter while on call, an important goal is to "plant a seed" by reinforcing or introducing of the idea that psychotherapy has great value for an older person. Effective grief recovery cannot take place without feeling heard.
- Continuous flexibility and interest in the "here and now" are an integral part of the therapeutic dialogue.

- It is important for clinicians who are usually trained well in "doing" to begin practicing "being." Allowing the patient to participate in the treatment planning, asking questions, and leaving room for ventilation and processing facilitates growth, empowerment, and resolution.
- Learning and personal growth can take place throughout the life span, and advanced age should not be a deterrent for clinicians in initiating a psychotherapeutic journey with geriatric patients.

References

1. Giroux C. The revolutionaries (poem). Sierra Sacramento Valley Med. November-December 2015; p.32.
2. Yalom ID. The gift of therapy. New York, NY:Harper Perennial; 2002.
3. Amyot A. "La psychothérapie analytique de la personne âgée" In: Doucet P, Reid W, "La psychothérapie psychanalytique" (French). Boucherville, QC: Gaëtan Morin Editeur Ltée. 1996.
4. Linehan MM. Cognitive-behavioral treatment of borderline personality disorder. New York: The Guilford Press; 1993.
5. James JW, Friedman R. The grief recovery handbook. New York: Harper-Collins Publishers; 2009. ISBN ISBN 978-0-06-185949-6.
6. Lynch TR, Smoski MJ. Individual and group psychotherapy. In: Blazer DG, Steffens DC, editors, Textbook of geriatric psychiatry. Arlington, VA: American Psychiatric Assoc Pub; 2009. p. 521–38.
7. Oslin DW. Evidence-based treatment of geriatric substance abuse. Psychiatr Clin N Am. 2005;28:897–911.
8. Verrier P, Bernier P. "La psychothérapie utilisant une médiation corporelle" In: Doucet P, Reid W, "La psychothérapie psychanalytique" (French). Gaëtan Morin Editeur Ltée; Boucherville, QC; 1996.
9. Laidlaw K. CBT for older people. An introduction. London: Sage; 2015.
10. Viorst J. The necessary losses. New York: Simon & Schuster; 1998. ISBN 0-684-84495-8.
11. Tatelbaum J. The courage to grieve. New York, NY: Harper and Row Publishers Inc.; 1980. ISBN 0-06-091185-9.
12. André C. Looking at mindfulness: 25 ways to live in the moment through art. New York, NY: Blue Rider Press; 2011. ISBN 978-0-698-40161-7.
13. Hanh TN. Peace is every step: the path of mindfulness in everyday life. New York: Bantam Books; 1991. ISBN 0-553-35139-7.
14. Williams M, Teasdale J, Zindel S, Kabat-Zinn J. The mindful way through depression. New York, NY: The Guilford Press; 2007. ISBN-13: 978-1-59385-128-6.
15. Burns DD. Feeling good. The new mood therapy. New York: Avon Books; Harper Collins Publishers; 2012. ISBN ISBN 10022–5299.
16. Chödrön P. The places that scare you: a guide to fearlessness in difficult times. Boston: Shambhala Publications Inc.; 2001. ISBN 1-57062-921-8.
17. Levine SB. Inventing the rest of our lives. New York: First Plume Printing; 2006. ISBN ISBN 0-452-28721-9.

5 Anti-oppressive Approach to Assessment

Albina Veltman and Tara La Rose

5.1 Background

Case Vignette It was Friday at 4:45 PM when Dr. S, who was catching up on some paperwork in her office after a long and challenging day of work on the geriatric psychiatry ward, received a page from the ward. She grudgingly called the ward to find out why she was paged. The charge nurse started to tell Dr. S about a geriatric patient, Mrs. M. Dr. S stated that she was fully aware of Mrs. M's issues without the charge nurse telling her the details of the current problem. Dr. S felt she had been dealing with issues related to this particular patient all week (and felt that most of the other patients on the ward were presenting with similar issues). Mrs. M was recently admitted to the ward and she had been agitated and aggressive since her admission, despite various attempts at medication management for these symptoms. The charge nurse asked Dr. S to come to see Mrs. M on the ward before she went home for the day. Dr. S, however, had made plans to pick up her daughter from an afterschool program by 5:15 PM, and she knew that if she went to the ward at that point, she would be late for picking up her daughter. Besides, Dr. S made plans to have dinner out that evening and do some shopping with her daughter. Having gone through a divorce last year, Dr. S was still trying to find a way to balance being a single mother with her challenging work on the geriatric psychiatry ward. In the previous 3 years, Dr. S had also been dealing with her parents' increased health issues, and she knew that she had to provide some care for them

A. Veltman, MD (✉)
Department of Psychiatry and Behavioural Neurosciences, McMaster University, Hamilton, ON, Canada
e-mail: veltmaa@mcmaster.ca

T. La Rose, MSW, PhD
Social Work Program, Trent University, Oshawa, ON, Canada
e-mail: taralarose@trentu.ca

A. Hategan et al. (eds.), *On-Call Geriatric Psychiatry: Handbook of Principles and Practice*, DOI 10.1007/978-3-319-30346-8_5

during the upcoming weekend. Frustrated with the charge nurse's request, Dr. S told her, "It's almost 5 PM on a Friday afternoon. I really don't see the point of me seeing Mrs. M now. Let's just increase her sedative medications. That should calm her down."

5.2 Reflective Questions Related to Case Vignette

1. What factors were contributing to Dr. S's reaction to the page and her decision with respect to management of Mrs. M's symptoms?
2. If Dr. S was practicing using an anti-oppressive framework, what are some of the factors that she would be considering with respect to interacting with Mrs. M's presentation?

A psychiatric assessment requires a holistic consideration of the patient's biological, emotional, social, and spiritual needs but must also consider the social and institutional context surrounding the patient. As in question 1 of the case vignette, the physician assessing the patient brings to the assessment process the lens of their own identity, attitudes, values, beliefs, and professional context; these phenomena must be made conscious and explicit in order to ensure that the patient remains at the center of the assessment. It is also important to keep in mind that individuals do not belong to just one social location. Our identities are complex and multiple, fluid rather than fixed [1].

Anti-oppressive practice (AOP) is an emerging concept in the field of medicine. Assessments based on AOP emphasize understandings of privilege, oppression, identity, context, and power as elements that enhance the meaning of traditional assessment criteria such as biological, psychological, and social characteristics. While this perspective may be a relatively recent one in medicine, nursing, social work, and psychology have considered AOP since the mid-1990s [2, 3]. The scholarship of AOP within these health professions acknowledges the interdisciplinary nature of psychiatric care, emphasizing holistic and context-informed understandings of patient needs, thereby expanding assessment beyond the traditional medical model approach [4].

AOP is a model of patient-centered care concerned with both the individual and institutional aspects of care. AOP has been defined as a commitment to social justice that includes:

- A clear theoretical and value base that promotes power sharing and egalitarianism
- An understanding of one's own social location and how it informs practice behaviors and relationships
- Specific practice behaviors and relationships that minimize power imbalances and promote equity and empowerment for patients [5]

AOP recognizes the presence of oppression and privilege in our interactions, and thus, taking responsibility as healthcare professionals for our privileges and educating ourselves about experiences different from our own become important aspects of effective practice. In addition, AOP involves taking action that challenges oppression in the institutions and contexts in which we experience privilege [6].

5.3 Aging and Anti-oppressive Practice

Age is one aspect of patient identity affecting patients' social standing, potentially contributing to vulnerability within the medical care system. Emergency medical care is often provided in high-stress/high-pressure environments [7, 8]. These environments promote assessments focused on threat to "life or limb," the "need for prompt attention," and detection of "common" or "most likely" clinical problems [8]. (See Chap. 16.) These pressures may mean that patients, particularly geriatric patients with complex presentations, may be treated with inadequate effort placed on participation or individualized care because of the need to "get the job done" [5]. These environmental contexts suggest that clinicians have a role to play in the creation of better healthcare, both on the basis of their own model of interaction with patients and in their negotiations with the institutions they serve.

Establishing a standard to measure deviance from the "norms" produces stereotypes of the "abnormal" in medical (including psychiatric) care [7]. This may lead geriatric patients to be described with terms emphasizing concepts like "dependency" and "frailty," which focus on physical incapacity, decline, and dysfunction, rather than their social identities that predated illness [7].

In contrast, some argue that "growing old" is a time when individuals may face changes and experience growth [9]. Older adults are a diverse group, bringing with them different understandings and interpretations of culture. Effective assessment includes consideration for the culturally specific practices and beliefs of patients, as well as changes to their beliefs and attitudes over time [10]. Older patients may fear that visiting a psychiatric clinician means that they are "crazy," while clinicians may maintain unrealistic attitudes about aging and see older persons as incapable of change [11].

Age-related vulnerabilities are numerous and include the view of biological (e.g., physical change, chronic illness, cognitive decline, sexual decline and diminution of physical attractiveness, death), psychological (bereavement, abandonment, institutionalization, forced dependency, facing regrets, and facing a foreshortened future), and social (societal devaluation, economic losses, loss of productivity, and loss of control, leadership, and authority) factors [9]. During on-call assessment, attending to those realities of aging is paramount while retaining the focus on the patient's current psychiatric and/or medical complaints. Therefore, assessment can be a process of helping patients develop a new understanding of self, opening the door to a new range of choices.

5.4 On-Call Psychiatric Care and Anti-oppressive Practice

The structure of medical care systems may facilitate elements of the stigma and oppression of patients, with heterogeneity shown across medical disciplines. In this vein, a recent survey of clinicians in Canada found differing levels of stigma about psychiatric illness across six major physician groups: the highest stigma ratings were among surgeons, followed by anesthetists, emergency rural physicians, and primary care physicians, whereas psychiatrists had the lowest stigma ratings [12]. Despite that, mental health clinicians do have the power in the medical system and the clinical tools at their disposal (e.g., mental health laws, adult protection legislation, diagnostic tools) to influence the goals, values, and desires of patients. Given these potential implicit and explicit expressions of power, on-call physicians need to be aware and practice situationally optimized "egalitarianism and power sharing" in interactions with patients, embracing actions and behaviors that support patient empowerment, decision making, and choice [5].

When traditionally marginalized populations attend psychiatric services, they may experience exclusion [5]. Factors such as gender, culture, and race are described as potentially producing disadvantage within medical settings [5]. Patients from various minority groups (e.g., patients with disabilities, patients who identify as LGBTQ, or patients who are racialized) all could face forms of oppression that are sometimes hidden and therefore difficult to identify [5], especially when these forms are concurrent and coupled with ageism and the realities of aging. Table 5.1 illustrates examples of some dimensions of diversity/identity and potential

Table 5.1 Dimensions of diversity/identity and types of oppression

Dimensions of diversity	Examples of types of oppression
Age	Ageism, elder/child abuse/neglect
Gender/gender identity/gender expression	Sexism, patriarchy, misogyny, chauvinism, transphobia, cisnormativity
Family or marital status	Sexism, patriarchy, misogyny, chauvinism, heteronormativity
Country of origin/creed/ethnicity	Xenophobia, racism, Eurocentrism, westernism, othering, cultural imperialism, ethnocentrism
Immigration/citizen status	Xenophobia, racism, colonialism, cultural imperialism
Socioeconomic background/class	Classism, elitism
Race/color	Racism, racialism, supremacism, colorism, othering
Sexual orientation	Homophobia, lesbophobia, biphobia, heteronormativity
Ability (physical and developmental)	Ableism, ablecentrism, disability oppression
Religion	Xenophobia, Islamophobia, anti-Semitism, Christocentrism
Mental health status	Mental health stigma, sanism, mentalism, pathologization
Place of residence	Regionality, regional stereotypes, "rural vs. urban"
Physical size/weight	Sizeism, weightism, thinnism, fat phobia

Note: Identities can form a system of interlocking oppressions

Table 5.2 Examples of elements of anti-oppressive practice

Goals and objectives	Management tips
Patient-centered goals and activities	Focus on patients' strengths and uniqueness, not on pathology
	Avoid judgments in the form of diagnostic categories and labels
	Listen to and take seriously what patients say about their own mental distress and experience – i.e., treating them as "experts in their own experience"
	Assure patients that they have the right to ask questions and to feel as they choose to feel
	Empower patients by involving them and their families in all decision making about their care and inviting them to participate in agency activities at all levels, including staff meetings and their own case conferences
	Sharing information with patients and their families and providing them with access to clinical records
Clinician-focused goals and objectives	Reflect on personal values, beliefs, and attitudes and how these may affect patients' assessments and treatment
	Reflect on the meaning of professional identity and its capacity to create distance between colleagues and patients
	Reduce the us-and-them distinctions between patients and professionals
	Not pretending competence and knowledge when they are not present; acknowledging what you do not know
Institutional goals and objectives	Reflect on the meaning of the institution to patients using the services
	Consider the effect of the physical environment on the experiences of patients, families, and staff
	Provide public access to information about policies and procedures, including complaint procedures
	Encourage transparency in the operation of the institution
	Establish egalitarian relationships with the communities served by the institution

Adapted from Refs. [2, 3, 13, 14]

associated types of oppression. AOP offers resources to challenge these realities by promoting activities and skills to challenge the status quo. Table 5.2 provides a summary of common examples of AOP elements in healthcare settings and may be helpful in answering the reflective questions from the case vignette presented earlier in the chapter [2, 3, 13, 14].

When patients enter into the process of receiving psychiatric care, systems of power, privilege, and oppression can be activated. Power and privilege take on unique forms at the intersection of age and psychiatric illness. When we add to this the challenges of receiving/providing care on an emergency on-call basis, the dynamics of power, privilege, and the potential for oppression can all become amplified. For many patients, emergency psychiatric care is often the point at which diagnoses are given and decisions are made to provide or deny certain types of care. Out of these decisions can flow a whole "tidal wave" of experiences, which may potentially reinforce patients' experiences of marginalization. Given the power present in these contexts, it is important to consider alternative ways of doing emergent work, ways that emphasize the positive aspects of crisis situations.

Using an AOP approach during on-call psychiatric assessment does not necessarily require additional time or energy. AOP techniques can actually save a clinician time in the long run, improving relationships with patients and their caregivers and enhancing the quality of the information obtained during assessment, furthering the clinician's understanding of the predisposing, precipitating, and perpetuating factors in an individual patient's presentation [13, 15, 16].

A model of assessment limited only to data collection, problem definition, and objective recommendations serves the needs of "management," but it likely represents an approach that departs from a patient-centered one [17]. Presenting a formal diagnosis to a patient without proper context can have an "iatrogenic effect," as labels can produce lasting outcomes that include stigmatization and may become the overarching understanding of the patient, eclipsing other issues and needs that may be better met in a social service sector agency [18]. While most psychiatric assessments tend to focus on the level of "ill-being" experienced by patients, an AOP assessment would also include an assessment of patients' "well-being" [18]. AOP assessments go beyond considerations of the patient's situation and problem to incorporate their strengths, coping strategies, personality, and life experience as well as the environmental resources from which the patient draws [2]. Clinicians who practice using an AOP framework may encourage patients to use their diagnosis strategically to improve their lives and to access needed resources, reminding patients they are more than their diagnosis [3].

AOP includes consideration of the clinician's interpretation and internalization of professional identity, their level of experience, tacit knowledge, and practice wisdom [2, 15], including their ideologies, worldviews, and personal values. The effect of the institutional setting on the assessment and the potential interventions available within this system are also a consideration in AOP assessment. This may include consideration of the employment context of the clinician (status as contract, temporary or permanent staff), the nature of the care facility and their attitude toward patients, the "mandate" of the service (community or hospital based, voluntary/involuntary, etc.), the laws and policies relating to services, as well as the funding structures influencing assessment and care [2].

The AOP process is inductive and built through a process of patient engagement [2]. Clinicians might consider this approach to assessment as a kind of unlearning in which they re-understand assessment not as a standardized pseudo-scientific activity but rather as an art form in which the process is understood as the skillful act of question posing [17] and as a process of eliciting stories from patients [13]. The questions asked and the way in which questions are asked shape the information provided by the patient [13] and also reveal a great deal about the question-poser and their priorities, goals, and values. The fastest kind of assessment is usually one that focuses on closed questions; this is also an assessment that has (generally) already determined what is important to know. Open-ended questions may take more time and may lead the assessment in directions that are unanticipated by the assessor. If concern with patient-centered care is the primary focus, then this type of questioning is likely to be the most effective and efficient approach to assessment. The stories gathered from patients afford clinicians opportunities to consider the importance of content, process, and context contained in the narratives shared. These stories may include pertinent information that may open the potential for AOP to proceed [13]. Patients are aware that there are "right stories" and "wrong stories" within healthcare; the stories told often need to match predetermined criteria in order for resources to be provided [19]. AOP assessments require clinicians to acknowledge the idea that patients may feel pressured to provide stories that reflect common/normative or dominant narratives [13, 19]. In this context, clinicians and patients may reinforce commonly held beliefs as those most likely to be believed and responded to positively. Applying an AOP framework means acknowledging that we need certain kinds of stories in order to get our job done, but it also requires us to accept that in looking for these stories, we may be missing many other stories that do not fit into our desired/needed narratives and which might suggest another course of action. Sometimes we may require "wrong stories" for the "right response" to be identified.

AOP approaches to mental health care consider the patient's social environment and the personal network surrounding the patient. This may mean inviting family members (including chosen family) to be a part of the process. Intimate people in the older patient's life are encouraged to take an active role in care, serving as consultants on the experiences of their loved one and sharing their perceptions of the effectiveness of their loved one's treatment [5].

Communication processes are important aspects of AOP since communication is the foundation of relationship building. Communication that is inclusive, that does not stigmatize patients, and that increases the patient's power and knowledge is fundamental [4, 16]. For example, avoiding the tendency to refer to patients as their symptoms ("auditory hallucinations in room ten"), their diagnosis ("bipolar in room ten"), or stereotypes about the types of patients ("bed blocker in room ten") is a great first step. Using critical reflexivity to shape practice is another important step [4, 16]. Also important in the AOP approach is providing explanations in plain language, in multiple languages if necessary, and providing written materials (especially for those with sensory and cognitive impairment) that support a continued development of patient knowledge.

Key Points

- Clinicians have a responsibility to educate themselves about the systems they work in and to understand who benefits and who suffers as a result of the structures and processes present within the system.
- Clinicians can either reinforce or challenge oppressions and disadvantages faced by patients with marginalized identities.
- Clinicians need to think concretely about the importance of identifying and managing various forms of oppression in their practice, including ageism, sexism, racism, ableism, and homophobia, which can occur concurrently, as concerns that directly affect many patients with psychiatric illness, including geriatric patients.

References

1. Training for Change – An Integrated Anti-Oppression Framework: A Tool for Trainers and Community Service Organizations. Rainbow health network. 2009. http://www.oaith.ca/assets/files/Publications/intersectionality/FrameworkARAO-Training.pdf. Accessed 4 Oct 2015.
2. Mullaly R. Challenging oppression: a critical social work approach. Oxford: Oxford University Press; 2002.
3. Baines D. Doing anti-oppressive practice: social justice social work. 2nd ed. Fernwood: Halifax; 2011.
4. Knott C, Scragg T. Reflective practice in social work. 3rd ed. Washington: Sage; 2015.
5. Larson G. Anti-oppressive practice in mental health. J Prog Hum Ser. 2008;19(1):39–54.
6. Clemens K. Anti-oppression toolkit. National Campus and Community Radio Association. 2013. http://www.ncra.ca/equity/ncra-anti-oppression-toolkit.pdf. Accessed 4 Oct 2015.
7. Martin GW, Younger D. Anti oppressive practice: a route to the empowerment of people with dementia through communication and choice. J Psychiatr Ment Health Nurs. 2000;7:59–67.
8. VanDerHeyden C, Sanders A. Emergency assessment of the older adult. In: Gallo J, Bogner H, Fullmer T, Pavez G, editors. Handbook of geriatric assessment. 4th ed. Toronto: Jones and Bartlett Publishing; 2006.
9. Gallo J, Bogner H. The context of geriatric care. In: Gallo J, Bogner H, Fullmer T, Pavez G, editors. Handbook of geriatric assessment. 4th ed. Toronto: Jones and Bartlett Publishing; 2006.
10. Mouton C, Esparza Y. Ethnicity and geriatric assessments. In: Gallo J, Bogner H, Fullmer T, Pavez G, editors. Handbook of geriatric assessment. 4th ed. Toronto: Jones and Bartlett Publishing; 2006.
11. Morgan AC. Psychodynamic psychotherapy with older adults. Psychiatr Serv. 2003;54(12):1592–4.
12. Ungar T, Knaak S, Szeto ACH. Theoretical and practical considerations for combating mental illness stigma in health care. Community Ment Health J. doi:10.1007/s10597-015-9910-4.
13. Fook J. Social work: critical theory and practice. 2nd ed. Thousand Oaks: Sage Publications; 2012.
14. Kinney M. Being assessed under the 1983 mental health act – can it ever be ethical? Ethics Soc Welfare. 2009;3(2):329–36.
15. Baines D. Doing anti-oppressive practice: building transformative politicized social work. Fernwood: Halifax; 2007.
16. Healy K. Social work methods and skills: the essential foundations of practice. New York: Palgrave MacMillan; 2012.
17. Hick S. Social work in Canada: an introduction. 3rd ed. Toronto: Thompson Publishing; 2014.
18. Heinonen T, Spearman L. Social work practice: problem solving and beyond. Toronto: Nelson Education; 2010.
19. La Rose T. Digital stories through the lens of multi modal analysis: a case study of Erahoneybee's Song about a Child Welfare Agency. J Hum Ser Technol. 2012;30(3/4): 299–311.

Decisional Capacity Assessments and Advance Directives

6

Usha Parthasarathi and Daniel L. Ambrosini

6.1 Background

Decisional capacity assessments are one of the most commonly sought consultation referrals to on-call psychiatrists. In hospital settings, one in six referral requests to a psychiatrist is to address decisional capacity [1]. Decisional capacity evaluations are often perceived to be more challenging and time-consuming than other types of consultations performed by psychiatrists (e.g., delirium and depression evaluations) [1]. Certainly, finding geriatric patients who are in a hospital setting incapable to make decisions is common, with prevalence estimates ranging from 20 to 50 % [1, 2]. There are various types of decisional capacity assessments including (1) capacity to consent to treatment; (2) capacity to consent for research; (3) capacity to drive; (4) capacity to live independently; (5) testamentary capacity; and (6) contractual capacity [3–5]. The most frequent capacity assessment referred to an on-call psychiatrist is for an assessment of capacity to consent to treatment. The following two vignettes highlight some of the issues that can arise in this context.

Case Vignette 1 The police brought Ms. G, an elderly woman, to the hospital. She was found in a neighborhood park in a state of distress and disoriented to time, place, and person. Her speech was nonsensical and she was observed to be mumbling

U. Parthasarathi, MBBS (✉)
Department of Psychiatry and Behavioural Neurosciences,
McMaster University, St. Joseph's Healthcare, Hamilton, ON, Canada
e-mail: uparthas@stjoes.ca

D.L. Ambrosini, LLB/BCL, MSc, PhD
Department of Psychiatry and Behavioural Neurosciences, Forensic Psychiatry Program,
McMaster University, West 5th Campus, 3rd Floor, D328, 100 West 5th, Box 585, Hamilton,
ON L8N 3K7, Canada

Legal Counsel, St. Joseph's Healthcare Hamilton, Hamilton, ON, Canada
e-mail: dambro@mcmaster.ca

A. Hategan et al. (eds.), *On-Call Geriatric Psychiatry: Handbook of Principles and Practice*, DOI 10.1007/978-3-319-30346-8_6

and appearing to be responding to hallucinations. The police were concerned that the woman may have been a recent victim of physical and sexual assault. The park where she was found was in a neighborhood that experienced a recent influx of sexual assaults toward elderly women. The emergency physician referred the woman for a consultation by the on-call psychiatrist and requested advice on patient's capacity to provide forensic evidence regarding the incident at the park.

Clinical Recommendation
Prior to starting any treatment, the physician needs to make a clinical judgment about the patient's decisional capacity to consent to treatment and would like to find out from the patient what actually occurred in the park for the purposes of collecting forensic evidence about the assault.

Case Vignette 2 Dr. J was the on-call psychiatrist for the hospital and was asked to assess Mr. B, a 75-year-old man who was brought to the hospital from his nursing home. Mr. B had a history of major depression and had recently expressed suicidal ideation. His wife of 50 years died from a heart attack 2 weeks earlier, causing Mr. B's mood to worsen. Earlier in the day, he attempted to lacerate his wrist. His son informed the clinical team that he was granted power of attorney (POA) for personal care. Before Dr. J could begin an assessment of Mr. B's mental state, his medical resident approached him and asked if he could enroll Mr. B in his research study. He was enrolling participants for a study examining clinical factors and biomarkers to differentiate major depression from grief reaction.

Clinical Recommendation
Dr. J needs to assess Mr. B's decisional capacity for consent to treatment and consider any direction provided by the legally authorized representative named in the POA. Mr. B's decisional capacity to consent to participate for research needs to be considered separately from his capacity to consent for treatment.

6.2 Decisional Capacity

During on-call shifts, some common psychiatric emergencies encountered with geriatric patients are related to delirium, major depression with suicidal ideation, major neurocognitive disorders, and substance abuse. Patients are by default presumed to be capable to make their own decisions, but decisional incapacity can often be intuited quickly after direct observation of the patient (e.g., confusion, disorientation, depression, psychosis, extreme anxiety, inability to make a decision, intoxication) [6]. Patients may lack insight into their psychiatric illness or their medical condition more broadly. Patients come to the attention of on-call clinicians at the behest of family members, caregivers, the public, the police, and other health-care agencies. Clinicians are often asked to assess patients who present with acute confusion, aggression, paranoia, and neglect. A lower educational level, chronic or acute medical illness, and cognitive impairment may be related to someone having diminished capacity in a geriatric population [5], but this is not definitive.

It is not always possible for on-call physicians to accurately assess whether a patient's current presentation is an actual change from their baseline state. This may be further complicated by limited access to caregivers, common during on-call hours, who would otherwise provide collateral information. Detecting changes in mental status may also be hampered by the limited information of prior mental health assessments during an on-call shift as a result of the inability to obtain health-care information due to privacy/information sharing restrictions and regulations [7]. Hence, conducting decisional capacity assessments during an on-call shift can also be challenging due to time and information constraints.

Many situations of diminished capacity are managed by medical teams without any formal determination of incapacity or appointment of a surrogate [8]. This often happens when patients have been compliant with treatment, and decisional capacity is questioned only when the patient refuses treatment or disagrees with a treatment plan, triggering a decisional capacity assessment. It is essential that clinicians determine a patient's decisional capacity for treatment prior to the medical treatment being initiated to ensure the consent was both informed and valid. A physician could be held liable if no consent was provided, if the treatment deviated significantly from that which was consented to, or if the consent to treatment was obtained through misrepresentation [9–11].

In many situations, a lack of decisional capacity may be readily apparent. Deciding whether a geriatric patient is capable of the decision at hand may have been undertaken by the primary clinical team, and documentation of the capacity findings may be available for the on-call physician to rely upon. It is important, however, that a physician does not presume decisional incapacity [12]. A formal assessment of capacity needs to be conducted when the patient's clinical presentation is unclear, there are underlying medicolegal issues, the issue has become contentious with others (e.g., family members), or status of decisional capacity appears to be transient in nature (e.g., in delirium with variable cognitive status).

Capacity to consent to treatment is foundational to the doctrine of informed consent. Capacity to consent has been defined as "the ability to understand significant benefits, risks, and alternatives to proposed health care and to make and communicate a health-care decision" [4]. Appelbaum and Gutheil [12] also define capacity as "a threshold requirement for persons to retain the power to make decisions for themselves." Decision-making capacities entail at least four components: (1) the ability to *understand* relevant information as it relates to the choice, such as the nature, purpose, and the potential risks and benefits of the proposed treatment as well as alternatives; (2) the ability to *appreciate* the relevance of treatment methods and their consequences for one's condition or situation; (3) the ability to *reason* about the different treatment options (consider and compare potential consequences of various options); and (4) the ability to *communicate* (express) a consistent choice [2, 12, 13].

Generally, a decisional capacity assessment involves the following steps: referral question clarification, general psychiatric assessment (including assessment of cognitive status), synthesis of data and case formulation, communication of findings to referring clinical service, and follow-up evaluation [8]. A physician may choose to evaluate a patient's decisional capacity using a combination of clinical judgment along with standardized capacity assessment tools. Valid clinical tools include, for example, the MacArthur Competence Assessment Tool for Treatment (MacCAT-T) [14], Aid to Capacity Evaluation (ACE) [15], and the Mini-Mental State Examination (MMSE) which have been found to correlate with clinical judgments of decisional incapacity [13].

Capacity and competency are terms sometimes used interchangeably, but there are subtle differences in their meaning [6]. Competency is a global assessment and a legal determination often made by a judge, whereas decisional capacity, on the other hand, is a functional assessment by a clinician regarding a particular decision. Decisional capacity is not static, and a decisional capacity determination can be performed by any physician who is responsible for the patient's care. A clinical finding of incapacity does not alter an individual's legal status, whereas a legal finding of incompetence does [5]. Table 6.1 summarizes a few common pitfalls and tips to consider during capacity assessments of geriatric patients [16].

6.3 Advance Directives

There are generally two types of advance directives: (1) instructional and (2) proxy directives. Instructional directives allow individuals to detail their instructions in the living will document, whereas proxy directives appoint a legally authorized representative (proxy) to make decisions on their behalf if the person becomes incapable. Psychiatric advance directives (PADs) are one type of document containing detailed information about patients' treatment preferences so their wishes are already recorded if they become mentally incapable in the future [17, 18]. In some cases, advance directives are overridden by health professionals, defeating their very purpose [19]. In one survey of legal and mental health professionals, less than half were willing to start using PADs [20]. Generally, it is good clinical practice for the on-call clinician working with a geriatric population to ask whether they may have an advance care planning tool that details their instructions or appoints a legally authorized representative.

There are circumstances when a physician may be required to conduct a capacity assessment quickly. In an emergency situation, diagnostic and treatment procedures are not delayed for a formal decisional capacity assessment to be performed. Even where a clinician has asked about the presence of an advance directive, there may not be enough time to locate the actual document. Generally speaking, emergency treatment may be provided where (1) a patient is unable to express his own preferences, (2) immediate action is required to prevent loss of life or limb, and (3) no surrogate decision-maker is available [21]. Where a patient is unable to communicate effectively, prior competent wishes must be taken into consideration and honored wherever possible [21].

Table 6.1 Common pitfalls and tips for on-call clinicians during capacity assessments of geriatric patients [16]

Pitfalls	Tips
• Appreciate that a finding of capacity or incapacity is not "all or nothing." Do not assume that, if a patient lacks capacity for one medical decision, he or she lacks capacity for all medical decisions. Be aware that capacity is decision specific. If physicians conceptualize a patient as globally lacking capacity, the patient is likely to not be allowed to make a variety of decisions that he/she is actually able to make • Appreciate that ineffective or inconsistent communication between a clinical team and patient may translate into a finding of incapacity. Presentation of information may vary on the basis of clinicians' knowledge, biases, and time constraints. Patients may require time to process information about their options and goals and to consult with family and friends • Appreciate that the process of engaging patients in a capacity assessment is of greater importance than the final outcome of the assessment. It is important to consider whether a patient lacks capacity even if he or she agrees with the physicians' recommendations [16]	• On-call physicians caring for geriatric patients should routinely consider decisional capacity in all clinical encounters • Use of narrative clinical interviewing along with additional valid clinical instruments are useful to assess capacity • Attempts should be made to maximize patient's functioning during a capacity assessment (e.g., offering written instructions or sensory aids such as eyeglasses or hearing aids) • If a decision of incapacity is determined, it is prudent to seek out who may become the legally authorized representative as early as possible • If an advance care planning document exists, it is important to identify and locate the legally authorized representative so physicians can receive instructions • If a capacity finding is equivocal, a reassessment or independent second opinion at a later time may be recommended • Document thoroughly in the clinical records how the capacity finding was determined and who the current legally authorized representative is, which can often change

Key Points

- The prevalence of decisional incapacity is common in geriatric populations and clinicians should monitor routinely.
- It is essential that clinicians determine an individual's mental capacity to make decisions about medical treatment prior to it being initiated.
- Clinicians should remain cognizant of the presence of advance care directives and attempt to honor prior capable wishes wherever possible.

References

1. Seyfried L, Ryan K, Kim S. Assessment of decision-making capacity: views and experiences of consultation psychiatrists. Psychosomatics. 2013;54(2):115–23.
2. Sessums L, Zembrzuska H, Jackson J. Does this patient have medical decision-making capacity? JAMA. 2011;306(4):420.
3. American Bar Association Commission on Law and Aging, & American Psychological Association. Assessment of older adults with diminished capacity: a handbook for psychologists. Washington, DC: Author; 2008.
4. Moye J, Marson D, Edelstein B. Assessment of capacity in an aging society. Am Psychol. 2013;68(3):158–71.
5. National Conference of Commissioners on Uniform State Laws. 1993. Uniform Health Care Decision. 2015.
6. Leo RJ. Competency and the capacity to make treatment decisions: a primer for primary care physicians. Prim Care Companion J Clin Psychiatry. 1999;1(5):131–41.
7. Christensen K, Haroun A, Schneiderman LJ, Jeste DV. Decision-making capacity for informed consent in the older population. Bull Am Acad Psychiatry Law. 1995;23(3):353–65.
8. Moye J, Marson D. Assessment of decision-making capacity in older adults: an emerging area of practice and research. FOC. 2009;7(1):88–97.
9. Glezer A, Stern TA, Mort EA, Atamian S, Abrams JL, Brendel RW. Documentation of decision-making capacity, informed consent, and health care proxies: a study of surrogate consent. Psychosomatics. 2011;52(6):521–9.
10. Derse AR. What part of "no" don't you understand? Patient refusal of recommended treatment in the emergency department. Mt Sinai J Med. 2005;724:221–7.
11. Anon. Case summaries: informed consent. In: Case summaries. 2015. http://www.lawandbioethics.com/demo/Main/LegalResources/C5/background01.htm. Accessed 30 Oct 2015.
12. Appelbaum P, Gutheil T. Clinical handbook of psychiatry and the law. Baltimore: Williams & Wilkins; 1991.
13. Appelbaum P. Assessment of patients' competence to consent to treatment. N Engl J Med. 2007;357(18):1834–40.
14. Grisso T, Appelbaum P. MacArthur treatment competence study. J Am Psychiatr Nurses Assoc. 1995;1(4):125–7.
15. Etchells E, Darzins P, Silberfeld M, Singer PA, McKenny J, Naglie G, et al. Assessment of patient capacity to consent to treatment. J Gen Intern Med. 1999;14(1):27–34.
16. Ganzini L, Volicer L, Nelson W, Derse A. Pitfalls in assessment of decision-making capacity. Psychosomatics. 2003;44(3):237–43.
17. Ambrosini DL, Crocker AG, Latimer E. Preferences for instructional or proxy advance directives in mental health: a mixed methods study. JEMH. 2012;6(1):1–19.
18. Ambrosini DL, Bemme D, Crocker AG, Latimer E. Narratives of psychiatric advance directives: qualitative study. J Ethics Ment Health. 2012;6(1):1–9.
19. Appelbaum PS. Advance directives for psychiatric treatment. Psychiatr Serv. 1991;42(10):983–4.
20. Ambrosini DL, Crocker AG, Perreault M, Israel M. Perceptions of psychiatric advance directives among legal and mental health professionals in Ontario and Quebec. JEMH. 2008;3(1):1–12.
21. Larkin GL, Marco CA, Abbott JT. Emergency determination of decision-making capacity: balancing autonomy and beneficence in the emergency department. Acad Emerg Med. 2001;8(3):282–4.

Use of Seclusion, Chemical and Physical Restraint

7

Lauren S. Barney, Sebastien Prat, and Usha Parthasarathi

7.1 Background

Aggression is a common clinical presentation in patients suffering from major neurocognitive disorders (NCDs) (formerly termed dementia). It is estimated that 96 % of patients diagnosed with major NCDs will display some form of aggression in their lifetime [1]. In psychiatric inpatient settings, it is estimated that 40 % of geriatric patients display aggression and violence during their hospital stay [2]. During an on-call shift, the psychiatrist is often consulted for management of agitation and aggression either in the inpatient units or in emergency department settings.

7.1.1 Agitation

Agitation is usually a precursor to an aggressive outburst. Agitation refers to a constellation of aimless and poorly organized clinical behavioral symptoms that often originate as a result of a patient experiencing physical or mental discomfort [3]. Agitation may present as motor restlessness, irritability, and inappropriate and usually purposeless verbal and motor activity [3]. If uncontrolled or untreated, agitation

L.S. Barney, BA, JD
St. Joseph's Healthcare Hamilton, West 5th Campus, Hamilton, ON, Canada

S. Prat, MD
Department of Psychiatry and Behavioural Neurosciences, McMaster University, Hamilton, ON, Canada

U. Parthasarathi, MBBS (✉)
Department of Psychiatry and Behavioural Neurosciences, McMaster University, St. Joseph's Healthcare, Hamilton, ON, Canada
e-mail: uparthas@stjoes.ca

A. Hategan et al. (eds.), *On-Call Geriatric Psychiatry: Handbook of Principles and Practice*, DOI 10.1007/978-3-319-30346-8_7

can translate into a verbal or physical aggression toward objects or persons; the patients may thus pose a danger to others [3, 4].

7.1.2 Aggression

Aggression has been defined as a hostile action directed toward other persons or objects or toward oneself. It presents as an overt act, involving the delivery of noxious stimuli to (but not necessarily aimed at) another object, organism, or self, which is clearly not accidental [4, 5]; 64 % of nursing staff working with geriatric patients in hospital settings reported having been physically assaulted by their patients [2, 6]. Although this behavior rarely results in severe injury, it has a negative impact on the staff and the ward milieu [2, 6]. Aggression can be of physical, verbal, or sexual nature [5]. Cohen-Mansfield and Werner have identified factors associated with aggressive behavior specifically in geriatric patients [4]. Cognitive impairment, poor quantity and quality of interaction with caregivers, and depressive symptoms were associated with physical aggression in these patients [4]. In addition to these factors, poor physical health was specifically associated with verbal aggression. Poor physical health and unremitted pain were the most significant predictors of aggression [4].

7.1.3 Etiology of Agitation and Aggression

The etiology of agitation and aggressive behavior in the geriatric population is multifactorial [2]. Common etiological factors for this behavior include pain and other physical discomfort such as dysregulated sleep, constipation, poor physical health, effects from polypharmacy, interpersonal conflicts, sensory overload, and other environmental factors [7].

7.1.4 Assessment and Management

Assess and manage the etiological factors if possible. Aggression and agitation in a geriatric patient should be managed conservatively with a patient-centered approach. Thwart the process of conversion of agitated behavior to aggression using supportive measures. Non-pharmacological and least restrictive measures should generally be used to control the disruptive behavior in a geriatric patient. However, in circumstances that the behavior presents an imminent threat to the safety of the patient or others in the unit environment, coercive measures such as isolation and/or restrain may be used as a protective intervention. Containment measures such as seclusion and restraint should only be used as a last resort in geriatric patients and that too only when other alternative approaches have been tried and failed [8]. Seclusion and restraint intervention is never regarded as a treatment per se [8].

7.2 Seclusion and Restraint and General Principles

7.2.1 Definition

Seclusion is defined as an involuntary confinement of the patient alone in a room or an area where the patient is physically prevented from leaving; a situation where a patient is restricted to a room or area alone and the staff physically intervenes to prevent the patient from leaving is also considered seclusion [8]. *Restraint* is defined as any manual method, physical or mechanical device, material, or equipment that immobilizes or reduces the ability of a patient to move his or her arms, legs, body, or head freely, or a drug or medication used as a restriction to manage the patient's behavior and/or restrict the patient's freedom of movement and is not a standard treatment or dosage for the patient's condition [8]. Restraints do not include devices such as orthopedically prescribed devices, surgical dressings or bandages, protective helmets, and other methods that involve the physical holding of a patient for the purpose of conducting routine physical examination or tests, to protect the patient from falling out of bed, or to permit the patient to participate in activities without the risk of physical harm [8]. Seclusion and restraint should only be used for the management of violent behavior that jeopardizes the immediate physical safety of the patient, a staff member, or others [8]. Seclusion and restraint should not be used for punishment, coercion, or threat [8].

7.2.2 Methods of Containment

Seclusion and restraint fall on a continuum of containment and restrictive measures to protect the patient, other patients, and staff members and to maintain the ward milieu stability. In an increasing restrictiveness order, containment measures include (1) manual restraint and oral medications, (2) loss of clothing, (3) intramuscular medication, (4) seclusion, and (5) restraint with constant observation [9]. In on-call and emergency situations, it would be prudent for the psychiatrist to be cognizant of this hierarchy to make the most appropriate clinical decision with least intrusive and restrictive measures. Clinical decision to use seclusion and restraint for management of violence or aggression in geriatric patients should be made thoughtfully and with significant caution. Both of these interventions are associated with significant negative patient and the staff experiences [2, 6–8, 10]. In geriatric patients, consider *alternative* methods for seclusion and restraint to manage aggression; these include (1) one-to-one observation, (2) time out, and (3) medications to control agitation [10, 11].

During an acute hospital admission, when compared to general adult patients, the geriatric patients are three times at higher risk of being physically restrained during their hospitalization [9, 12]. Geriatric patients with impaired memory, judgment, and comprehension often have difficulty adapting to the hospital setting. At a particular risk for restraint use are patients whose behavior (e.g., confusion, agitation, impulsivity) is judged to be "unsafe" (e.g., contributing to falls or interfering with treatment or medical devices). Other hospitalized geriatric patients at risk are those who have experienced stroke or traumatic brain injury with cognitive deficits resulting in impulsivity, wandering, confusion, impaired judgment, agitation, and aggression [6, 9, 12].

Seclusion and restraint approach is associated with adverse outcomes, particularly in geriatric patients [2, 6–8, 10, 13]. The use of physical restraints has been associated with significant mortality and morbidity [8, 11, 13, 14]. Some of the serious adverse events associated with the use of restraints include dehydration, choking, circulatory and skin problems, loss of strength and mobility, incontinence, and injury from other patients [11, 13]. Physical injury and death due to restraints have been related to patient actions, improper application of restraints, or failure of restraints [11, 13]. Asphyxiation, aspiration, cardiac arrest, and strangulation have been the leading causes of deaths related to restraints [13]. With restraint in the prone position, a simple flexion of the head onto the chest, a partial or complete external airway obstruction, or neck compression has been implicated in causing restraint asphyxia [13]. Restraining a patient in the supine position has been associated with deaths due to aspiration [13]. The risk of aspiration is elevated with decreased level of consciousness, either due to physical condition or due to medications.

Aggressive behavior typically involves behavioral arousal and psychological stress and is associated with massive release of adrenal catecholamines, otherwise known as the "catecholamine rush" [13]. This can cause abnormal cardiac rhythm and may result in death in predisposed patients from arrhythmia [13]. Extreme physiological exertion in response to a psychological stress can cause severe metabolic acidosis and can result in death. Patients on psychotropic medications, particularly in geriatric cohort, are at a high risk for mortality due to sudden death. Psychotropic medications such as antipsychotics and antidepressants are known to cause prolongation in QTc interval, and many of these agents also have inherent anticholinergic effects that can increase body temperature [11, 13, 15]. Therefore, in a restraint situation, geriatric patients suffering from aggression (e.g., due to agitated delirium) are of particular risk for fatal hyperpyrexia, when factors, such as poorly ventilated room, dehydration, and abnormal serum electrolytes, in combination with physiological effects of psychotropic interplay can increase the body temperature to dangerous levels [14]. Death related to rhabdomyolysis has also been documented in a restraint situation. Rhabdomyolysis may result from extreme physical exertion seen in a restraint situation and has been associated with the use of benzodiazepines, chlorpromazine, hyponatremia, and a full sheet restraint [14]. Prolonged restraint and, hence, immobility can result in thromboembolism that can lead to fatal outcome [14].

Therefore, it is recommended that physical restraint be used sparingly as a clinical intervention in geriatric population. If used, it is essential that need for such a restraint be evaluated constantly and the duration of the restraint used is as brief as possible. Patients should be constantly monitored for any adverse physiological changes, and restraint be terminated at the earliest indication of worsening of physical, psychological, or physiological status of the patient. Consider a patient's premorbid physical and mental status, and choose the most appropriate and the least restrictive containment measure for management of aggression in a geriatric patient.

Patients can have long-term psychological consequence from experiencing physical restraint. Reports suggest patients associate their experience in physical restraint as traumatic and can exhibit fear, anxiety, and rage [8–14]. They may experience confusion and bewilderment at being restrained. Long-term consequences include mistrust of healthcare professionals, nightmares, and avoidance [11, 13]. This may place these patients at a higher risk for aggression in the future and perpetuate the cycle of seclusion and restraint. Therefore, it is important that the clinicians provide the patients feedback and explanation of the rationale and expectations of behavior following their restraint episode. The use of restraints or seclusion must be well documented, patient's psychiatric and physical condition carefully monitored, and all changes and progress of their status recorded [15]. Clinicians, caregivers, and peer support personnel should be available on an ongoing basis to address any questions from patients related to their experience during restraints. This allows for continuation of therapeutic rapport and a better outcome.

Antipsychotic medications may be used as restraints in geriatric patients with delirium or major NCDs who become combative and endanger themselves and others. When possible, offer oral medications in lieu of injectables [15, 16]. Consider low-dose atypical antipsychotics as a first-line medication for use as chemical restraint in geriatric population, particularly patients suffering from parkinsonism symptoms [15, 16]. Caution is advised with the use of benzodiazepines in geriatric patients. Benzodiazepines increase the risk of ataxia, oversedation, and asphyxiation [15, 16]. Anticholinergic medications may cause an acute exacerbation of psychiatric symptoms and may cause oversedation. Oversedation in geriatric patients can be potentially dangerous as it may lead negative outcomes including dehydration, falls, respiratory depression, aspiration pneumonia, and death [14, 16]. Therefore, if possible, avoid prescribing anticholinergic and benzodiazepine as a chemical restraint for an agitated geriatric patient [16]. Start low-dose and go low on medication doses. Be cognizant of age-related physiological changes in drug absorption and metabolism in a geriatric patient, and adjust the dose accordingly (see Chap. 3). Prior to prescribing chemical restraint, consider other physical comorbid conditions and other concomitant medications. The following are a few suggestions for medications to be used as chemical restraint in geriatric patients: olanzapine IM 2.5 mg, haloperidol IM 0.25–0.5 mg, risperidone ODT 0.5–1 mg, or quetiapine 25–50 mg PO (if the patient is cooperative with oral administration). If necessary, use the most minimum dose of benzodiazepine such as lorazepam 0.5 mg [16]. Monitor closely for any adverse effects or sudden deterioration of physical or psychological status of the patient.

Tips to approach and manage an agitated geriatric patient	
	When approaching an agitated geriatric patient move and speak quietly, slowly, and directly
	Stay relaxed and position yourself safely when addressing the patient
	Redirect patient to a less stimulating or frustrating activity, discontinue an activity
	Do not argue with a patient about their behavior
	Be flexible, and modify treatment interventions
	Provide the patient with clear expectations of interactions and treatment
	Facilitate safety by removing items that could cause injury, arranging for constant observation, or involving family (if calming and reassuring to patient)
	Place patient in a common area where staff can frequently visualize patient and behaviors
	Assess and treat etiological factors for aggression from a biopsychosocial approach
	Review the medication effects and medication side effects on cognition
	Avoid medications that can aggravate acute confusion in the geriatric patients (e.g., hypnotics, sedatives, antianxiety agents, tricyclic antidepressants, other medications with anticholinergic side effects)
	Offer low dose of additional medication in addition to regular medication
	Suggest visual cues such as calendars and memory aids to reduce confusion and agitation
	Recommend that staff frequently reorient the patient
	Suggest to the staff to move the patient's room near the nursing station
	Consider discontinuation of lines and tubes and perhaps using long sleeve clothing (or knit sleeve to limit access to lines and tubes)
	Arrange for continuous observation by staff
	Recommend family staying with the patient, if appropriate.
	If all the above approaches fail, consider a *brief* seclusion and restraint

Fig. 7.1 Tips to approach and manage an agitated geriatric patient during an on-call event

Seclusion for an agitated geriatric patient may be considered in situations where other alternative methods of containment have either failed or are contraindicated. Seclusion can be effective in controlling agitation by immediate removal of the patient from causative stimuli. It also provides immediate protection to the staff and other patients on the unit by isolating the agitated patient. It is estimated that seclusion is used as an intervention in 25.6 % of an emergency department [7]. In some geriatric patients, a brief period of seclusion with constant observation may be preferable to the use of restraints, due to limitations of chemical and physical restraints in this population as described previously. However, seclusion approach has its own set of adverse effects. Seclusion may exacerbate confusion and agitation in patients with major NCDs [14, 17]. Neglect, inappropriate monitoring, and longer duration in isolation have been associated with deaths of patients in seclusion [17]. Figure 7.1 presents a few tips on how to approach and manage an agitated geriatric patient during an on-call event.

7.3 Legal Doctrines of Seclusion and Restraint Practices

Seclusion and restraint practices are governed by legal and ethical doctrines. The following information is meant to provide a brief overview of seclusion and restraint provisions under legislation in the USA, Canada, and the UK.

7.3.1 The United States

Title 42 of the Code of Federal Regulations, Chapter IV, Part 482, regulates the administration of hospitals under the Medicare program. At §482.13 the regulation states that "all patients have the right to be free from physical or mental abuse, and corporal punishment. All patients have the right to be free from restraint or seclusion, of any form, imposed as a means of coercion, discipline, convenience, or retaliation by staff. Restraint or seclusion may only be imposed to ensure the immediate physical safety of the patient, a staff member, or others and must be discontinued at the earliest possible time" [18].

The use of seclusion or restraint should be the least restrictive method and should only be used when less restrictive methods are ineffective in protecting the patient or staff from harm [19]. Orders for seclusion or restraint cannot be standing orders or PRNs [20] although in an on-call setting this would likely not be the case at any rate.

When using the order for seclusion or restraint to manage violent or self-destructive behavior, unless superseded by state law, the order may only be renewed every 4 h for a maximum of 24 h [21]. Interestingly, the 4-h renewal provision applies to all adults over the age of 18 years old. No special consideration was given to geriatric patients. However, Part 483 of the same Chapter deals with seclusion and restraint in long-term care settings.

7.3.2 Canada

In Ontario, under the Mental Health Act, R.S.O. 1990, c. M.7, restraint is defined as a means to "place under control when necessary to prevent serious bodily harm to the patient or to another person by the minimal use of such force, mechanical means or chemicals as is reasonable having regard to the physical and mental condition of the patient."

When a patient is restrained, the clinical team has a legal obligation to carefully document a description of the means of restraint and a description of the patient's behavior leading up to the restraint in the patient's record of personal health information. When a chemical restraint is used, the clinical team must also document the type of medication and dosage used [22]. In Manitoba similar provisions exist under the civil mental health legislation [23], while in other provinces and territories, the term restraint is often used but never clearly defined.

7.3.3 The United Kingdom

In the UK, section 64G of the Mental Health Act outlines *emergency treatment for patients lacking capacity or competency*. We highlight this section because in some on-call geriatric situations, the patient lacks capacity and competency. The section lists the following criteria for *emergency treatment*:

1. The person must believe that the patient lacks the capacity to consent or is not competent to make a treatment decision.
2. The treatment must be immediately necessary.
3. If it is necessary to use force to treat the patient
   (a) The treatment needs to be given in order to prevent harm to the patient.
   (b) The use of such force is a proportionate response to the likelihood of the patient's suffering harm and to the seriousness of that harm [24].

A treatment is deemed immediately necessary if (1) it is either immediately necessary to save the patient's life, (2) it is immediately necessary to prevent a serious deterioration of the patient's condition and is not irreversible, (3) it is immediately necessary to alleviate serious suffering by the patient and is not irreversible or hazardous, and (4) it is immediately necessary, and represents the minimum interference necessary to prevent the patient from behaving [24].

Key Points

- Non-coercive de-escalation should be the intervention of choice in the management of acute agitation and threatening behavior in geriatric patients.
- Seclusion and restraint should be used as a last resort containment measure when alternative methods have been unsuccessful in managing imminent threat of violence.
- Beware of the risks associated with seclusion and restraint practices and monitor accordingly.

References

1. Jackson JL, Mallory R. Aggression and violence among elderly patients, a growing health problem. J Gen Intern Med. 2009;24(10):1167–8.
2. Almvik R, Rasmussen K, Woods P. Challenging behaviour in the elderly – monitoring violent incidents. Int J Geriatr Psychiatry. 2006;21(4):368–74.
3. Patel V, Hope T. Aggressive behaviour in elderly people with dementia: a review. Int J Geriatr Psychiatry. 1993;8(6):457–72.
4. Cohen-Mansfield J, Werner P. Predictors of aggressive behaviors: a longitudinal study in senior day care centers. J Gerontol B Psychol Sci Soc Sci. 1998;53(5):300–10.
5. Ryden M. Aggressive behavior in persons with dementia who live in the community. Alzheimer Dis Assoc Disord. 1988;2(4):342–55.
6. O'Callaghan C, Richman A, Majumdar B. Violence in older people with mental illness. Adv Psychiatr Treat. 2010;16:339–48.
7. Leger JM, Moulias R, Vellas B, Monfort JC, Chapuy P, Robert P, et al. Causes and consequences of elderly's agitated and aggressive behaviour. Encéphale. 2000;26(1):32–43.

8. Centers for Medicare and Medicaid Services. Department of Health and Human Services. Medicare and medicaid programs; hospital conditions of participation; patient's rights. Final rule. Fed Regist. 2006;71:71377–428. https://www.cms.gov/Regulations-andGuidance/Legislation/CFCsAndCoPs/downloads/finalpatientrightsrule. Accessed Dec 2015.
9. Palazzolo J. Restraint and seclusion in psychiatry in the elderly: review of the literature. Ann Depress Anxiety. 2015;2(2):1044.
10. Evans LK, Cotter VT. Avoiding restraints in patients with dementia: understanding, prevention, and management are the keys. AJN. 2008;108(3):40–9.
11. Wang WW, Moyle W. Physical restraint use on people with dementia: a review of the literature. Aust J Adv Nurs. 2005;22(4):46–52.
12. Said AA, Kautz DD. Reducing restraint use for older adults in acute care. Nursing. 2013;43(12):59–61.
13. Mohr WK, Petti TA, Mohr BD. Adverse effects associated with physical restraint. Can J Psychiatry. 2003;48(5):330–7.
14. Evans L, Strumpf N. Tying down the elderly. A review of the literature on physical restraint. J Am Geriatr Soc. 1989;37(1):65–74.
15. Mohr P, Pecenak J, Svestka J, Swingler D, Treuer T. Treatment of acute agitation in psychotic disorders. Neuro Endocrinol Lett. 2008;26(4):327–35.
16. Sellers B, Aldeen A. Focus on chemical restraint in the ED/ACEP. http://www.acep.org/education/continuing-medical-education-(cme)/focus-on/focus-on-chemical-restraint-in--the-ed/. Accessed 3 Dec 2015.
17. Way B, Banks S. Use of seclusion and restraint in public psychiatric hospitals: patient characteristics and facility effects. Psychiatr Serv. 1990;41(1):75–81.
18. 42 CFR Ch. IV (10–1–14 Edition), §482.13 (e).
19. 42 CFR Ch. IV (10–1–14 Edition), §482.13 (e)(2)(3).
20. 42 CFR Ch. IV (10–1–14 Edition), §482.13 (e)(6).
21. 42 CFR Ch. IV (10–1–14 Edition), §482.13 (e)(8)(1)(A).
22. Mental Health Act, R.S.O. 1990, c. M.7, s. 53.
23. The Mental Health Act, C.C.S.M. c. M110, s. 29(4).
24. Mental Health Act 1983, c. 20, s. 64G (1)-(4).

8 Palliative Care and the Dying Patient

Margaret W. Leung

8.1 Background

Palliative care dates back to the Middle Ages where places of *hospitium* (Latin for hospitality) provided places of rest for travelers and pilgrims, many of whom were ill and searching for miracles of cure. Modern palliative care grew out of St. Christopher's Hospice in London in the 1960s where caring for the dying involved a multidisciplinary approach. Palliative care focuses on symptom and stress relief for patients living with a serious illness at any stage with the goal of improving quality of life for patients and their families [1]. There is considerable overlap between geriatrics and palliative care [2]. Both fields optimize patient care by addressing the medical, psychological, and social needs through involvement of the patient, their families, and the larger community. Marked by multiple comorbidities, frail older adults experience progressive functional decline. Palliative care offers the opportunity through advanced care planning to live each day as well as possible with the understanding that goals of care are not curative but focus instead on comfort with an emphasis on maximizing quality of life.

Case Vignette Mr. P was an 82-year-old man with a history of major neurocognitive disorder due to Alzheimer disease. He lived at an assisted living facility where he required assistance with all his activities of daily living. He had lost 10 lb in the previous 3 months and was hospitalized three times in the previous 6 months for recurrent aspiration pneumonia. He was readmitted with another episode of pneumonia. The primary medical team consulted palliative care to determine what the family wanted done in the possibility of Mr. P's imminent death during the on-call practice of the upcoming weekend.

M.W. Leung, MD, MPH
Department of Palliative Care Services, Kaiser Permanente,
1600 Eureka Road, Roseville, CA 95661, USA
e-mail: margaret.w.leung@kp.org

A. Hategan et al. (eds.), *On-Call Geriatric Psychiatry: Handbook of Principles and Practice*, DOI 10.1007/978-3-319-30346-8_8

8.2 Patient-Centered Care and Medical Decision-Making

A common reason for consulting palliative care is to help patients identify goals of care after they have received news from their clinician that their disease has advanced to the point that either treatments are harmful (e.g., a cancer patient cannot continue chemotherapy because of renal failure) or that supportive measures are the only treatments indicated (e.g., massive stroke causing aphasia, paralysis, and dysphagia). Identification of goals of care involves a series of conversations to elicit patient values, wishes, and preferences to guide care.

The Serious Illness Conversation Guide offers prompted questions to begin exploring goals of care with patients who have life-threatening diseases [3]. The conversation begins with exploring patients' understanding of their illnesses. Most patients struggle to contextualize their serious illnesses especially when living with chronic diseases where the disease trajectory can be unpredictable. Corrections or clarifications may be needed before moving to the next step of assessing goals and values. Some patients may prefer communication with details, while others favor a broad overview. Others may prefer to have a family member be the primary decision-maker. A curiosity approach to exploring what gives life meaning permits patients to share what life is like beyond the disease, what relationships they value, and what brings them joy. Fears about the future are frequently raised and can overshadow hope. Clinicians can respond with a "balanced realism" that aligns with patient's hopes and also acknowledges planning for period of poorer illness and death [4]. Once patient goals are established, clinicians recommend a care plan that aligns with those goals. This plan includes what will be done (e.g., intensive symptom management, nonabadonment) and what will not be done (e.g., cardiopulmonary resuscitation, feeding tube, more chemotherapy).

Documentation in the medical chart of the patients' goals of care ensures that multiple clinicians are providing care consistent with the patients' goals. An advance directive identifies whom the patient would want to designate as a healthcare proxy or surrogate decision-maker in the event the patient becomes incapacitated to make medical decisions. The advance directive also specifies the patient's preferences for life-sustaining therapy although the language can be vague and difficult to apply in specific situations. Some US states use a Physician's Order for Life-Sustaining Treatment (POLST) that indicates the patient's desired level of care (e.g., resuscitation, artificial nutrition, rehospitalization). The POLST is distinct from the advance directive with the former referring to specific orders for current treatment and the latter specifying patient's preference for future treatments [5].

Case Vignette (Continued) The palliative care team assessed the family's understanding of the patient's illness. Mr. P's daughter was concerned that her father's quality of life had diminished rapidly because he was bedbound. After reviewing the trajectory of the major neurocognitive disorder, the palliative care team and daughter agreed that Mr. P would not have wanted to continue to be hospitalized. In light of his deteriorating clinical picture and low likelihood of sustained recovery, the primary medical team discussed goals of care with the patient's family members.

The patient's daughter was appointed the surrogate decision-maker in light of Mr. P's decisional incapacity. The palliative care team discussed a change to comfort measures only.

8.3 Ethical Principles in Palliative Care

The US legal system and standard clinical practice have provided recommendations for three ethical principles related to end-of-life care. (1) Clinicians often feel uncomfortable withdrawing care rather than withholding because the former is an active process. There is no ethical distinction between withdrawing and withholding care [6] because any type of therapy should be based on the benefits and burdens. (2) Numerous US court cases affirm that withdrawing care is not equivalent to killing a patient [7]. Patients have the right to refuse unwanted medical treatment, and removal of life-sustaining treatment would allow patients to die naturally from their underlying illness. (3) Lastly, the intentions of clinicians to provide comfort at the end of life with large doses of medications may be questioned. The doctrine of "double effect" distinguishes the intent to kill from the intent to palliate, with the possibility of hastening the patient's death [8]. With regular communication to patients and families and frequent assessment of pain and suffering, clinicians can follow clinical guidance that supports their clinical judgment. Moreover, studies suggest that using analgesia and sedatives do not hasten death [9].

8.4 Symptom Relief with a Focus on End-of-Life Care

During the dying phase, communication with families is an essential component of providing excellent care to a dying patient alongside intensive symptom management. Families will need preparation and education about good end-of-life care. Frequent, timely, consistent, and empathic communication are vital strategies to support families through this process. One framework to improve communication between families and the medical team caring for dying patients called "VALUE" provides opportunity for increased proportion of time for families to speak: *v*aluing statements made by family members, *a*cknowledging emotions, *l*istening to family members, *u*nderstanding the patient as a person, and *e*liciting questions from family members [10].

Recognizing that uncontrolled symptoms can severely impair the quality of life of a terminally ill patient, palliative care can offer strategies to alleviate symptoms. Be clear to the patient and family about the intent of the intervention (e.g., "We recommend increasing the morphine to better control his shortness of breath."), ask about understanding of actions and concerns, and address spoken and unspoken concerns (e.g., "The medication changes we make will not hasten his death. Our goal is to achieve a peaceful death.") [11].

Of the major symptoms, pain and dyspnea are the two most commonly encountered symptoms managed in the dying phase [12, 13], and management of such symptoms

Table 8.1 Opioid management of dyspnea and pain

	Equivalent dose (IV)	Duration of effect (h)	Typical adult doses (IV)	Special notes
Morphine	10 mg	3–4	2–10 mg	Avoid in renal and liver disease
Fentanyl	100 mcg	0.5–2	25–100 mcg	Safe in renal failure because it has no active metabolites
Hydromorphone	1.5 mg	3–4	0.2–2 mg	Metabolite hydromorphone-3-glucuronide can accumulate between hemodialysis treatments but can be effectively removed during dialysis

also can become the chief complaint in a geriatric psychiatric patient at the end-of-life care stage. Effective pain management begins with a thorough pain assessment. The World Health Organization's pain ladder guides clinicians on the pharmacological management of pain, beginning with the use of nonopioids such as acetaminophen or nonsteroidal anti-inflammatory agents and escalating adjunctive opioids as needed for persistent pain [14]. In end-of-life care, opioids such as morphine or hydromorphone are the medication of choice to treat both pain and dyspnea. To help manage these symptoms effectively, involve internists or hospitalists who are familiar with dosing and routes of administration. Table 8.1 provides a summary of commonly used opioids.

Dyspnea is the subjective sensation of breathlessness. Potential causes include lung tumor burden, pulmonary edema, pneumonia, pleural effusions, or heart failure. Non-pharmacological strategies to treat dyspnea include repositioning or blowing cool air from a fan. Opioids are the primary medication to treat dyspnea and they indirectly decrease anxiety associated with breathlessness. Some clinicians worry that administering opioids will cause respiratory depression when opioids are used to treat pain. There is no evidence to show that oxygenation levels change with opioids [15]. The use of supplemental oxygen, corticosteroids, diuretics, and bronchodilators can individualize treatment based on the underlying cause of dyspnea.

Delirium is frequent at the end of life affecting up to 88 % of patients [16]. It predicts the approach of death within days to weeks [17] and often becomes an irreversible and terminal event. The Confusion Assessment Method is one of the most commonly used screening tools for delirium [18]. Two common causes of terminal delirium are opioid toxicity and dehydration. Signs of myoclonus and escalating pain refractory to titration of opioids suggest that opioid rotation may be necessary to reduce both pain and delirium. Methadone and fentanyl are the preferred opioids in patient with terminal delirium [19]. Dehydration can lead to toxic accumulations of medications including opioids. Oral rehydration or a time-limited trial of parenteral fluids may relieve symptoms if they do not worsen symptoms of dyspnea or edema. Although there are no specific medications indicated for

Table 8.2 Medical management of terminal delirium

	Dosing (PO, IV, SL)	Special notes
Haloperidol	0.5–5 mg every 30 min as needed	Available as an injection
Chlorpromazine	12.5–25 mg every 30 min as needed	Intravenous form can cause hypotension if given too quickly; available rectally
Lorazepam	0.5–5 mg every hour as needed	Can treat opioid-related myoclonus

Table 8.3 Medical management of terminal secretions

	Dosing	Special notes
Scopolamine	1–3 patches (1.5 mg each) every 72 h	Can increase/cause delirium risk
Glycopyrrolate	1–2 mg orally two to three times daily, or 0.1–0.2 mg intravenous/subcutaneous/intramuscular every 4–8 h	Does not cross blood-brain barrier, so potentially useful in cases of delirium
Atropine drops	1 drop every 4–6 h sublingual as needed	Use 1 % ophthalmic solution

terminal delirium, haloperidol and chlorpromazine have the most evidence (see Table 8.2) [20]. The addition of benzodiazepines such as lorazepam can be beneficial if agitation remains uncontrolled even at higher doses of antipsychotics.

Patients who no longer are able to swallow or expectorate saliva will collect secretions at the back of the throat. The noisy gurgling, often referred to as "death rattle," heard each time the patient breathes can be distressing for families, although patients are often unconscious at this point and thus are not distressed. Families can be reassured that patients are not suffocated by the secretions and can be repositioned to a lateral recumbent position. In most cases, anticholinergic medications reduce secretions (see Table 8.3).

8.5 Notification of Death

Death, even when it is anticipated, is stressful for families and the medical team [11]. When called to pronounce a death, check-in with other clinicians such as nurses to see whether the family is present and how they are responding. Chaplaincy or social work may provide important support as needed. Encourage the family to stay if they feel comfortable viewing the last physical exam to confirm death. Clearly and empathically communicate that their loved ones has died without use of euphemisms for "death."

Ideally, the optimal time to discuss arrangements such as organ donation and autopsies is prior to death. Grieving families may be too distraught to make a well-informed decision immediately after death. Autopsies can be limited to certain parts of the body. Autopsies can provide for family a better understanding of what led to death, as well as benefit the larger society by adding to medical knowledge. An autopsy may be required by law such as when foul play may have caused death. Jurisdiction on type of coroner's cases varies by legal jurisdiction.

Bereavement support services for both the family and the medical team are an essential part of providing palliative care, sometimes lasting months to years after a patient dies. Families participate in various tasks and rituals to express their grief including accepting the reality of loss, adapting to a world without the deceased, and reintegrating the past with the present [21]. Clinicians also have bereavement needs and if not addressed appropriately can compromise their care and lead to complications like compassion fatigue [22, 23].

Case Vignette (Continued) During Mr. P's hospitalization, his breathing became labored with frequent gurgling noises. During the night, he frequently attempted to get out of bed. The on-call psychiatrist was urgently requested to see Mr. P for agitation. His agitation was likely a manifestation of delirium, with multifactorial risk factors, including hypoxia and infection, and further complicated by advanced neurocognitive disorder. The psychiatrist reviewed the chart and discussed with the staff and family who was present. The palliative care team had already discussed with the daughter that the patient was entering the dying phase. The palliative care clinician explained to the daughter and documented in the chart that morphine (2 mg IV every hour) as needed would help his air hunger and sublingual atropine solution (1 drop sublingually every 4 h) would be used to decrease his oral secretions. The on-call psychiatrist further recommended scheduling haloperidol (1 mg subcutaneously every 6 h) to control his agitation due to terminal delirium. Chaplaincy had offered additional support to the daughter. Mr. P died peacefully during the night.

Key Points

- Palliative care supports patients with serious illness through intensive symptom management and exploration of goals of care.
- Explore with patients and families their understanding of the illness and goals in order to offer recommendations that align with patient goals and quality of life.
- Pain and dyspnea are common symptoms in the dying process that can be managed intensively with opioids.

References

1. Center for Advanced Palliative Care. https://www.capc.org/about/palliative-care/(2015). Accessed 15 Oct 2015.
2. Finucane TE, Nirmalasari O, Graham A. Palliative care in the ambulatory geriatric practice. Clin Geriatr Med. 2015;31:193–206.
3. Bernacki R, Block S. Communication about serious illness care goals: a review and synthesis of best practices. JAMA Int Med. 2014;174:1994–2003.
4. Back A, Arnold RM, Quill TE. Hope for the best, and prepare for the worst. Ann Int Med. 2003;138(5):439–44.
5. Flint LA, Sudore RL, Calton B. Documenting goals of care and treatment preferences in the hospital: a case-based discussion. In: Pantilat S, Anderson W, Gonzale M, Widera E, editors. Hospital-based palliative medicine: a practical, evidence-based approach. Hoboke: Wiley; 2015. p. 133–42.
6. American Medical Association. Code of Medical Ethics of the American Medical Association. http://www.ama-assn.org/ama/pub/physician-resources/medical-ethics/code-medical-ethics/opinion220.page. Accessed 15 Oct 2015.
7. Luce J, White DB. A history of ethics and law in the intensive care unit. Crit Care Clin. 2009;25:221–37.
8. Gillon R. The principle of double effect and medical ethics. Br Med J. 1986;292:193–4.
9. Sykes N, Thorns A. The use of opioids and sedatives at the end of life. Lancet Oncol. 2003;4:312–8.
10. Curtis JR, Engelberg RA, Wenrich MD, Nielsen EL, Shannon SE, Treece PD, et al. Studying communication about end-of-life care during the ICU family conference: development of a framework. J Crit Care Med. 2002;17:147–60.
11. Hallenbeck J. Palliative care in the final days of life: "They were expecting it at any time". JAMA. 2005;293:2265–71.
12. The Study to Understand Prognoses and Preferences for Outcomes and Risks of Treatments (SUPPORT): a controlled trial to improve care for seriously ill hospitalized patients. JAMA. 1995;274:1591–8.
13. Hall P, Schroder C, Weaver L. The last 48 hours of life in long-term care: a focused chart audit. J Am Geriatr Soc. 2002;50:501–6.
14. Ferris FD, von Gunten CF, Emanuel LL. Ensuring competency in end-of-life care: controlling symptoms. BMC Palliat Care. 2002;I:5.
15. Clemens KE, Klaschik E. Symptomatic therapy of dyspnea with strong opioids and its effect on ventilation in palliative care patients. J Pain Symptom Manag. 2007;33:473–81.
16. Lawlor PG, Fainsinger RL, Bruera ED. Delirium at the end of life: critical issues in clinical practice and research. JAMA. 2000;284:2427–9.
17. Morita T, Tsunoda J, Inoue S, Chihara S. Survival prediction of terminally ill cancer patients by clinical symptoms: development of a simple indicator. Jpn J Clin Oncol. 1999;29:156–9.
18. Adamis D, Sharma N, Whelan JP, Macdonald AJD. Delirium scales: a review of current evidence. Aging Ment Health. 2010;14:543–55.
19. Moyer DD. Terminal delirium in geriatric patients with cancer at the end of life. Am J Hosp Palliat Care. 2011;28:44–51.
20. Jackson KC, Lipman AG. Drug therapy for delirium in terminally ill patients. Cochrane Database Syst Rev. 2004;(2):Art No: CD004770.
21. Knight SJ, Emanuel L. Processes of adjustment to end-of-life losses: a reintegration model. J Palliat Med. 2007;10:1190–8.
22. Vachon M. Staff stress in hospice/palliative care: a review. Palliat Med. 1995;9:91–122.
23. Sanso N, Galiana L, Oliver A, Pascual A, Sinclair S, Benito E. Palliative care professionals' inner life: exploring the relationships among awareness, self-care, and compassion satisfaction and fatigue, burnout, and coping with death. J Pain Symptom Manage. 2015;50:200–7.

9 Safe Clinical Handover

Mariam Abdurrahman and Claudia Garcia

9.1 Background

Handover is the process of communicating pertinent patient information and transferring clinical responsibility among clinicians [1, 2]. Frequently, handover tends to be a reductionist process in which clinical information is abridged to a diagnosis, laboratory results, and a discrete list of "actionable items," thus resulting in the transmission of incomplete or inaccurate information which may potentially result in adverse events [2, 3]. Furthermore, in some clinical care settings, the design of the space where handover occurs and the characteristic interruptions promote a suboptimal handover process.

On-call handovers during patient care occur across multiple clinical contexts including:

- Shift-to-shift handovers such as on-call handover in the inpatient unit and shift changes in the emergency department (ED)
- Site-to-site transitions of care facilitated by on-call staff when discharge occurs after hours, during the weekend, or statutory holidays
- Discharge to the community clinician and home/residential setting by on-call clinicians when discharge occurs after hours during the weekend or statutory holidays

In addition, multiple layers of handover occur within multidisciplinary settings, among various disciplines of clinicians. Thus, handover presents any number of

M. Abdurrahman, MD, MSc, Dip (GHEI) (✉)
Department of Psychiatry, St. Joseph's Health Centre, Toronto, ON, Canada
e-mail: mariam.abdurrahman@medportal.ca

C. Garcia, MD
Post-graduate Medical Education, Department of Psychiatry, University of Toronto, Toronto, ON, Canada

A. Hategan et al. (eds.), *On-Call Geriatric Psychiatry: Handbook of Principles and Practice*, DOI 10.1007/978-3-319-30346-8_9

opportunities for medical errors. Transitions of care refer to the movement of patients among clinicians, healthcare settings, and home as their clinical state evolves [3].

9.2 Shift-to-Shift Handover

Shift transitions present a high-risk period for patient safety due to variable handover practices, miscommunication, time and space constraints, changes in staff-to-patient ratio (particularly during overnight and weekend on-call period with the reduction in staff allocation), handover interruptions, poor formal handover coverage in medical trainee curricula, and incomplete team attendance at handover in multidisciplinary on-call settings.

It is also important to consider internal human factors [4, 5] such as the cognitive bias of undervaluation, sometimes manifested in the perception of geriatric patients as less medically acute or "inactive patients." This bias may potentially be problematic in trauma-focused settings such as the ED where the modus operandi is generally rapid intervention for rapid turnover (see Chap. 16). Geriatric patients are often treated for their chief presenting complaint and notable incidental medical problems, thus creating a relatively narrow "lens of care" and increasing the risk of handover omissions.

9.2.1 The Inpatient Ward

During an episode of acute care, a patient may potentially be treated by a number of clinicians in multiple settings, with final disposition occurring through primary care and/or specialized outpatient care [5]. At each stage, there is an inherent risk of medical error, notably during on-call hours. On-call shift handovers in the inpatient setting can be enhanced by conducting handover in a systematic fashion, starting with the orientation of new trainees to principles of safe handover and proceeding with the methodical use of a standardized handover template during each handover: on-call handover in the morning and at the end of the day, new admissions and transfers, and discharge back to community clinician and family [1, 4, 6, 7].

At the level of medical trainees, consistent use of a standardized template on the ward can minimize missing information. This is important with the recent and growing trend of resident duty hour restrictions as this will result in increased handovers per unit of time. Residency programs will need to provide formal competency-based handover training to ensure that handover is valued and employed consistently. The issue of consistency is underscored on considering the breadth of omissions during inpatient handovers [1, 8, 9] (see Table 9.1).

Although a universal best practice process has yet to be identified, the *S*ituation, *B*ackground, *A*ssessment, and *R*ecommendation (SBAR) technique is widely used

Table 9.1 Key items omitted during inpatient handovers [1, 8, 9]

Item	Details
Alerts	Name alerts, medication alerts, safety alerts
Clinical status	Changes in clinical status
Decisional capacity	Patient capacity and current substitute decision makers, existence of legal documentation (power of attorney), pending changes in decisional chain
Laboratory results	Pending laboratory results, trending laboratory parameters, omission of laboratory tests ordered, and reason for ordering
Medication	Episodic medications given during on-call hours, medication refusals, altered medication dosage
Medicolegal status	Psychiatric detention status, including changes to/from voluntary to involuntary status
Advanced directives	Code status (resuscitation documentation)
Vital signs	Transient but notable changes in vitals, e.g., overnight spikes in temperature

[3, 8, 10, 11]. Situational debriefing models like SBAR provide a framework for standardized communication. The ISOBAR variation is a particularly useful iteration in that it places the patient's *identity* (rather than the clinical diagnosis) in primary position, in addition to reinforcing the transfer of information and accountability [11, 12]. The ISOBAR model has been further modified in this chapter to provide a more robust framework, the ISCOBAR which gives additional emphasis to the responsibility and risk management components of handover [5] (see Fig. 9.1 for the ISCOBAR model).

The inpatient ward is a multidisciplinary setting, thus requiring a common language of communication among disciplines when patients are reviewed. Thus, team rounds are an essential avenue to discussing patient progress and engaging in a team-level on-call handover process at the start of each day. For each patient discussed at team rounds, the discussion should include, at the very least, the items elucidated in Fig. 9.1. Most members of the clinical team typically work in shifts and service blocks or periods, which constitutes another layer of handover. Although this is an unavoidable structure affecting the work flow, it is possible to optimize handover by approaching the process systematically and including items listed in Fig. 9.1, adjusted for the specific clinical discipline and stratified for patient acuity. For the on-call psychiatrist, the elements noted in Fig. 9.1 constitute essential information to be transmitted at the end of each call shift.

Some centers are also piloting the use of patient navigators and transitional care facilitators [10, 13, 14] to further minimize gaps during transitions. Other techniques in use include electronic sign-outs (e-sign outs) to maintain the continuity of information flow and facilitate timely updates, particularly when multiple consulting services are involved. Centers using e-sign out use it as an adjunct to face-to-face handover and typically utilize a standardized template to document pertinent handover information, although no specific template has been studied for generalizability.

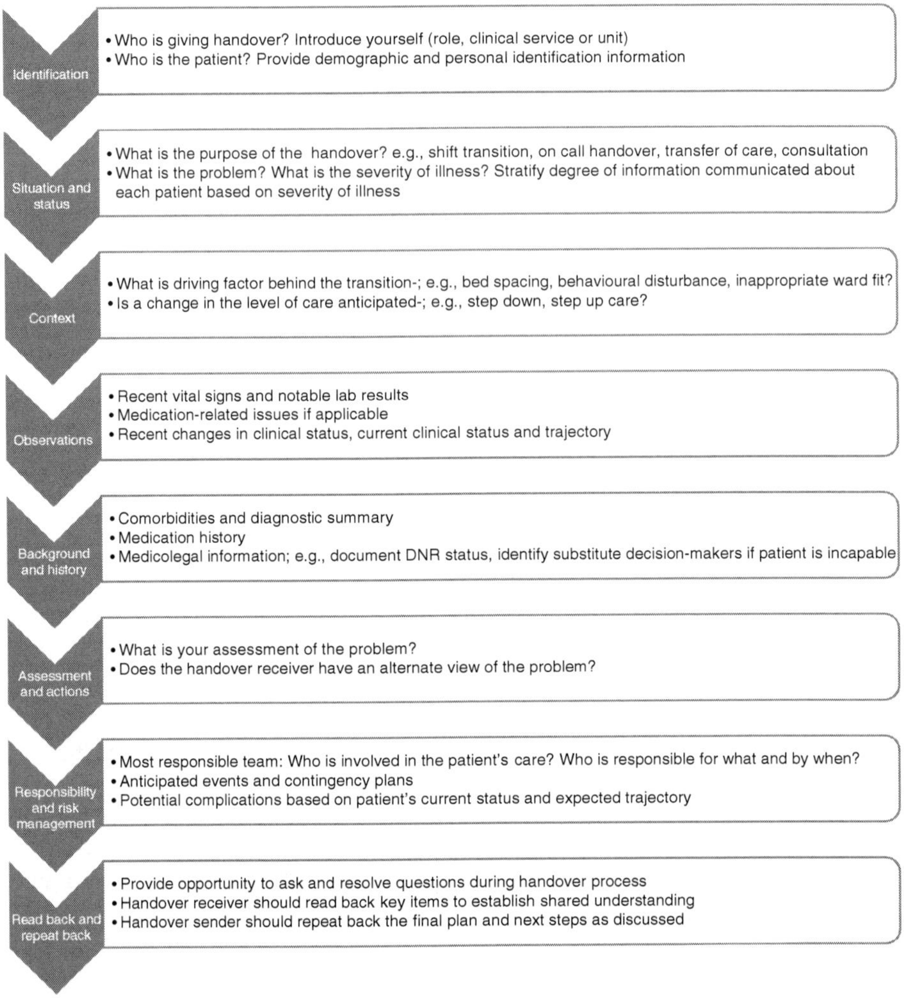

Fig. 9.1 ISCOBAR, a modified handover checklist and protocol (*Note*: The modified protocol illustrated above accounts for both the principles and action items recommended for effective handover content and process, to be adapted based on the particular clinical context. The *sender* is the party responsible for transmitting patient data and releasing the care of the patient to the *receiver*, who in turn receives the information and accepts accountability for care of the patient [5])

9.2.2 The Emergency Department

With most episodes of acute care typically originating in the ED, it is a critical location for exercising safe clinical handover practices. The high-paced setting of the ED elevates the risk of medical error by virtue of gaps in information flow that occur with multitasking and shift changes [4, 9, 14]. Information transfer in the ED is rapid and constant, yet prone to error at multiple levels of handover, including at

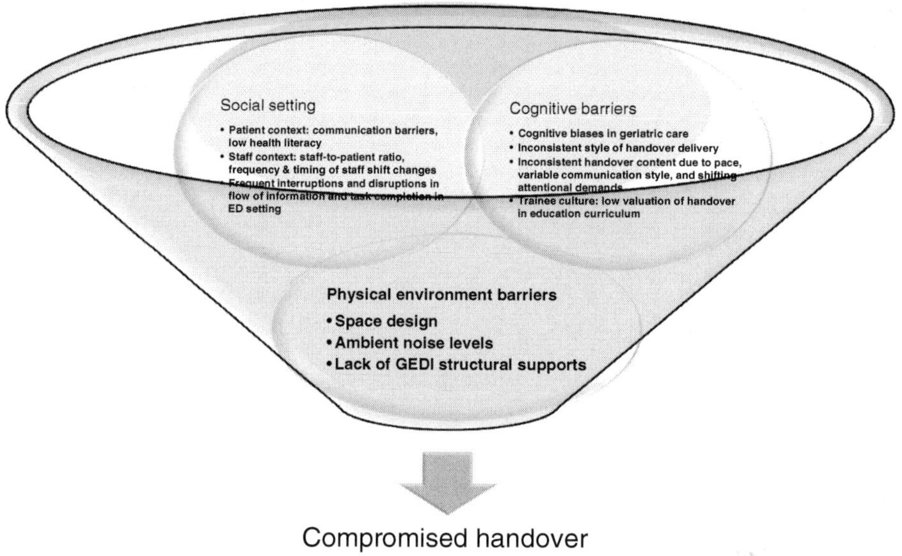

Fig. 9.2 Key barriers to effective handover in the emergency department setting [12–14] (*Note*: GEDI denotes geriatric emergency department intervention)

shift change, at transfers for diagnostic investigations, and at the consultation liaison psychiatry interface with other clinical services.

ED handovers also notably occur in a challenging space that introduces barriers to optimal on-call handover as illustrated in Fig. 9.2. Furthermore, gaps also occur during various ED activities, such as documentation, reviewing cases with trainees, teaching activities, and the utilization of electronic resources and other decisional supports [4]. Recognition of the cognitively demanding nature of the ED setting and the intrinsic barriers of the ED environment (see Fig. 9.2) is essential in considering any approach to safe ED handover [12–14]. Viewing the ED shift handover as an on-call handover is essential to enhancing a culture of patient safety.

On a more practical level, the approach to handovers in the ED setting should include consideration of three basic elements: person, place, and time [7–10, 15] (see Fig. 9.3). The *person* element requires consideration of who the patient is and who is involved in their care in the community so that the discharge communication loop is complete. In EDs with the capacity and resources, a shift toward a geriatric ED intervention model of care is highly recommended [13], as a dedicated nurse or social worker liaison facilitates care transitions, thus enhancing continuity and safety.

The *place* element addresses the fact that geriatric patients are frequently not asked about their domicile context; however, place is an essential element in the final ED pathway of discharge handover. The concept of discharge as the final handover in an episode of care is further discussed in the Discharge section. Discharge from ED should ideally consider goodness of fit of the residential context for the patient's functional needs. Discharging patients to home with inadequate assessment of the degree to which the home environment can support discharge

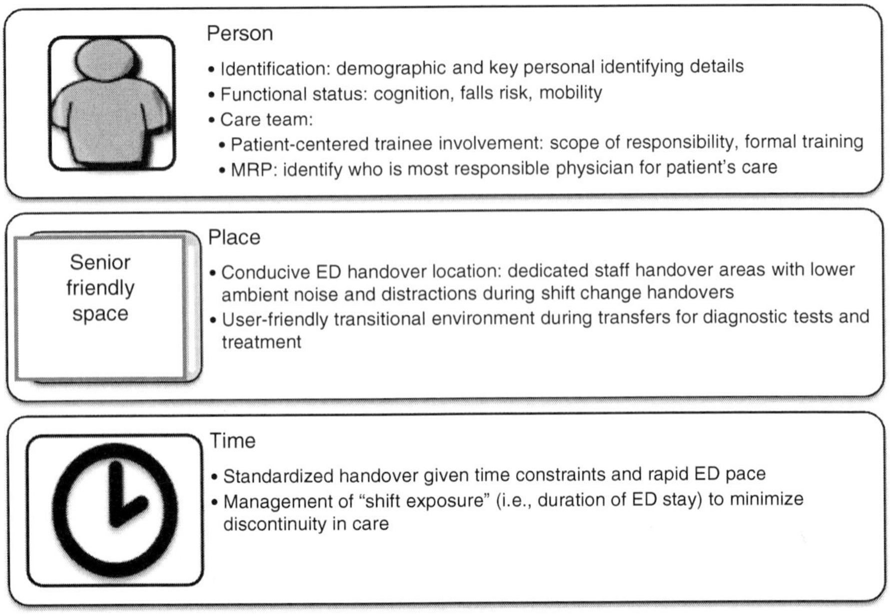

Fig. 9.3 Basic elements of handover communication in the emergency department [7–10, 15]

recommendations increases the risk of adverse events. A failure in handover related to place is an important contributor to readmission, particularly in geriatric patients with chronic or complex medical conditions and socioeconomic adversities [16] such as those described in Chap. 27.

Place also necessitates consideration of the various diagnostic and treatment areas that one ED visit may encompass as these transitions may introduce gaps in handover communication. In terms of time, increased ED visit durations expose patients to increased handovers by way of multiple staff shift changes, thus exposing them to increased handover hazards. Electronic sign-outs provide one way of enhancing handovers in that e-sign outs provide the capacity for updates concurrent with evolving patient care [5], a feature invaluable during frequent transitions.

9.3 Site to Site: Institutional Transfers and the On-Call Handover

Case Vignette: Omissions in an Institutional Handover Mr. J was a 67-year-old male with schizoaffective disorder, transferred from a long-term care facility (LTCF) to the ED for assessment of acutely increased hallucinations. The LTCF sent his medication administration list and emergency family contact information, but failed to hand over information about other symptoms including recent dysuria. On arriving at the ED, Mr. J was medically cleared although his urine culture had to be repeated due to contamination of the original specimen. In the interim, Mr. J was referred to the on-call psychiatric consultant for assessment, but the on-call psychiatrist was not advised of the pending urine culture. Mr. J did not exhibit an altered level of consciousness. His psychotropic medications were adjusted by the psychiatrist, and he was discharged back to the LTCF as the ED advised the on-call psychiatrist that there were no medical concerns. Thus, Mr. J was discharged back to the LTCF with the change in psychotropic medications noted but no documentation of the pending urine culture, which later returned positive for an infection. Soon after discharge, Mr. J returned to the ED with increased hallucinations and was then determined to be delirious due to urinary tract infection.

Transitions in care location may occur within an institution and between institutions such as transfers from hospital to LTCF and vice versa or transfers between hospitals. At each transition, risks associated with handover are readily apparent in the variation of handover practices across units and institutions. Key approaches are similar to those already discussed, with modifications based on the transfer locations. Family and/or external caregiver involvement is essential in these transitions. Furthermore, added attention is required to ensure accurate handover of information related to functional status as this could potentially result in dangerous outcomes as illustrated in the case vignette.

The ED to LTCF transition illustrated in the vignette presents a concerning source of handover breakdown given the frailty of the geriatric population. Relative to their community-dwelling counterparts, the LTCF population utilizes the ED more frequently [17] (see Chap. 20). While both the ED and LTCF perform investigations and initiate treatment plans that directly affect care at the other site, patients are frequently transferred with inadequate inter-institutional communication and documentation [17]. This gap can be detrimental and could be avoided by implementing a standardized transfer protocol specific to this transitional point. The transition can also be enhanced by using dedicated transitional care facilitators whose involvement begins at the sending site and continues through to the receiving location. Handover during inter-institutional transfers should at the very least include items described in Fig. 9.4 [8, 10, 11, 15, 18].

9.4 The Discharge Handover

The discharge process can present a particularly precarious layer of handover particularly when discharge occurs during the on-call period, notably during the weekend and statutory holidays. Key discharge risks occur with regard to medication, pending laboratory results, other pending investigations, and coordination of follow-up care [18–22]. This is particularly challenging when discharge disposition is made during the on-call shift because of the limited time-sensitive period for coordinating an optimal care plan. Medication discrepancies in particular have been

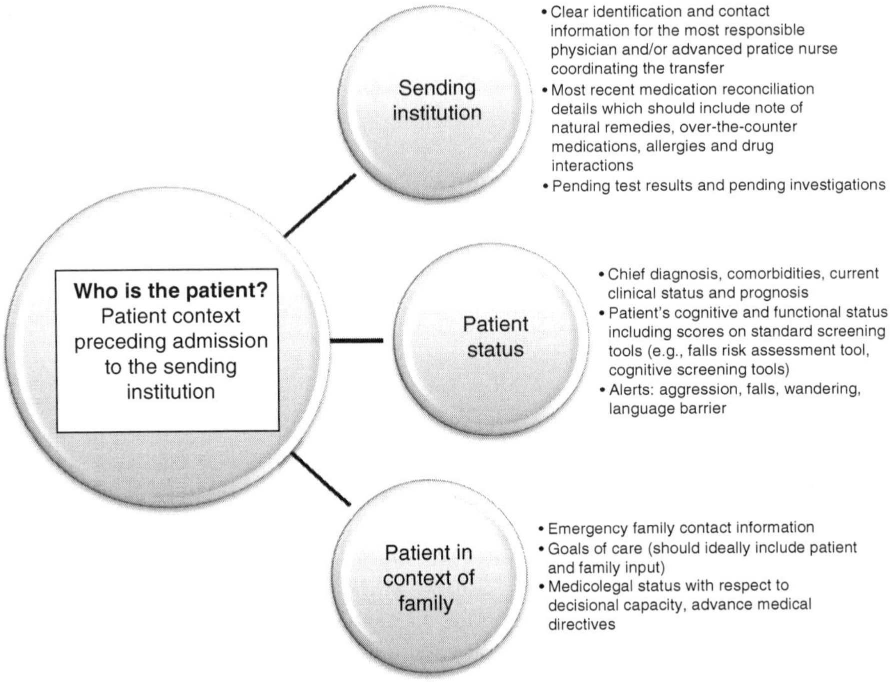

Fig. 9.4 Essential handover content in inter-institutional transitions of care [8, 10, 11, 15, 18]

shown to be prevalent, with elevated rates of rehospitalization as a result of such discrepancies [20–23]. Medication reconciliation with documentation of the rationale for changes is essential in managing medication-related adverse events. Medication changes frequently occur during on-call hours but are not always transmitted during on-call handover and may not be reconciled if patient discharge occurs during or soon after the on-call shift.

In the case of ED visits, the frequency of care transitions can make it challenging to generate accurate documentation to community clinicians on completion of the ED visit. The use of a standardized ED visit letter that is auto-populated with relevant clinical data directly from electronic records or completed manually by ED staff may help bridge the gap. The concept is similar to the "patient letter" described below and can be used to rapidly notify community providers of key aspects of the ED visit.

Increasingly, hospitals are adopting intranet patient lists and electronic clinical records that auto-populate standardized discharge templates and allow rapid updates in a secure manner. As well as giving details of the location and consultant team responsible for the patient, it provides a summary of current problems and outstanding management issues [24].

To minimize medication-related adverse events on discharge, if the discharge plan is implemented during the on-call shift, the consulting physician should reconcile medications by reviewing preadmission medications and final in-hospital medications before issuing a discharge prescription. The discharge or transfer note should provide an itemized summary of medications continued, held but resumed, discontinued, or new, and the rationale [20, 23]. The discharge prescription and after-care plans should ideally be reviewed with the patient and caregivers in a discharge meeting. To further enhance the discharge process, some hospitals provide patients with a "patient letter" summarizing their admission, upcoming appointments, and discharge prescription.

In summary, clinical handover can present a hazard in the continuity and safety of patient care, particularly during the on-call shift. Key handover problems include missing, incomplete, or inaccurate information, which may potentially result in adverse events. However, handover risks can be minimized by remaining cognizant of the patient care setting and the handover risks inherent to each setting, ensuring the consistent use of a situational handover model, and ensuring that handover is valued among all staff, including trainees. The Key Points further summarize principles of promoting safe clinical handover.

Key Points

- Clinical handover is the process of communicating pertinent patient information and transferring clinical responsibility between clinicians.
- On-call handover presents a process with inherent opportunities for medical error.
- Geriatric patients may experience a significant number of transitions in care during the course of an acute care visit.
- Many transitions may occur in an episode of care, yet handover is frequently incomplete, particularly when handover occurs during on-call hours.
- Handover risks can be minimized by remaining cognizant of the patient care setting and the handover risks inherent to each setting.
- Situational handover models allow for more complete on-call handovers.
- The role of medical trainees should be enhanced by prioritizing on-call handover in their curriculum.
- Standardized on-call handover processes and templates should be used to minimize handover errors.
- Electronic sign-outs present a useful adjunct tool for prompt updates in patient status.
- Discharges present a handover interface in which key risks include medication errors, pending laboratory results and investigations, and failure to communicate follow-up plans adequately to patients, caregivers, and community clinicians.
- Medication reconciliation with documented rationale for medication changes is essential at transition points and should account for any changes made during on-call shifts as these are often overlooked.
- Discharge risks can be managed through the use of standardized discharge templates, "patient letters," and concurrent communication with the community clinician during the course of an episode of acute care.

References

1. Devlin MK, Kozij NK, Kiss A, Richardson L, Wong BM. Morning handover of on-call issues: opportunities for improvement. JAMA Intern Med. 2014;174(9):1479–85.
2. Manser T, Foster S. Effective handover communication: an overview of research and improvement efforts. Best Pract Res Clin Anaesthesiol. 2011;25(2):181–91.
3. Joint Commission Center for transforming healthcare: improving transitions of care: hand-off communications. 2014. http://www.centerfortransforminghealthcare.org/assets/4/6/handoff_comm_storyboard.pdf. Accessed 3 Sep 2015.
4. Laxmisan A, Hakimzada F, Sayan OR, Green RA, Zhang J, Patel VL. The multitasking clinician: decision-making and cognitive demand during and after team handoffs in emergency care. Int J Med Inform. 2007;76:801–11.
5. World Health Organization Collaborating Centre for patient safety solutions: communication during patient hand-overs. 2007. http://www.ccforpatientsafety.org/common/pdfs/fpdf/presskit/PS-Solution3.pdf. Accessed 20 Jul 2015.
6. Payne CE, Stein JM, Leong T, Dressler DD. Avoiding handover fumbles: a controlled trial of a structured handover tool versus traditional handover methods. BMJ Qual Saf. 2012;11: 925–32.
7. Farhan M, Brown R, Woloshynowych M, Vincent C. The ABC of handover: a qualitative study to develop a new tool for handover in the emergency department. Emerg Med J. 2012;29(12):941–6. doi:10.1136/emermed-2011-200199.
8. Agency for health care research and quality: patient safety primers: handoffs and signouts. 2014. http://www.psnet.ahrq.gov/primer.aspx?primerID=9. Accessed 4 Aug 2015.
9. Borowitz SM, Waggoner-Fountain LA, Bass EJ, DeVoge JM. Resident sign-out: a precarious exchange of critical information in a fast-paced world. In: Henriksen K, Battles JB, Keyes MA, Grady ML, editors. Advances in patient safety: new directions and alternative approaches (vol. 2: culture and redesign). Rockville: Agency for Healthcare Research and Quality; 2008. p. 1–21.
10. Joint Commission Center for transforming healthcare: hot topics in healthcare- transitions of care: The need for a more effective approach to continuing patient care. 2012. http://www.centerfortransforminghealthcare.org/assets/4/6/handoff_comm_storyboard.pdf. Accessed 3 Sep 2015.
11. NSW health: implementation toolkit – standard key principles for clinical handover. 2009. www.archi.net.au/e-library/clinical/nsw-handover. Accessed 25 Sep 2015.
12. Porteous JM, Stewart-Wynne EG, Connolly M, Crommelin PF. iSoBAR – a concept and handover checklist: the national clinical handover initiative. Med J Aust. 2009;190 Suppl 11:152–6.
13. Welch S. The geriatric emergency department. In: quality improvement and patient safety. American College of Emergency Physicians. 2015. http://www.acep.org/content.aspx?id=87577. Accessed 16 Jul 2015.
14. American College of Emergency Physicians: Geriatric Emergency Department Guidelines. 2014. http://www.acep.org/geriEDguidelines/ Accessed 28 Aug 2015.
15. Australian Commission on Safety and Quality in Health Care. Clinical handover: critical communications. Med J Aust. 2009;190 Suppl 11:108–9.
16. Center for Healthcare Quality and Payment Reform. Using medical homes to reduce hospital readmissions. 2013. http://www.chqpr.org/readmissions.html. Accessed 25 Sep 2015.
17. Wilber ST, Gerson LW, Terrell KM, et al. Geriatric emergency medicine and the 2006 Institute of Medicine reports from the Committee on the Future of Emergency Care in the U.S. health system. Acad Emerg Med. 2006;13:1345–51.
18. Snow V, Beck D, Budnitz T, et al. Transitions of care consensus policy statement: American College of Physicians, Society of General Internal Medicine, Society of Hospital Medicine, American Geriatrics Society, American College of Emergency Physicians, and Society for Academic Emergency Medicine. J Hosp Med. 2009;4(6):364–70. doi:10.1002/jhm.510.

19. Mixon AS, Neal E, Bell S, Powers JS, Kripalani S. Care transitions: a leverage point for safe and effective medication use in older adults- a mini-review. Gerontology. 2015;61(1):32–40. doi:10.1159/000363765. Epub 2014 Sep 30.
20. Coleman EA, Smith JD, Raha D, Min SJ. Posthospital medication discrepancies: prevalence and contributing factors. Arch Intern Med. 2005;165(16):1842–7.
21. Kripalani S, LeFevre F, Phillips CO, Williams MV, Basaviah P, Baker DW, et al. Deficits in communication and information transfer between hospital-based and primary care physicians: implications. JAMA. 2007;297(8):831–41.
22. Tsilimingras D, Bates DW. Addressing post-discharge adverse events: a neglected area. Jt Comm J Qual Patient Saf. 2008;34(2):85–97.
23. Lenert LA, Sakaguchi FH, Weir CR. Rethinking the discharge summary: a focus on handoff communication. Acad Med. 2014;89(3):393–8.
24. British Medical Association: Safe handover: safe patients. Guidance for clinical handover for clinicians and managers. 2014. http://bma.org.uk/-/media/files/pdfs/practical%20advice%20at%20work/contracts/safe%20handover%20safe%20patients.pdf. Accessed 25 Sep 2015.

Part II

On-Call Geriatric Psychiatry and Clinical Problems: The Chief Complaints

The Chief Psychiatric Complaints

10

Ana Hategan, James A. Bourgeois, Karen Saperson, and Simon Chiu

10.1 Background

When requested to see a patient during an emergent or crisis situation while on call, there is essential basic information that the consulting physician may need to obtain from nursing staff before seeing the patient (either over the phone or in person) in order to determine whether medical orders are required prior to the physician's arrival and prior to performing the bedside assessment and intervention for the respective chief complaint(s) (see Fig. 10.1).

As shown in Fig. 10.1, the on-call *bedside* geriatric psychiatric assessment comprises several elements, which should be an essential part of the care of geriatric patients and a prerequisite for appropriate intervention. Monitoring for drug-disease and drug-drug interactions is imperative as a first step in the evaluation process.

A. Hategan, MD (✉) • K. Saperson, MBChB
Department of Psychiatry and Behavioural Neurosciences, Division of Geriatric Psychiatry, Faculty of Health Sciences, Michael G. DeGroote School of Medicine, McMaster University, Hamilton, ON, Canada
e-mail: ahategan@stjosham.on.ca

J.A. Bourgeois, OD, MD
Department of Psychiatry/Langley Porter Psychiatric Institute, Consultation-Liaison Service, University of California San Francisco Medical Center, San Francisco, CA, USA

Consultation-Liaison Service, University of California San Francisco Medical Center, San Francisco, CA, USA

S. Chiu, MD, PhD
Department of Psychiatry, Lawson Health Research Institute, University of Western Ontario, London, ON, Canada

A. Hategan et al. (eds.), *On-Call Geriatric Psychiatry: Handbook of Principles and Practice*, DOI 10.1007/978-3-319-30346-8_10

On-call psychiatric assessment and management

Information obtained *before* seeing the patient

Does the patient have a diagnosis of prior/current psychiatric illness?; What is the patient's behavior?; Is the patient dangerous to himself/herself or to others?; What is the reason for his/her hospitalization?; What is his/her current medication list, and if any recently started or discontinued medications?; Has there been any recent change in his/her level of consciousness?; Has there been any previous similar episodes?; What are the patient's vital signs?; What is the patient's allergy status?; Has the patient been deemed incapable to make treatment decisions, and if incapacitated, who acts as the proxy decision maker?; What is the patient's code status?; What is the patient's legal hospitalization status?

Medical orders authorized *before* seeing the patient

Verbal order for appropriate level of monitoring for the situation (e.g., close observation).
Verbal order for chemical restraints or as-needed medication before the patient can be safely assessed, or in cases of dangerousness.
Verbal order for seclusion or physical restraints in acutely dangerous behavior to the patient and/or others.

***Beside* assessment and management**

Selective chart review and history
Review of vital signs
Selective physical examination (as the patient cooperates or tolerates)
Selective mental status examination
Review of recent laboratory/neuroimaging examination
Review of working diagnosis
Review of differential diagnosis
Management of the chief psychiatric complaint

Fig. 10.1 General strategies for the on-call physician in the provision of geriatric psychiatric assessment and management

A complete list of the patient's prescription and nonprescription medications should be reviewed. If a new medication was recently prescribed or discontinued, drug-drug interactions must be reviewed.

Delirium, major neurocognitive disorders (NCDs) (formerly termed dementia), depressive disorders, and other psychiatric disorders are common in the older population. Maintaining high vigilance for symptoms of depression is essential since geriatric patients may not endorse depressed mood per se, but instead present with cognitive disturbance as well as nonspecific, vague complaints as fatigue, constipation, and anorexia, with subsequent weight loss, which may mimic physical illnesses. Although the on-call principles of psychiatric examination of the geriatric patient are described in Chap. 1, integrated elements of such assessment should include review of findings of psychiatric, cognitive, and functional assessment tools. Being familiar with common screening tools used specifically in the geriatric population for identifying various psychiatric syndromes is essential for on-call practice. Performance-based screens, usually completed by clinicians other than the on-call physician, can be readily available to the on-call physician to incorporate into their medical practice.

It is important to know that cognitive tests can have multiple utilities. The Montreal Cognitive Assessment (MoCA), Mini-Mental State Examination (MMSE), Mini-Cog Test, and the Addenbrooke's Cognitive Examination-Revised (ACE-R) are validated brief screening tests for major or mild NCDs [1]. Other brief performance-based screening instruments shown to be useful in identifying medical patients with cognitive dysfunction are the Short Blessed Test, Brief Alzheimer's Screen, Ottawa 3DY, and Frontal Assessment Battery (FAB) [2, 3]. Poor performance on the FAB in conjunction with the presence of behavioral abnormalities could be an important factor in the diagnosis of frontotemporal NCD. These tests all require a cooperative patient. These instruments do not assess the impact of cognitive dysfunction on social or occupational activities of daily living, which are also performance-based measures (e.g., Kohlman Evaluation of Living Skills (KELS) – an in vivo standardized test designed to determine a patient's ability to function in basic living skills [4]) and which have been promoted as important criteria to distinguish demented and non-demented populations [2]. It is important to know that scoring perfectly on any cognitive screening test does not preclude the diagnosis of delirium, or major or mild NCDs. The fluctuating course of delirium can allow for "lucid intervals" in which some delirious patients may have the ability to perform well, whereas highly educated patients with major NCDs may score perfectly but have deficiencies in insight, judgment, and other areas of cognitive function. Additionally, patients may score suboptimally on a screening test because of language or education level barrier, but have good performance when tested in greater depth [5].

Determining the areas of functional impairment helps with the diagnosis. There is a great deal of interdependency among patients' social, financial, and functional status. Low socioeconomic status may play a role in undernutrition and the ability to purchase medications. A critical issue to assess patients being evaluated on call is the concern about driving ability due to a medical condition. Patients given prescription drugs known to have pharmacologic effects and/or side effects that can impair the ability to drive should be advised not to drive until their individual response is known or the side effects no longer result in impairment. Physicians have a mandatory or discretionary duty to report patients whom they believe to be unfit to drive to the relevant licensing agency, depending on the jurisdiction involved. There is no test which has sufficient sensitivity or specificity to be used as a single determinant of driving ability. However, abnormalities on the MoCA, MMSE, clock drawing, and Trails B tests should trigger further in-depth testing of driving ability [6]. Moderate to severe major NCDs, or an inability to independently perform multiple instrumental activities of daily living (IADLs) or any of the basic activities of daily living (ADLs) due to cognitive impairment, are contraindications to driving [6].

Medical decisional capacity determination is an essential part of geriatric psychiatric care (see Chap. 6). Studies have shown that MMSE scores less than 20 out of 30 points appear to increase the likelihood of decisional incapacity [7]. Therefore, the MMSE or MoCA could be used to quantitate cognitive function as part of an assessment of a patient with questionable medical decision-making capacity, which should then trigger a formal capacity assessment (specific to the clinical issue at hand) when a patient's score is low. Aligning patients' medical decisions with their belief system is essential throughout care plan decision steps.

A summary of the screening tools used in the psychiatric examination of geriatric patients is presented in Table 10.1 [1, 2, 4, 8–18].

Table 10.1 Geriatric screening tools used in the psychiatric examination [1, 2, 4, 8–18]

Psychiatric assessment tools	Geriatric depression: (a) PHQ-9 [8] (self-administered tool) or PHQ-2 [9] (performed by an interviewer); (b) GDS, available in 5-item [10], 15-item [11], and 30-item versions; (c) BASDEC [12]
	Harmful or hazardous drinking: (a) CAGE [13], (b) MAST-G [14], (c) ARPS [15]
	Behavioral disturbance of major neurocognitive disorders: (a) Cohen Mansfield Agitation Inventory [16]; (b) Neuropsychiatric Inventory [17]
Cognitive assessment tools	Cognitive impairment: (a) MoCA; (b) MMSE; (c) Mini-Cog test (it combines three-term registration and recall with clock drawing); (d) clock drawing test (which is less influenced by educational level and culture, as is MMSE or MoCA) [1]; (e) other cognitive screening tools: ACE-R, Short Blessed Test, Brief Alzheimer's Screen, and the Ottawa 3DY [1, 2]; (f) CAM, which distinguishes delirium from major neurocognitive disorders [18]
Functional assessment tools	Kohlman Evaluation of Living Skills (KELS) [4]. Functional performance is assessed at two levels: (a) IADLs (e.g., driving or ability to use public transportation, shopping, meal preparation, telephone skills, housework, laundry, medication administration, handling finances) and (b) ADLs (e.g., bathing, dressing, transferring, feeding, toileting, continence)

Note: *ACE-R* Addenbrooke's Cognitive Examination-Revised, *ADLs* Activities of Daily Living, *ARPS* Alcohol-Related Problems Survey, *BASDEC* Brief Assessment Schedule Depression Cards, *CAGE* Cut-Annoyed-Guilty-Eye, *CAM* Confusion Assessment Method, *GDS* Geriatric Depression Scale, *IADLs* Instrumental Activities of Daily Living, *KELS* Kohlman Evaluation of Living Skills, *MAST-G* Michigan Alcoholism Screening Test – Geriatric Version, *MMSE* Mini-Mental State Examination, *MoCA* Montreal Cognitive Assessment, *PHQ-2* Patient Health Questionnaire-2, *PHQ-9* Patient Health Questionnaire-9

10.2 The On-Call Chief Psychiatric Complaints

The chief psychiatric complaints occurring in geriatric patients in crisis presenting during on-call, after-hours shifts and in any urgent institutional setting are discussed below. We incorporate case vignettes representative of plausible scenarios in geriatric patients to address on-call assessment and management strategies.

10.2.1 The Confused Patient

Case Vignette The nursing home staff asked you to urgently see Mr. A, a 79-year-old male with Parkinson's disease, who became suddenly confused, agitated, and attempted to leave the facility. He has had fluctuating vivid and frightening visual hallucinations of rodents running into his room after an anti-Parkinson medication, pramipexole, was newly started. He was also taking carbidopa/levodopa for 10 years, in the absence of previous depression or cognitive impairment. Upon your assessment, you determined that Mr. A was suffering from an acute onset of cognitive impairment, perceptual disturbances, and psychomotor agitation following initiation of a dopamine agonist, in keeping with a diagnosis of medication-induced delirium. You discontinued pramipexole. Although there was a partial benefit with the discontinuation, his symptoms remained distressing, and a trial of low-dose quetiapine 12.5 mg at bedtime was started. His confusion fully resolved in 1 week.

Confusion is a cognitive dysfunction, for which the on-call physician is frequently requested to see a patient in various institutional settings. However, confusion is also highly under-recognized in the emergency department (ED), and emergency-based case finding is an opportunity to identify and intervene early for this potentially reversible condition.

"Confusion" is a common synonym for delirium. However, confusion is also a symptom of major or mild NCDs, major depression, or psychotic disorders. Because delirium is often a psychiatric and medical emergency, it must be clinically differentiated from other psychiatric syndromes. This can be challenging, especially when such psychiatric syndromes occur concurrently (e.g., delirium superimposed on major or mild NCD). Until another cause is identified, the confused geriatric patient should be assumed to have *delirium*, which is often reversible with treatment of the underlying systemic medical disorder.

As illustrated in Fig. 10.2, some common risk factors for delirium include metabolic disorders, infections, and medications [19, 20]. Potentially reversible causes of major or mild NCDs include thyroid dysfunction, vitamin deficiencies, human immunodeficiency virus infection, normal-pressure hydrocephalus, and depression, whereas major irreversible causes include Alzheimer's disease, other neurodegenerative conditions (e.g., frontotemporal and Lewy body NCDs, Parkinson's disease, Huntington's disease), and vascular NCD. It is essential to identify and treat potentially reversible causes of delirium episodes occurring "within" an irreversible NCD such as Alzheimer's disease, because this may lead to periods of some short-term improvement.

Most causes of confusion in the geriatric patients can usually be identified based on the complete history, medication review, physical including mental status examination, laboratory examination, and with longitudinal reevaluation. Identifying delirium requires a high index of suspicion. Delirium typically has an acute onset in disturbances of attention and consciousness and a fluctuating course, and in most cases, these hallmarks of delirium allow for recognition [21]. Because delirium is associated with high morbidity and mortality, under-recognition can be problematic especially with age 80 years or older, preexisting NCD, visual impairment, and/or hypoactive subtype of delirium [22]. The rates can be as high as 50 % in geriatric hospitalized medical patients [19, 22]. Below, we will focus on the evaluation and management of delirium due to its acuity during on-call and crisis situations.

10.2.1.1 Assessment of Delirium

(a) Use Brief Bedside Tools to Screen for Delirium The Confusion Assessment Method (CAM) is a validated tool for frontline clinicians that can be used to identify the presence of delirium even if a preexisting NCD is established. The CAM includes four features: (1) acute onset and fluctuating course, (2) inattention, (3) disorganized thinking, and (4) altered level of consciousness. The presence of

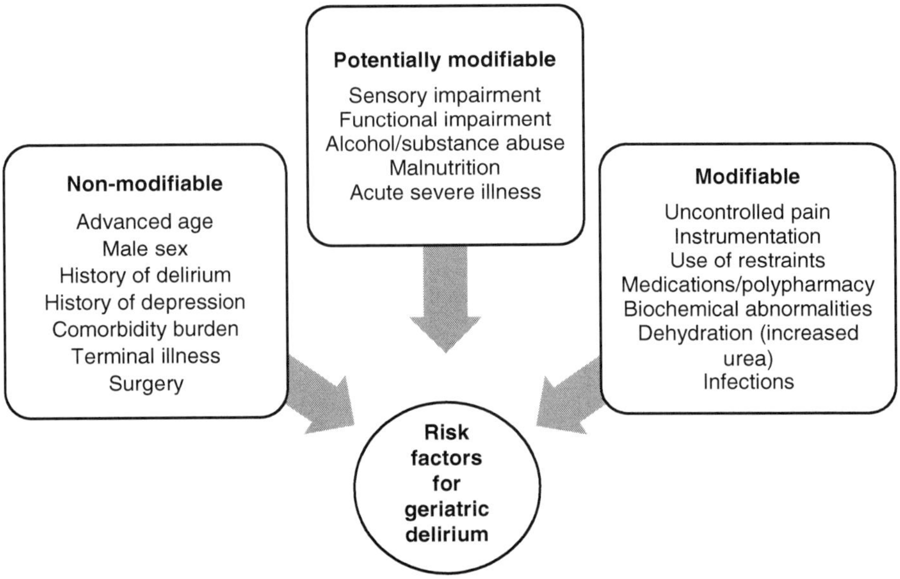

Fig. 10.2 Common risk factors for geriatric delirium [19, 20]

delirium is indicated by a CAM algorithm that includes features 1 *and* 2, *plus* either 3 *or* 4 [18]. The MoCA or MMSE are not by themselves definitive in screening for delirium or differentiating it from major or mild NCDs. For test of inattention, assess the patient by reciting, backwards, days of the week or months of the year, or by serial subtractions of the same number from a starting point, and by observing for problems focusing, staring off into space, or losing track of questions (see also Table 18.1 for identification of delirium).

(b) Obtain Collateral Information from Staff or Caregivers Obtain information (e.g., nursing notes, comments of family members) over the previous 24 h, especially if there was any acute change from baseline cognition, behavior, and function.

(c) Differentiate Delirium from Other Conditions with Similar Symptoms Assessment of delirium includes examining levels of arousal, cognition (i.e., orientation, attention, memory), psychomotor activity, and perceptual disturbances. Remember that falling asleep during the daytime, staring off into space, decreased motor activity, and lethargy, usually seen in hypoactive delirium, are abnormal in geriatric patients with major NCDs. Major or mild NCD is the most likely predisposing factor for geriatric delirium, and recurrent delirium should raise the suspicion for preexisting NCD.

Unlike the rapid onset of delirium, the onset of major NCD is usually insidious and not associated with fluctuations in mental status (except for NCD with Lewy bodies, which has fluctuations in cognition as one of the core features). A change from baseline is often key to confirming the diagnosis of delirium in those with major or mild NCD. Acute- and new-onset visual hallucinations, behavioral disturbances such as "picking at the air" or disrobing, and poor attention or distractibility during assessment can be helpful features in distinguishing delirium from major NCDs. Patients with major NCDs can present with comorbid depression (e.g., mood change, anhedonia, insomnia, anorexia, psychomotor change), who then can develop delirium as a result of "failure to thrive."

Therefore, these three syndromes (delirium, major NCD, and depression) can present with an overlap in some features (e.g., anorexia, insomnia, and psychomotor change). Notably, a patient with major depressive disorder will present such features for at least 2 weeks and will not be associated with dramatic changes in attention (although depressed patients may have *some* attentional disturbances especially on formalized testing) or level of consciousness, unlike delirium, which features fluctuating mental status disturbances. Figure 10.3 illustrates some differences among delirium, major NCD due to Alzheimer's disease, and depression [21].

(d) Assess for Current Psychiatric Symptoms Ask the patient about the presence of vivid dreams, nightmares, or poor sleep quality during the previous night, although some patients may have little recollection of the night before. Assess for sleep-wake disturbance, anxiety, mood disturbances, and agitation (hyperactive subtype) or apathy (hypoactive subtype); note that hypoactive delirium can resemble depression.

Delirium	Alzheimer's disease	Depression
• Acute onset	• Insidious onset	• Subacute onset
• Psychomotor changes, mood changes, sleep (circadian) disturbances	• Apathy, agitation, sundowning, weight loss	• Psychomotor changes, anhedonia, anxiety, sleep disturbance, weight loss
• Fluctuating cognitive loss	• Stable short-term (i.e., no daily fluctuations) cognitive loss (but progressive over time)	• Stable cognitive loss
• Patient may minimize cognitive deficit	• Patient may minimize cognitive deficit despite impaired memory and executive function	• Patient may express subjective complaints of cognitive impairment that exceed objective deficit
• Performance characterized by short attention span	• Guesses and wrong answers during testing	• "I don't know, I can't" responses
• Aphasia and apraxia	• Aphasia and apraxia	• Language and motor skills clinically intact
• Usually reversible, but can also be prolonged or chronic	• Irreversible	• Reversible

Fig. 10.3 Clinical differences among delirium, Alzheimer's disease, and depression [21]

(e) Assess for Subtle Manifestations of Delirium New-onset incontinence, mild disorientation, hypersensitivity to environmental stimuli, hypervigilance, dysphagia, dysarthria, refusal to mobilize, or falls can represent subtle manifestations of delirium, which then can progress to include more dramatic agitation, anxiety, and/or psychotic symptoms [22].

(f) Assess the Capacity to Consent to Specific Tasks, Including Medical Investigations and Treatments The fluctuating course of delirium can allow for "lucid intervals" in which the patient's decisional capacity may appear to be generally preserved. This circumstance is challenging in that patients may not later remember the informed consent discussion accomplished during a brief "lucid interval" occurring during more symptomatic periods. Because of this, they may not be able to give informed consent until the entire delirium episode is clearly over. The assessment of *financial decision making* should be deferred unless there is an urgent necessity to accomplish this.

10.2.1.2 Management of Delirium

(a) Correct the Underlying Causes Common causes for delirium can be prescription or over-the-counter medications, such as analgesics (e.g., opioids such as meperidine, nonsteroidal anti-inflammatory drugs), anticholinergics (e.g., benztropine, oxybutynin, diphenhydramine), or dopamine agonists (e.g., levodopa, pramipexole, ropinirole); these should be switched to less delirium-provoking agents if possible, discontinued, or have the doses decreased under observation. Other delirium-provoking drugs (e.g., corticosteroids, beta-blockers, antimicrobials, antineoplastics, antiseizure medications, benzodiazepines in susceptible patients) should be tapered, switched, or discontinued. Checking for pain and constipation should be routine in the on-call management of delirious patients, whereas performing a post-void residual bladder scan can identify urinary retention quickly.

Clinical Recommendation

As in Mr. A's case, when there are medical conditions that necessitate review of newly started, possibly delirium-provoking medications, consider dosage tapering or discontinuation of nonessential medications.

(b) Treat the Psychiatric Symptoms When asked to assess a patient for distressing agitation, aggression, psychotic symptoms, or sleep disturbance due to delirium in which non-pharmacological approaches (e.g., environmental modification, restraint-free care with sitter for constant supervision) solely did not suffice, psychopharmacological treatment may be required. (See Table 18.1 for non-pharmacological management of delirium.) Antipsychotic medications are the treatment of choice for short-term duration until delirium resolves. Close monitoring is required because antipsychotics can be associated with adverse neurological effects, such as

extrapyramidal symptoms (EPS) or neuroleptic malignant syndrome (NMS) – which *itself* causes delirium, particularly in Parkinson-sensitive populations. In cases of confirmed NMS, all antipsychotics need to be held until the creatine phosphokinase (CPK) has been normalized for 2 weeks, and then a less D_2 blocking antipsychotic agent can be cautiously given if an antipsychotic is still required, with continued surveillance for recurrence of NMS (e.g., serial CPK monitoring). Antipsychotics can produce a particular type of EPS called akathisia (motor restlessness) that can aggravate the hyperactive, delirious patient.

Haloperidol, a typical antipsychotic, is recommended in delirium clinical practice guidelines mostly based on clinical experience and a large evidence base; haloperidol lacks hypotensive, anticholinergic, and sedating effects at low doses, but may lead to EPS at doses above 3 mg a day in the geriatric patients [19]. Initial oral dosing range of haloperidol is 0.25–1 mg, once or twice daily, with additional doses every 4 h as needed (peak effect, 4–6 h) [19, 23]. The dose can be titrated as needed, and severely agitated patients may require higher dosage. Haloperidol is not recommended if there is a preexisting Parkinson's disease or Lewy body NCD [23, 24]. Baseline electrocardiogram (ECG) is recommended to rule out corrected QT (QTc) prolongation syndrome, ventricular arrhythmias, and torsades de pointes, particularly for the intravenous administration of haloperidol. Although rare in geriatric patients, these cardiac adverse events are typically associated with additional risk factors (e.g., female sex, genetic predisposition, bradycardia, hypokalemia, hypomagnesemia) and after 24-h cumulative haloperidol dosages of 2 mg or more [23–25]. For prolongation of QTc intervals to greater than 450 ms or greater than 25 % over baseline ECG, consider cardiology consultation and antipsychotic dosage decrease or discontinuation [23].

Various other antipsychotics (which have different receptor activities and side effect profiles, and thus should *not* be thought of as completely interchangeable) can be used for delirium treatment. Initial oral dosing ranges of commonly used atypical antipsychotics in delirium include risperidone, 0.25–0.5 mg once or twice daily; olanzapine, 1.25–5 mg once daily; and quetiapine, 12.5–25 mg once or twice daily, whereas very limited data exist for the use of other atypical antipsychotic agents [19, 22, 23]. While quetiapine has less EPS potential and more sedative and hypnotic qualities than most other antipsychotics, it also has significant alpha-1 blockade and risk for orthostatic hypotension. Ziprasidone can prolong the QTc interval. Aripiprazole is rarely associated with QTc prolongation, making it a desirable option particularly in geriatric patients who may have multiple risk factors for QTc prolongation. Alternative routes of administration, such as subcutaneous, intramuscular, or intravenous, can be offered in patients refusing or unable to use orally administered agents; intravenous administration of haloperidol, approved for use in Canada but not in the USA by the Food and Drug Administration (FDA), is usually the first choice in critical care settings [24, 25].

Benzodiazepines such as lorazepam, 0.5–1 mg, with additional doses every 4 h as needed, are first-line treatment for delirium that is associated with seizures, withdrawal from alcohol or benzodiazepines/hypnotics, and for delirium due to NMS [19].

Caution should be exercised when using benzodiazepines in the delirious patient due to risk of paradoxical excitation, respiratory depression, falls, sedation, and worsening cognitive impairment [19] (also see Sect. 10.2.7 on the addicted patient).

Clinical Recommendation
The goal for the pharmacological treatment of delirium should be an *alert* patient who is manageable, rather than a sedated patient, and the medication should be tapered and discontinued as soon as possible after recovery from delirium.

Tapering to discontinuation of the antipsychotic treatment should be considered when the patient has been symptom-free for 1 week [26]. Some patients may be predisposed to recurrent or prolonged/chronic delirium (e.g., end-stage liver disease, cancer), and longer-term (even indefinite) antipsychotic treatment may be required in these circumstances. For delirium at the end of life, the goal is to minimize suffering and discomfort in patients in palliative care.

Physical restraints should be applied only in exceptional circumstances when there is serious risk of bodily harm to self or others; other interventions including medications were ineffective in ensuring safety; and when the benefits outweigh the risks of restraints. Direct, constant monitoring, reevaluation, and documentation are necessary to justify the continued use of physical restraints. (Also see Chap. 7.)

(c) Implement a Safe Discharge Premature or inadequately planned discharges may lead to rehospitalization or increased safety risks at home. Some patients wishing to leave hospital against medical advice without having their emergency care needs addressed may require involuntary detention under the psychiatric commitment statute specific to the local jurisdiction.

Clinical Recommendation
When the on-call physician is asked to see a delirious patient who requests to leave the hospital, the decision to discharge should be guided by clinical judgment rather than the patient's desire to go home, particularly if there are not adequate supports at home.

Those deemed mentally incapacitated to consent to treatment may need to be formally reassessed after being treated. Delirium in older, compared to younger, patients is associated with more severe cognitive impairment, morbidity, and mortality. Therefore, it is important to list "delirium" on the patient's medical profile (including on the hospital discharge summary and problem list) and ensure that the patient's primary care physician (PCP) is alerted to the history of an episode of delirium in order to assume an active role in post-delirium care, including post-recovery cognitive evaluation, delirium recurrence surveillance, medication adjustments, and risk factor management [20].

10.2.2 The Violent Patient

Case Vignette Mr. B, a 77-year-old male with a history of major NCD due to Alzheimer's disease (MoCA was 14 out of 30 points 2 months earlier), was admitted to a psychiatric ward for increasing agitation and exit-seeking behavior at the skilled nursing facility where he had been living for 6 weeks. His PCP started him on a memory enhancer, donepezil, 6 weeks previously, but the staff noted increasing agitation thereafter. You were the on-call physician and asked to assess Mr. B because he was aggressive toward another patient during the night. In speaking with the staff and reviewing the chart, you identified a behavioral pattern that Mr. B had been wandering on the ward particularly in the early evening, appearing to be perplexed while trying to find his room. The identified trigger for his current event was that Mr. B sat on another male patient's bed and became combative during altercation with that patient.

Aggressive behavior may be a symptom of several psychiatric disorders, such as neurocognitive (e.g., delirium, major NCDs), psychotic, bipolar, substance use, anxiety, and/or personality disorders, but it can also be a warning sign of an underlying critical systemic medical illness (e.g., stroke, hypoglycemia, pulmonary embolism, myocardial infarct). It can also be a manifestation of medication-induced adverse events (e.g., dopamine agonists, psychostimulants). Agitation can increase the potential for physical aggression and injury due to lack of behavioral control and lead to severe medical complications (e.g., exhaustion, rhabdomyolysis, renal failure, death) in the geriatric patient. "Sundowning" due to major NCDs refers to a specific pattern of agitation, with worsening of agitation in the late afternoon or early evening. Possible contributing factors for sundowning include decreased light exposure, timing of medications, and dysfunctional sleep-wake cycles.

10.2.2.1 Assessment

An episode of aggressive behavior must be defused before assessment and management can take place. A decision should be made about whether to first review the medical chart or evaluate the patient, depending on the severity of the agitation. Aggression due to delirium will be associated with other typical features of delirium (e.g., altered level of consciousness, circadian disturbance, fluctuating mental status, abnormal electroencephalogram). Aggression due to a major NCD will manifest typically in the moderate to severe stages of the disease and can include swearing, screaming, shouting, making threats, pinching, scratching, hitting, hair-pulling, biting, and behaving in a sexually inappropriate manner (see Chap. 17 for further details on neuropsychiatric symptoms of major NCDs).

(a) Aim for Safety First in all Instances of Aggression Adopt a nonconfrontational approach. The reader is referred to Fig. 10.4 for emergency safety measures that clinicians need to promptly implement when assessing an aggressive patient during an on-call event.

Aim for safety	***Give the patient space and control the environment.*** Clinicians involved should stop doing whatever appears to be associated with the behavior (e.g., attending to personal care, changing a dressing), remove any obvious stressors (e.g., noise, equipment, pain), and move out of range. Remove items that a patient can grab (e.g., exposed jewelry, scarf, loose hair, ties, stethoscope, pen). Wear your hospital identification breakaway chain. View the patient initially from a distance, then approach the patient cautiously to perform the evaluation, if cooperative. If there is significant psychomotor activity, assume that the situation may be dangerous and be prepared before approaching the patient. Approach the patient slowly, use direct language, and remain calm in voice and demeanor. Ask the patient to describe the situation.
	Know how to access the security arrangements at that facility. Ensure there is sufficient trained staff members available to help control the patient physically. Announce your intention in advance of any action. Remain at least 3 feet away from the patient, stand sideways so that you can remove yourself from a potentially combative patient, and do not turn your back on the patient until you are at least 15 feet away. In the emergency room, patients are usually searched for weapon possession before evaluation, but do not assume this has been done. Call hospital security to perform a search when necessary. Depending on the situation, if you suspect the patient has a weapon, call police right away for any disarming of patient. Never ask the patient to hand you a weapon, and never attempt to take a weapon from the patient. Assess the patient in a quiet, open area, while positioning yourself nearest to the exits.
	Implement a calm and empathic approach, while meeting the patient's immediate need as appropriately as possible. Attempt to settle a tense situation by using the patient's preferred name and by not arguing or disagreeing. Attempt to empathize ("I can see you are upset. Can I help you?"). Listen carefully to their reply and investigate any claims or accusations. Attempt to divert the attention, particularly if there could be an element of major neurocognitive disorder involved. Offering the patient something to eat (a sandwich) helps to restore behavior in many cases, but do not give the patient food items that may be thrown at you (hot food/beverage, cutlery).

Fig. 10.4 Emergency safety measures for assessing and reducing patient violence

(b) Evaluate the Event and Search for a Precipitant After implementing the emergency safety measures, assess the patient's mental status, including sensorium (e.g., alert, drowsy), orientation level (e.g., temporal and spatial disorientation), behavior (e.g., calm, agitated), speech (e.g., pressured, slurred, loud, threatening), and thought processes (e.g., coherent, illogical). Read the medical chart, and follow-up with the staff and the patient to determine further assessment and management. Any interventions should develop based on the existing treatment plan.

Documentation by staff by way of a standardized *Behavior Chart* can be helpful in mapping and understanding events to prevent recurrence. This should include the "ABC approach" [27]:

A. The *Antecedent* – what happened before the event?
B. The *Behavior* – what behavior occurred?
C. The *Consequences* – what response was there from others?

The A or antecedent is most important and is a description of the events immediately preceding the aggressive event, such as "Mr. B was disoriented on the ward and could not find his room." It is important to search for the trigger, or "activating factor," e.g., "Mr. B sat down on Mr. X's bed." Overall, facilitate assessment for major NCDs and delirium and/or bipolar or other psychiatric disorders known to precipitate aggression. In cases of aggression due to suspected overdose, follow management protocols for the specific substance.

(c) Do Not Hesitate to Call Other Medical Consultants if Acute Physical Problems Are Suspected Review vital signs taken over the past 24–48 h and rule out medication or substance withdrawal. Tapering or discontinuing medication believed to cause symptoms may not immediately relieve the agitation; thus, a psychotropic agent may be required initially. Lithium therapy requires particular caution in geriatric patients. Even if the serum level is 0.6 or 0.8 mmol/L (or mEq/L), which is in the "normal" range in a younger patient, it may actually be neurotoxic in a geriatric patient, likely due to age-associated changes in the blood–brain barrier which alter lithium uptake into the brain. Another common problem is insidious decrease in renal function in older lithium patients, requiring a renal panel with every serum lithium level. Toxic lithium levels may require intravenous fluids or even urgent renal dialysis. Abrupt discontinuation of certain medications may have deleterious effects (e.g., carbidopa/levodopa in Parkinson's disease can induce NMS), while initiating other medications (e.g., cholinesterase inhibitors, as in Mr. B's case) can trigger or exacerbate aggression.

(d) Duty to Inform (Protect or Warn) If the patient made significant and specific threats against a particular person or group of persons, and when there is an element of imminence, in many jurisdictions, the clinician who elicits the dangerousness data has the duty to inform the police and/or the intended, "identifiable" victim to protect that person [28]. Document concerns and the actions taken clearly and concisely in the chart. Give verbal sign-out of this information to the next on-call physician or the attending physician.

Clinical Recommendation
In the event of informing, the information disclosed should be limited to that which would provide protection. Consult with hospital risk management and legal team, and/or the ethics committee as necessary, especially for clarity of clinician duties under the laws of the local jurisdiction.

(e) Always Remember to Support the Staff Members and Others Involved Arrange a time to allow them to reflect on their role in the incident in a safe and supportive manner, and enunciate their concerns.

10.2.2.2 Management

(a) With the "ABC" in Mind, Plan the Ongoing Management Aim for a consistent approach with consideration of the possibility of patient's misunderstanding of their surroundings (particularly in cognitively impaired patients), divergent communication skills and language barriers, and biases both in the patient and the staff.

(b) If the Problem Persists, Encourage the Patient to Take Medication to Help Regain Self-Control If necessary, consider chemical restraint in the least restrictive manner possible. The last resort of mechanical restraint requires one-to-one supervision, and

the facility's policy must be followed rigorously – especially the need for a written medical order, physician rounding, frequent reassurance, and a clear plan of observation and release timeframe (see Chap. 7). The short-term use of typical antipsychotic medications, such as haloperidol (0.5–2 mg), STAT (immediately), and PRN (pro re nata, or as-needed), and atypical antipsychotic medications, such as risperidone (0.5–1 mg), olanzapine (2.5–5 mg), or aripiprazole (2–10 mg), with small doses repeated often, is suggested for severe aggression or agitation. Careful monitoring for signs of medication effectiveness or the development of Parkinsonian features (e.g., restlessness, tremor, rigidity, stooped posture) is essential. (Also see Chap. 3.)

Clinical Recommendation
The initial dose of antipsychotics used to treat severe aggression or agitation is substantially reduced for geriatric patients. As a rule, "start low, go slow, and stay low." In some cases, a dose more typical of a younger adult patient may be needed, but this should be approached only incrementally.

In patients with major NCDs with severe agitation without psychotic features, antidepressants such as trazodone or selective serotonin reuptake inhibitors (SSRIs) (e.g., citalopram, sertraline), anticonvulsants (e.g., valproate, carbamazepine), and short or intermediate acting benzodiazepines (e.g., lorazepam) can be used [27]. If carbamazepine is started, monitor for adverse events such as sedation, hyponatremia, cardiac toxicity, and drug-drug interactions because carbamazepine is a strong enzymatic inducer. If valproate is used, monitor for liver-associated enzymes, ammonia, and platelet count. Carbamazepine and valproate therapeutic drug monitoring levels should be routinely accomplished. If a benzodiazepine is started, use should be limited to brief periods in most cases [27].

(c) Document the Events Clearly and Frequently This is done particularly in the ongoing management.

10.2.3 The Psychotic Patient

Case Vignette Ms. C, a 75-year-old female, retired from her secretarial job 10 years previously, never married, socially isolated, and living in an apartment with her five cats, was reluctantly brought to the emergency room by her niece because of bizarre behavior. You were the on-call psychiatrist. Collateral information from the niece revealed that Ms. C had always been "odd and eccentric," mistrustful of others, and had never gotten along with her neighbors. There was no family history of psychiatric disorders. She had bilateral hearing loss but refused to wear hearing aids. She actively smoked and did not use alcohol. She did not take any prescribed medications or over-the-counter remedies, except acetaminophen occasionally for headaches. While you interviewed Ms. C, she endorsed beliefs that a young couple upstairs were spying on her, released laser beams and gas (which she could see and smell) through a vent in the ceiling to "knock her out," and took her to the building's basement to "perform tests." She claimed that they inserted "a chip" in her arm to monitor her location. She showed you a bruise on her arm as proof of the tests. She stated she could hear them through the walls, saying "let's get rid of her." These symptoms began at least 6 months previously. She did not have any memory problems and was fully independent for IADLs and ADLs. Ms. C was cooperative with MoCA (score of 30 out of 30 points) and clock drawing test (normal). Computed tomography of head showed age-related atrophy and no vascular changes. Routine blood work was normal. She was fully oriented and alert. Your diagnosis was very-late-onset schizophrenia-like psychotic disorder.

Delusions, hallucinations, impaired reality testing, and sometimes decreased impulse control can be manifestations of a psychotic disorder. However, psychotic symptoms can be associated with various diagnostic categories including delirium, major NCDs, schizophrenia, delusional disorder, depressive and bipolar disorders, drug-induced disorders, and a range of medical-neurologic conditions (e.g., seizure disorders, brain tumors, Parkinson's disease). More than 50 % of patients with major NCD of the Alzheimer's type manifest psychotic symptoms during the course of this progressive illness [29]. In addition, several commonly prescribed medications can also produce psychotic symptoms in geriatric patients (e.g., dopamine agonists, anticholinergics, corticosteroids). The frequent coexistence of psychotic symptoms occurring in patients with major NCDs who may have other comorbid medical conditions and can be taking multiple medications complicates an already complex treatment situation in a geriatric patient.

Therefore, geriatric patients are at increased risk for developing psychotic symptoms due to multiple factors: age-related cortical changes in areas such as temporal or frontal lobes, age-related pharmacokinetic and pharmacodynamic changes, polypharmacy, cognitive changes, comorbid physical illnesses, social isolation, and sensory deficits (e.g., hearing loss) [30].

10.2.3.1 Assessment

(a) Determine the Underlying Etiology of the Psychotic Symptoms Review the patient's chart to include medical history, medications and over-the-counter remedies, and most recent investigations (e.g., complete blood count, electrolytes, renal panel, liver-associated enzymes, ammonia, glucose, calcium, magnesium, albumin, lipid profile, thyroid-stimulating hormone, vitamin B_{12}, folate, urinalysis, and neuroimaging findings). Perform or review recent cognitive screening tests (e.g., MoCA) to rule out cognitive impairment. Obtain collateral information regarding the patient's risk factors for late-onset psychotic disorder, including premorbid personality traits. In Ms. C's case, the risk factors were female sex, hearing impairment, social isolation, abnormal premorbid personality, and abnormal social functioning. Review the psychiatric history as this may reveal past episodes of psychotic or depressive disorder that may predispose geriatric patients to psychotic symptoms.

Clinical Recommendation
There may be more than one causal factor contributing to the emergence of psychotic symptoms. For instance, psychiatric disorders like schizophrenia or major depression may coexist with major NCDs and/or acute causes of psychotic symptoms (e.g., medication-induced delirium). Treating or mitigating predisposing factors (e.g., optimizing sensory function) may be considered prior to pharmacological intervention.

(b) Consider Differential Diagnosis Psychotic symptoms can manifest across a spectrum of disorders that must be considered in the differential diagnosis prior to initiating appropriate pharmacological intervention.

Medical conditions such as thyroid disease, diabetes mellitus, vitamin B_{12} and folate deficiency, electrolyte imbalance, dehydration, sleep deprivation, as well as chronic illnesses such as Parkinson's disease, Huntington's disease, multiple sclerosis, and amyotrophic lateral sclerosis have all been associated with psychotic symptoms [29]. Delirium, subtle seizure disorders, or structural brain lesions must be ruled out as well. Nearly 40 % of Parkinson's disease patients develop psychotic symptoms, and the incidence increases with age; psychotic symptoms may result from the systemic disease process, emerging comorbid major NCD or major depression, or the dopaminergic medications used to treat Parkinson's disease [29]. Complex, formed, and mobile visual hallucinations (often of people, animals, or objects) occur in over 20 % of patients receiving dopaminergic agents and appear to be dose related [29]. NCD associated with Parkinson's disease vs. NCD associated with Lewy bodies are clinically "more similar than different"; the major difference is in the timing of symptom onset (with motor symptoms preceding cognitive decline in Parkinson's disease and vice versa in Lewy body NCD).

Psychosis in *delirium* is different than in late-onset schizophrenia; misinterpretations, illusions, and visual hallucinations are more common, whereas delusions in delirium are usually transient and poorly systematized.

Psychosis in *major NCDs* differs from late-onset schizophrenia in that paranoid beliefs are often simple and visual hallucinations are more common. For instance, delusions (i.e., fixed, false beliefs) must be differentiated from misperceptions due to sensory or cognitive impairment (e.g., seeing a shadow on the wall could be mistaken for an intruder in the house). Delusional reports of theft by a geriatric patient may seem plausible at first and can delay recognition of a psychotic symptom.

Visual and somatic hallucinations may be more common in older than in younger patients, particularly when the psychosis is secondary to a medical condition (e.g., Parkinson's disease). Visual hallucinations must be differentiated from *illusions* and *visual release hallucinations* (or Charles Bonnet syndrome), which are caused by vision impairment. Hallucinations must be differentiated from *sleep hallucinations* due to hypnagogia/hypnopompia, a transition to and from sleep (daytime sleep episodes or at night) which may be attended by multiple sensory experiences ranging from barely perceptible to vivid hallucinations. Visual hallucinations must also be differentiated from *rapid eye movement (REM) sleep behavior disorder*, which involves abnormal behavior during the REM sleep phase. REM sleep behavior disorder is most often associated with age, Parkinson's disease, multiple system atrophy, and major or mild NCD with Lewy bodies [31].

Auditory hallucinations must be differentiated from *tinnitus* or *carotid bruits* in the geriatric patients [29]. *Musical hallucinations*, in which a sound is perceived as instrumental music or songs, represent a rare disorder of auditory hallucinations most commonly caused by hypoacusis [32].

Adverse drug reactions and dosages must be reviewed when evaluating *medications* as causative agents for psychosis (e.g., antiparkinsonian drugs, anticholinergics, antihistamines, antidepressants).

Psychotic symptoms in *major depressive* or *bipolar disorder* are usually mood congruent, with common themes of persecution, guilt, nihilism, or grandiosity. The presenting symptoms of psychosis may differ in quality and intensity in older patients compared with younger patients. Differentiating *early-onset schizophrenia* from *very-late-onset schizophrenia-like psychotic disorder* is essential. Table 10.2 illustrates a comparison of their distinct characteristics [33].

Table 10.2 Clinical characteristics of early-onset vs. very-late-onset schizophrenia-like psychotic disorder (adapted from reference [33])

Clinical characteristics	Early onset (<40 years)	Very-late onset (>65 years)
Female predominance	–	++
Paranoid type	+ (often elaborate)	+ (often elaborate)
Partition delusions	–	+
Negative symptoms	++	–
Thought process disorder	+	–
Hallucinations	+ (especially auditory)	++ (multiple modalities: visual, tactile, olfactory, auditory)
Neuropsychological impairment:		
Learning	++	?++
Retention	–	?++
Progressive cognitive impairment	–	++
Brain structural abnormalities (e.g., strokes, tumors)	–	++
Premorbid functioning	++	–
Family history of schizophrenia	+	–
Sensory deficits (auditory, visual)	–	++
Risk of tardive dyskinesia	+	++
Daily antipsychotic dosage	++	+

Note: –, less common or absent, + common, ++ very common or marked, ?++ probably very common, but limited published data exist

10.2.3.2 Management

(a) Implement Urgent Measures for Self-Protection and to Prevent Harm to Others This is because psychotic behavior can result in physical aggression, accidents, suicide, or physical impairment due to refusal to treatment.

(b) Provide Immediate Treatment Geared Toward the Specific Cause of Psychosis and Tailored Based on Comorbid Conditions For psychosis associated with medical conditions, treatment of the underlying etiology will eventually lead to clearance of the psychotic symptoms. Frequently, environmental and psychosocial interventions (e.g., provide hearing amplifiers or hearing aids) are first-line treatments, with the judicious use of pharmacotherapy as needed.

Antipsychotics are often used to manage psychotic symptoms (hallucinations and delusions) and are started at low doses and up-titrated until there is clinical benefit. (See Chap. 3 for details regarding on-call pharmacotherapy principles.)

Clinical Recommendation
Typical antipsychotics such as haloperidol tend to increase tremor and worsen psychomotor retardation. The atypical antipsychotics like quetiapine and clozapine can effectively treat Parkinson-related psychotic symptoms because of their low EPS potential due to low degree of D_2 blockade. If the assessment reveals that depressive symptoms are the dominant-presenting problem, a trial of antidepressants may precede the introduction of antipsychotic medications in psychotic geriatric patients. Depressive disorders with psychotic symptoms may benefit from early use of electroconvulsive therapy (ECT).

10.2.4 The Suicidal Patient

Case Vignette While consulting in the psychiatric ED, you met Mrs. D, 78-year-old Caucasian female, brought in by ambulance after her spouse found her lying unresponsive on the bathroom floor next to empty bottles of two antidepressants and a blood pressure medication and with alcohol on her breath. Her spouse reported that Mrs. D had been worried about the upcoming wedding party for their daughter's oldest child, as their ex-son-in-law and his new wife (for whom he left their daughter) would be in attendance. Mrs. D started an argument with her spouse "for no apparent reason" and was very upset earlier in the day as he was heading out grocery shopping. You identified that the suicide risk factors were older age, white race, psychiatric illnesses (likely alcohol abuse, anxiety, and/or depression), medical illness (hypertension), negative life stressor (her child's divorce), and borderline personality traits (recently being angry and impulsive). You interviewed Mrs. D shortly after she was deemed medically stable. She was hopeless, extremely anxious, pessimistic about the future, and demanded to go home. You determined that Mrs. D was at-imminent risk of suicide and admitted her to the hospital on a psychiatric commitment order.

The after-hours, on-call physician will often be called to assess a geriatric patient's suicidal ideation and behavior. One or more psychiatric disorders are virtually ubiquitous among geriatric patients with suicidal ideation and/or behavior, and medical trainees frequently encounter suicidal patients in the course of their training rotations. Therefore, enhancing clinician knowledge and skill in working with patients at risk for suicide is crucial. Many types of self-harm behavior can be encountered in patients during an on-call shift, including ED patients with command auditory hallucinations to harm themselves, patients with personality disorders presenting with pathological defense mechanisms, older adults with malingering looking for a temporary shelter or food, psychiatric inpatients struggling to keep from taking their own lives, or medical inpatients and nursing home residents looking for a way out of physical pain. Establishing the etiology of the suicidality, ensuring provision of the immediate stabilization necessary for safety of the patient, and initiating appropriate treatment are paramount.

10.2.4.1 Assessment

(a) Use a Stepwise Approach Use a stepwise approach that starts with a general question and becomes more specific with each successive question. It is important to ask the patient about:

- *Hopelessness* or *thoughts of death*
- Explicit *thoughts of suicide*
- Specific *suicide plan* and how close the patient is to carrying out this plan
- *Intention* to carry out suicide plan
- *Means* for carrying out suicide plan
- Whether the patient thought what would happen *after his/her death*
- Presence of *command hallucinations* (e.g., hearing voices telling the patient to do things) and whether the voices tell the patient to kill or injure himself/herself or someone else
- Prior history of *suicide attempts* (the strongest predictor of death by suicide [34])
- *Family history* of suicide completion
- *Current/past psychiatric treatment*, as an inpatient or outpatient, and whether there has been medication, and which treatment has helped the patient most
- *Stressors* or *losses* happening in the patient's life or causing the patient to worry a lot and how long they have been going on
- *Active substance abuse* (e.g., ask "how much alcohol do you drink a day?" instead of "do you drink alcohol?")

Clinical Recommendation
Suicide risk assessment necessitates establishing a clinical rapport with the patient and conducting an assessment in a sensitive manner, utilizing a biopsychosocial framework.

(b) Complete the Survey of the Risk Factors Complete the survey of the risk factors that increase risk of suicide in the geriatric patient. These include the presence of one or more psychiatric disorders (especially depressive, psychotic, and substance use disorders; risk is higher with multiple comorbidities), personality disorders (e.g., borderline, narcissistic), negative life events (e.g., separation, divorce, death of a spouse), medical illness, pain (experienced or anticipated), functional impairment, and being an older white male [35]. Symptoms of borderline personality disorder such as mood dysregulation, impulsivity, and aggression are independent risk factors for suicide and self-harm behavior.

(c) Survey the Protective Factors Survey the protective factors or resiliency of the patient, which may mitigate the risk of suicide. These include recognizing meaning and purpose of life, adopting meaningful daily routines, active interests and social roles, caring for others and/or pets, maintaining social contact with family and friends, and exhibiting better healthcare practices including moderate alcohol consumption [35].

(d) Perform or Review Recent Findings of a Physical Examination Perform or review recent findings of a physical examination including evaluation of the patient's mental status. This will guide the on-call psychiatric consultant to exclude underlying medical cause to the symptom presentation (e.g., acute, untreated pain), understand the severity of the depression, identify the presence of psychotic symptoms of command auditory hallucinations, and whether the patient has recently been angry, demanding, or manipulative, which can be suggestive of substance abuse or personality disorders. General appearance is key. Note the patient's speech, eye contact, and motor activity. Depressed patients may have a blunted affect, avoid eye contact, and have psychomotor retardation, whereas patients in manic episodes may have agitation, pressured speech, and increased psychomotor activity. Note that akathisia (motor restlessness) can increase the risk of suicide. Refusal to eat, take life-sustaining medications, or follow medical advice can be forms of self-injurious behaviors often referred to as "indirect self-destructive behaviors," which can serve as a way of either communicating one's distress or an effort to hasten death. Some have proposed that indirect self-destructive behaviors are due to poor impulse control and physical isolation rather than depression per se [36, 37]. Screening tools for depression that could explain the patient's suicidality, such as the Patient Health Questionnaire-9 (PHQ-9), Patient Health Questionnaire-2 (PHQ-2), and Geriatric Depression Scale (GDS), represent rapidly administered tools that may provide important additional information [38]. For patients with aphasia, consider using a point-board, or a board with the scale and yes/no next to the items, and have patient point out correct answer.

(e) Determine Whether the Patient is "At-imminent Risk of Suicide" Determine whether the patient is "at-imminent risk of suicide" (within hours for committing suicide), if the patient [38]:

(i) Expresses the *intent* to die
(ii) Has a clear *plan*
(iii) Has *access* to lethal means (e.g., a gun, prescribed medications for overdose)

Giving away belongings, rewriting a will, and making the rounds to express goodbye to people should increase suspicion of suicide risk. Factors that further increase risk of an imminent suicide are [38]:

(iv) Hopelessness
(v) Pessimism about the future
(vi) Increased anxiety
(vii) Command hallucinations directing suicide

Patients are at "short-term risk" if they are likely to commit suicide within days to weeks and at "long-term risk" if they have sufficient risk factors associated with an eventual death by suicide [38]. Any patient deemed at-imminent risk for suicide should be hospitalized immediately for treatment.

(f) Determine Whether the Suicide Assessment Is Part of a Request for a Physician-Assisted Death The on-call physician may be asked to assess a patient without a depressive disorder who contemplates suicide, particularly in jurisdictions where physician-assisted suicide has been legalized. Associated factors include illnesses that cause continuous pain or interfere with a patient's autonomy and dignity, and patient-perceived limited quality of life. Referral to appropriate social and/or clinical services for a thorough evaluation is necessary. Standard protocols for this include multiple physician assessments (which may include a psychiatric assessment and absence of a current mood disorder).

(g) Upon Discharge, Provide Communication to the Patient's Healthcare Clinicians Also, promote provision of interdisciplinary team-based care to ensure recurrent assessment of suicide risk and resiliency factors. Maintaining detailed clinical notes is crucial.

10.2.4.2 Management

(a) Keep the Patient Safe Search patient's belongings for potentially dangerous objects to patient or others. The patient may not leave medical facility without a formal psychiatric evaluation. Those at high risk of suicide should be admitted to a specialized psychiatric service for further assessment, treatment, and suicide prevention strategies. For patients who refuse such an evaluation, it may be necessary to involuntarily hold them in the ED until a complete psychiatric and safety evaluation is performed, followed by an involuntary (or "civil") commitment if necessary. Maintain one-to-one observation if clinically indicated. If the patient is safe for discharge home, arrange outpatient psychiatric follow-up, discuss the plan with patient's PCP, and document patient's contact information and additional emergency information. Note that current data on the use of "no-harm contracts" within the scope of acute management of suicide risk is equivocal and thus not recommended [35].

(b) Initiate Treatment for Major Depression and/or Alcohol Use Disorder, Comorbid Anxiety, or Agitation as the Initial On-Call Management Aggressively treating

agitated states may resolve a suicide crisis. Although this section emphasizes patient's safety, please refer to Sections 10.2.5 and 10.2.6 regarding actual depression and anxiety management. As indicated, referral to specialized outpatient services for psychotherapy is recommended.

Clinical Recommendation

Clinical interventions that have been empirically shown to help reduce or resolve suicidal ideation, behavior, and/or death among geriatric patients support combination antidepressant pharmacotherapy and empirically supported psychotherapies (e.g., cognitive, interpersonal, or psychodynamic psychotherapies) [39, 40].

(c) Other Strategies Refer the depressed, socially isolated, or otherwise at-risk geriatric patients to a telephone distress outreach and support program, collaborative/shared care programs for ongoing management, and consider means restriction (e.g., restricting access to alcohol and firearms, detoxifying gas ovens, restriction of medication pack sizes).

10.2.5 The Depressed Patient

Case Vignette You were the psychiatrist on call and asked by your emergency physician colleague to see Mr. E for depression. Mr. E, an 85-year-old male with a prostate cancer with bone metastases, presented to the hospital for "failure to thrive." He complained of anhedonia, insomnia, anergia, anorexia, 35-lb weight loss, and a passive death wish. Upon examination, he denied being depressed but endorsed being lonely, tired of living, and ready to die. He attributed his insomnia to bone pain and the rest of his symptoms to his cancer. However, his anhedonia was one element that increased your confidence in a diagnosis of major depressive episode.

Depression is common in geriatric population, but there are suboptimal rates of clinical detection, explained in part by the fact that geriatric patients are less likely to endorse the word "depressed" or low mood and are more likely to present with somatic symptoms, and other medical conditions can confuse the diagnosis of depression [35]. Depression in geriatric patients usually presents as a gradual/subacute onset with mild cognitive impairment, mood being worse in the morning with improvement toward the end of the day and is present for at least the previous 2 weeks. It may be differentiated from delirium which presents as an acute onset with fluctuating symptoms that worsen toward the end of the day (see Fig. 10.3). To aid accurate diagnosis, it is better to describe the actual signs and symptoms rather than just say that the patient "appears depressed."

Clinical Recommendation
Recognizing geriatric depression is imperative because it is associated with poor functional status, physical symptoms (e.g., somatization), cognitive impairment, disability, increased utilization of healthcare resources, and medical mortality and suicide.

The on-call physician can be consulted in critical situations in which depression is suspected in some patients, and a high alertness to recognize and accurately diagnose depression is a required skill. As in Mr. E's case, clues to suspect geriatric depression include the following [41]:

- Persistent complaints of fatigue, weight loss, multiple diffuse symptoms, or persistent complaints of pain (e.g., headache, gastrointestinal, and joint pain)
- Food refusal, neglect of personal care, treatment refusal, or "failure to thrive"
- Recent bereavement with unusual and extreme symptoms (e.g., active suicidal ideation, guilt not related to the deceased, psychomotor retardation, mood congruent delusions)
- Apathy, withdrawal, or isolation
- Persistent sleep difficulties
- Persistent complaints of memory difficulties
- Frequent calls and visits to healthcare professionals, often for ill-defined, nonspecific complaints
- Recurrent or prolonged hospitalization or delayed rehabilitation
- Hospital discharge refusal

10.2.5.1 Assessment

(a) Use Age-Appropriate Depression Screening Tools This is applicable in patients in whom there is any concern for depressive disorder. The *PHQ-2* [9] is performed by an interviewer who asks the patient: "Over the past 2 weeks, how often have you been bothered by either of the following problems? (i) Little interest or pleasure in doing things; (ii) feeling down, depressed, or hopeless." Other screening tools for geriatric inpatients with mild or no cognitive impairment include the self-rating *GDS*, the self-rating *SELFCARE scale*, and the *Brief Assessment Schedule Depression Cards* (*BASDEC*). The *Cornell Scale for Depression in Dementia*, which is an observer-rated instrument, is recommended for patients with moderate to severe cognitive impairment [41].

(b) Conduct a Biopsychosocial Assessment This assessment follows a positive screen for depression, which include:

- Review of diagnostic criteria for types of depression as outlined in the Diagnostic and Statistical Manual, 5th edition (DSM-5) [21] (e.g., minor or major depressive

disorder; bipolar I or II disorder, current depressive episode; persistent depressive disorder – formerly dysthymic disorder; adjustment disorder with depressed mood)
- Estimate of severity, including the presence of melancholic, psychotic, and/or catatonic symptoms
- Risk assessment for suicide (see Section 10.2.4 for a method for directly asking patients about suicidal ideation, intent, and plan)
- Review of current stressors and life situation (e.g., grief, losses)
- Personal and family history of depressive or bipolar disorder
- Review of medications and substance use
- Review of functioning and/or disability and social support
- Physical examination and laboratory investigations looking for evidence of medical illness that could contribute to or mimic depressive symptoms (e.g., hypothyroidism)
- Mental status examination, including assessment of cognitive function

(c) Obtain Collateral Information Information can be obtained from the patient's family, or the staff from the retirement home or nursing home, who often have an in-depth knowledge of the patient's usual status and coping skills.

10.2.5.2 Management

(a) Consider Treatment with Antidepressants This is for symptoms of major depression. Antidepressants should be used when indicated, even in patients with multiple comorbidities and serious illnesses. Comorbid psychiatric disorders, particularly generalized anxiety and substance use disorders, should be identified and appropriately treated as they will adversely influence the outcome of depressive disorder. Note that minor depression of less than 4 weeks' duration and adjustment disorder with depressed mood are initially treated with supportive psychosocial interventions; however, brief use of anxiolytics/benzodiazepines or hypnotics for sleep disturbance in patients with severe life stressors may be considered. If symptoms persist after resolution of the stressor or for more than 4 weeks after initiation of the psychosocial interventions, revise the diagnosis and consider antidepressant medication or more specific psychotherapy [41].

Management considerations when initiating antidepressant treatment in geriatric patients are presented in Fig. 10.5 [41–43]. (Also see Chap. 3.)

Clinical Recommendation
Select an antidepressant with the lowest risk of drug-drug interactions (e.g., sertraline, citalopram, escitalopram, venlafaxine, bupropion, mirtazapine) and the lowest anticholinergic properties. Monitor for suicidal ideation and risk when initiating an antidepressant.

Recommend	Monitor	Avoid
• Choose an AD with the lowest risk of drug-drug interactions (e.g., sertraline, citalopram, escitalopram, venlafaxine, bupropion, mirtazapine). • Select ADs with the lowest anticholinergic properties. • Add an AD in depressed patients with bipolar disorder previously stabilized on a mood stabilizer [41]. • Consider use of lithium, antipsychotics, and ECT (although these are not geriatric-age specific indications). Consider an urgent referral for ECT treatment in cases of: acutely suicidal patients, required rapid response to maintain safety, depressed patients with psychotic features, AD intolerance, or a history of unstable medical conditions.	• Monitor for suicidal ideation and risk when initiating an AD. • Check sodium levels before switching to another AD because of poor response or tolerance, or when displaying symptoms of hyponatremia (e.g., fatigue, malaise, delirium). Document the need to check sodium levels 1 month after initiating SSRIs/SNRIs, especially if concurrent medication use that can cause hyponatremia (e.g., diuretics) [41]. • If SSRIs/SNRIs are used, monitor for serotonin-related side effects (e.g., agitation) and acute hemorrhagic stroke or other active bleeds. If citalopram is used, especially when concomitantly used with psychotropics known to extend QTc (e.g., quetiapine), monitor for QTc values; citalopram should be discontinued if persistent QTc >500 msec [42]. • If TCAs are used, monitor for postural hypotension, cardiac symptoms, anticholinergic side effects, and serum drug levels. • If benzodiazepines must be used to prevent acute withdrawal, consider a review and gradual discontinuation when feasible. • Mood stabilizers require monitoring over time for possible short-term and longer-term adverse events.	• Avoid initiating fluoxetine, paroxetine, fluvoxamine due to CYP450 drug-drug interactions. • Avoid initiating citalopram in patients with known personal or family history of QTc prolongation. • Avoid SSRIs/SNRIs in active cerebral or other bleeds, history of SIADH, current hyponatremia. • TCAs should not be used as a first-line treatment due to their side effect profiles (e.g., sedation, orthostatic hypotension, anticholinergic side effects, QTc prolongation, and ventricular arrhythmias [43]. • Avoid initiating TCAs in patients with history of conduction abnormalities on ECG or postural hypotension. • Avoid TCAs due to their high lethality risk in overdose. • Avoid adding on benzodiazepines due to side effects in the elderly.

Note: AD, Antidepressant; CYP450, cytochrome P450; ECG, electrocardiogram; ECT, electroconvulsive treatment; SIADH, syndrome of inappropriate antidiuretic hormone; SNRIs, serotonin norepinephrine reuptake inhibitors; SSRIs, selective serotonin reuptake inhibitors; TCAs, tricyclic antidepressants.

Fig. 10.5 On-call management considerations for antidepressant initiation in geriatric patients [41–43]

(b) Observe the Patient for Signs of Deterioration This is for cases where there are other underlying or masked medical problems (Fig. 10.5).

10.2.6 The Anxious Patient

Case Vignette Ms. F, a 78-year-old female, lived on her own, had a long-standing history of generalized anxiety disorder, and was seen frequently over the previous few weeks by her PCP for increased worries around her physical health following a fall at home. You were the on-call psychiatrist who saw her now in the ED for unexplained complaints of dizziness and shakiness. Her sleep and appetite have recently deteriorated, with some mild weight loss. She had asthma, hypothyroidism, and type 2 diabetes mellitus. Zopiclone 7.5 mg at bedtime for insomnia was added 1 week previously by her PCP with no response. Ms. F told you that she stopped her citalopram 20 mg daily 2 months previously, without her physician's knowledge, because she read that medication could contribute to the risk of falls. You corroborated the information with her PCP over the phone. You determine that the treatment for her physical illnesses was optimal. You evaluated the severity of her anxiety symptoms and whether there were any behavioral changes. She did not meet criteria for a diagnosis of major depressive disorder. Generalized Anxiety Disorder-7 (GAD-7) score was 15 (indicative of severe anxiety). You decided to resume her citalopram, provided psychoeducation about treatment, including relaxation techniques, and suggested frequent follow-up with her PCP, particularly within the first month of treatment or dose change, to encourage adherence and monitor response to treatment. You recommended concurrent cognitive behavioral therapy (CBT) if Ms. F would be interested. You suggested her treatment with zopiclone should be of short duration and be discontinued by her PCP when appropriate.

Severe anxiety can be disabling and can be associated with substance overdose/intoxication or withdrawal, suicidal behavior, and impaired judgment. Anxiety can also be a symptom of acute physical illness, which can result in significant morbidity or mortality if not treated appropriately.

10.2.6.1 Assessment

(a) A thorough assessment is warranted even if the patient is calm and relaxed by the time of the on-call clinician's arrival.

(b) Rule Out Underlying Medical Problems Carefully examine the patient who describes dizziness, fainting, or fear of dying because these symptoms can mimic physical illness (e.g., hypoglycemic episodes). If the patient is pacing, fidgety, and unable to stand still, consider akathisia, which is associated with antipsychotics and, to lesser degree, antidepressants. Akathisia can occur at any time during the treatment, although is more likely to occur at initiation or increase of the medication dose. Under-recognition of akathisia could lead to increasing the dosage of the antipsychotic or SSRI, exacerbating the problem.

Clinical Recommendation

Akathisia may be differentiated from anxiety as being a restlessness/agitation, especially in the lower extremities, that stems from the muscles instead of from the mind, and patients may feel worse if asked to stand still or sit. Pronounced rhythmic or regular movements are more characteristic of akathisia, whereas complex behaviors are more characteristic of psychomotor agitation.

The medical history and medication list and dosages are important to review. For example, misuse of bronchodilators, dopamine agonists, and thyroid replacement drugs, drug-drug interactions from concurrent use of medications, or recent addition or discontinuation in medications may be responsible for the onset of anxiety. Abrupt discontinuation of benzodiazepines or antidepressants can induce withdrawal that can manifest as anxiety, irritability, dizziness, lethargy, and headache, particularly those with shorter half-lives such as alprazolam and moclobemide.

(c) Order Vital Signs Do this frequently, if feasible, even if the staff already took vital signs, as this may have a calming effect on the patient.

(d) Obtain a Drug and Alcohol History This includes caffeine-containing and over-the-counter products (e.g., cold remedies). Herbal medications often contain stimulants and sympathomimetics (e.g., ephedrine) and can precipitate anxiety, especially in high doses. If substance abuse is suspected, order a urine toxicology screen and treat accordingly. Some patients who abuse substances can either exaggerate or fabricate symptoms in order to gain access to more drugs, or can self-medicate an underlying anxiety disorder. Therefore, discuss with the staff if the patient's behavior before seeing the patient has been consistent with anxiety.

(e) Conduct a Full Psychiatric and Physical Examination in a Patient with No Prior History of Anxiety The physical examination should be directed toward evaluating the patient's somatic complaints and any preexisting medical conditions that could contribute to anxiety to rule out a possible medical cause, if any. On mental status examination, cognition, insight, and judgment may appear impaired, but sensorium is generally clear. Psychotic symptoms can trigger secondary anxiety.

10.2.6.2 Management

(a) Taper or Discontinue a Medication or Substance That Could Have Induced Anxiety Withholding the offending drug may alleviate the symptoms. Anxiety due to substance abuse/withdrawal should be approached as clinically indicated. If akathisia is suspected, attributed to antipsychotic and/or antidepressant, consider lowering the dose of the antipsychotic (or change to an antipsychotic with lower D_2 blockade, e.g., quetiapine) and/or antidepressant (or change to a different class of antidepressant). If not improved, consider adding a benzodiazepine, low-dose propranolol, or the alpha-adrenergic drug clonidine, especially if the patient is in great distress [44]. These medications can have adverse effects, including confusion and gait instability; therefore, initial treatment should be for 5–10 days and followed by a gradual reduction in dose, although some may require continued treatment for the duration of antipsychotic or antidepressant treatment. Akathisia usually disappears when antipsychotic or antidepressant treatment is discontinued.

(b) Initiate Anxiolytic Medication, If Necessary

Clinical Recommendation
Reassuring the patient, identifying the cause for anxiety, and teaching basic CBT/relaxation techniques (e.g., deep diaphragmatic breathing) are adequate interventions before considering a medication. (See Chap. 4.)

Anxiety secondary to psychotic symptoms may benefit from additional scheduled or PRN small doses of antipsychotic medications. Benzodiazepines can be effective agents for the treatment of acute anxiety. Hepatic dysfunction and medications can inhibit the metabolism (i.e., oxidation) of certain benzodiazepines. However, lorazepam, oxazepam, and temazepam are least affected by these interactions and, thus, favorable choices in geriatric patients. Caution is required when prescribed because benzodiazepines act synergistically with other central nervous system depressants (alcohol, opioids, and barbiturates). Important adverse events to consider when administering benzodiazepines in geriatric patients are gait disturbance, increased risk of falls and fractures, respiratory depression, drowsiness, cognitive impairment, disorientation, delirium, depressive symptoms, and paradoxical disinhibition. If signs of paradoxical disinhibition occur, benzodiazepines should be discontinued. Second-line pharmacological therapies should be considered, including low-dose antipsychotics, especially if behavioral dysregulation is severe.

(c) Other Supportive Strategies Provide a secure, nonstimulating environment for the patient, with intermittent observation. Allow the anxious patients to express their concerns, as this may alleviate their anxiety.

10.2.7 The Addicted Patient

Case Vignette Mr. G, a 68-year-old retired police officer, was seen in the ED for upper abdominal pain due to alcohol-related erosive gastritis. He had a history of hypertension, type 2 diabetes mellitus, and osteoarthritis. He endorsed drinking a bottle of wine every evening on his own at home. He had no other psychiatric history. He was not sure he wanted to stop drinking but worried that it would further complicate his already compromised physical health. Never previously a problem, he admitted to a growing dependence on alcohol especially after a number of events that disrupted his life: his retirement and the death of his son (his only child) due to an inadvertent cocaine overdose 3 years previously and then the break-up of his long marriage a year later. He was financially secure, had a couple of male friends, and pursued an interest in model trains. He was not interested in attending Alcoholics Anonymous because he stated he did not share their ideology. Before being discharged home from the ED, Mr. G received brief alcohol counseling, and he had agreed to pursue an outpatient treatment program for alcohol harm reduction. He stated that he read about naltrexone and acamprosate and asked the emergency physician whether he should be taking one of them for his alcohol problem. You were the on-call psychiatrist and your opinion about this was sought.

Addictions in geriatric patients are most commonly due to benzodiazepines/hypnotics and alcohol, unlike younger patients who abuse a wide range of drugs. But this may soon change to include other drugs because of the growth of the geriatric population and cohort changes (e.g., the aging of middle-aged abusers of other substances). Due to the high prevalence of sleep disturbances in geriatric patients, benzodiazepines and other hypnotics are frequently prescribed, sometimes resulting in abuse. Chronic pain is by far the most common reason for nonmedical use of prescription pain medications later in life [45].

The on-call physician must differentiate between low-risk drinking, at-risk or problem drinking, and alcohol dependence when evaluating a geriatric patient. Contrary to low-risk drinking, any illicit substance use is considered to have greater risk than benefit.

Clinical Recommendation
According to the National Institute on Alcohol Abuse and Alcoholism, the recommended consumption of alcohol, or the low-risk drinking limit, in those aged 65 years or older is lower than for younger adults and is no more than one standard drink per day, or seven drinks per week, and no more than three or four drinks on any drinking day [46]. A standard drink is defined as a 5-ounce glass of wine, a 12-ounce bottle of wine cooler, a 12-ounce can of beer, a 1.5-ounce shot of hard liquor, or a cocktail with 1.5-ounce shot.

Factors contributing to the lower drinking limits for older adults compared with younger adults include:

- Decreased lean body mass and body water volume
- Diminished efficiency of hepatic metabolism
- Increased brain sensitivity to alcohol
- Increased medical comorbidity
- Increased alcohol-drug interactions due to polypharmacy

Older adults engaging in problem, or at-risk use, are drinking at a level that does not yet meet the criteria of dependence, and thus clinicians may underestimate the risks of this level of consumption. Geriatric patients often present to medical attention with subtle or confusing symptoms, which can suggest a pattern of substance misuse, especially alcohol abuse. Some red flags for substance abuse problems in geriatric patients are daily use of alcohol, physical stigmata of chronic alcohol use (e.g., mild tremor, enlarged and tender liver), nutritional deficiencies, labile vital signs (e.g., fluctuating blood pressure and tachycardia, suggestive of alcohol withdrawal), anemia or thrombocytopenia (i.e., suggestive of chronic alcohol use), liver chemistry abnormalities (e.g., elevated transaminases/gamma-glutamyl transpeptidase), new seizure activity, depression, anxiety, sleep disorders, or neurocognitive disorders, "aftershave/mouthwash syndrome" (to mask the odor of alcohol), history of frequent trauma, falls, fractures, or accidental injuries, and frequent use of ED services [46, 47].

10.2.7.1 Assessment

(a) Use of Screening Tools This may help detect geriatric substance use in on-call practice, which helps initiate provision of appropriate management [13–15, 48, 49] (see Table 10.3).

Table 10.3 Select brief screening tools for geriatric substance use [13–15, 48, 49]

Screening instrument	Description
CAGE questionnaire	A 4-item question tool: (1) Have you ever felt you should *c*ut down on your drinking? (2) Have people *a*nnoyed you by criticizing your drinking? (3) Have you ever felt bad or *g*uilty about your drinking? (4) Have you ever had a drink first thing in the morning (*e*ye opener) to steady your nerves or get rid of the hangover? The cutoff positive score is 2 affirmative answers [13], but some suggest only 1 affirmative answer when screening the older patients [14]
Michigan Alcoholism Screening Test – Geriatric Version (*MAST-G*)	A 24-item tool that includes elderly-specific consequences, with a cutoff of 5 affirmative responses. Its length may hinder routine use even in shortened form [14]. Both the CAGE and the MAST-G are sensitive to capturing alcohol use disorders in the elderly, but neither the CAGE nor the MAST-G distinguishes recent from remote drinking behavior
Alcohol Use Disorders Identification Test (*AUDIT*)	A 10-item tool that focuses on consumption; it has a cutoff score of 8, but is less sensitive than the CAGE [14]
Alcohol-Related Problems Survey (*ARPS*)	An 18-item, self-administered tool developed for use in geriatric patients with medical comorbidity or who used medications that placed them at risk for adverse events; it detects hazardous and harmful drinkers usually not identified by the three screens CAGE, MAST-G, and AUDIT [15]. Time to administer is 10 min. Although this tool is not designed for emergency care settings, efforts are needed to include geriatric-specific consequences and meaningful consumption thresholds in a brief, easily applied screen in such acute settings
Screener and Opioid Assessment for Patients with Pain (*SOAPP*)	A brief, self-administered tool used to assess suitability of long-term opioid therapy for chronic pain patients [48]
Current Opioid Misuse Measure (*COMM*)	A brief, self-report measure of current aberrant drug-related behavior [49]

(b) Obtain a Careful History This includes recent and past use of alcohol, tobacco, anxiolytic, hypnotic, and other psychoactive drugs (including prescribed to the patient, prescription medications from others borrowed or otherwise diverted, and over-the-counter medications). Questions about total amount of alcohol consumption are less useful than questions about frequency, pattern, and consequences of excessive drinking. It is also important to assess for any comorbid psychiatric disorders. Depressive or anxiety disorders are very common in patients who are alcohol dependent and often contribute to social isolation [35]. Symptoms of substance abuse are often missed in geriatric patients because of their multiple comorbid conditions that may present atypically or nonspecifically in later life.

(c) Laboratory Tests The most useful laboratory tests to confirm alcohol-abuse problems are gamma-glutamyl transpeptidase (GGT), mean corpuscular volume (MCV), and carbohydrate-deficient transferrin. The serum GGT measurement is one of the most widely used laboratory tests for heavy alcohol use. However, nonalcoholic liver disease, hyperthyroidism, and use of anticonvulsants can elevate

GGT levels [47]. MCV is less sensitive than the GGT measurement, but elevated MCV and GGT levels should raise suspicion about alcohol abuse [47]. Carbohydrate-deficient transferrin test is used to screen for excessive alcohol consumption. A urine toxicology screen is the best test to confirm problems with other drugs.

(d) Assess the Need for Medical Detoxification A history of severe withdrawal delirium and the presence of medical comorbidities such as coronary artery disease, seizure disorder, hypertension, and diabetes mellitus increase the morbidity of alcohol withdrawal and warrant inpatient detoxification. As they become medically ill, geriatric patients can decrease or cease their heavy alcohol consumption over days or weeks, which can precipitate withdrawal. Therefore, collateral information is necessary for a careful review of alcohol consumption just before hospitalization.

Hospitalized geriatric patients may be particularly vulnerable to alcohol or benzodiazepine withdrawal if clinicians are unaware of the use of these substances. Alcohol withdrawal can range from unnoticeable or mild to severe and life threatening symptoms, which may require on-call acute intervention. The severe symptoms associated with alcohol withdrawal include autonomic hyperactivity (e.g., sweating, tachycardia, hypertension), psychomotor agitation, insomnia, nausea, vomiting, anxiety, hand tremor, transient visual, tactile, or auditory hallucinations, delirium, seizures, and coma [21]. However, confusion, rather than tremor, may be the predominant early clinical sign of geriatric alcohol withdrawal [22]. Fluctuations in vital signs are less helpful in monitoring withdrawal in older patients, necessitating the use of standard withdrawal assessment scores, such as the Clinical Institute Withdrawal Assessment for Alcohol (CIWA-Ar) Scale [50]. Benzodiazepine withdrawal symptoms are similar to alcohol withdrawal symptoms and are also potentially life threatening. Opioid withdrawal has distinct symptoms including dysphoric mood, insomnia, diarrhea, nausea, vomiting, muscle aches, lacrimation, rhinorrhea, pupillary dilation, piloerection, sweating, yawning, and fever [21]. (Also see Table 16.2 for early vs. late nonpsychiatric symptoms of opioid withdrawal.)

10.2.7.2 Management

(a) Treatment for Alcohol Use Disorders *Treatment for alcohol withdrawal delirium.* Alcohol withdrawal delirium (or delirium tremens) typically occurs 2–10 days after alcohol cessation or decreased use and should be part of the differential diagnosis in any confused geriatric patient. (Also see Section 10.2.1 on the confused patient.) Benzodiazepines remain the mainstay of pharmacological management. Shorter acting benzodiazepines such as lorazepam are the agents of choice in geriatric patients, due to uncomplicated metabolism and shorter half-life, leading to ease of dose adjustment.

Clinical Recommendation

Note that the symptom checklist of a withdrawal screening tool such as the CIWA-Ar contains features common to delirium related to general medical conditions, and therefore these symptoms may be solely attributed to alcohol withdrawal, triggering the excessive use of benzodiazepines [51].

Antipsychotics may be considered when other medical causes of delirium complicate alcohol withdrawal; however, they may lower the seizure threshold and must be used with careful monitoring. Antipsychotics can also be added to benzodiazepines if agitation, perceptual disturbances, or disturbed thinking cannot be adequately controlled with benzodiazepines alone. Geriatric patients should be frequently reevaluated for the control of symptoms and the development of excessive sedation with benzodiazepines. Benzodiazepines should be tapered following alcohol withdrawal rather than abruptly discontinued. Administration of thiamine is recommended to prevent or treat Wernicke encephalopathy or Wernicke-Korsakoff syndrome.

Treatment for Alcohol Dependence Naltrexone and acamprosate have both been US FDA and Health Canada approved for the treatment of alcohol dependence. Naltrexone 50 mg daily appears safe in older patients and is helpful in reducing cravings, avoiding relapse to heavy drinking, and achieving/maintaining abstinence [46]. Acamprosate has proven effective in the maintenance phase of abstinence [46]. Acamprosate has not been studied in geriatric patients, but caution is needed when creatinine clearance is less than 50 mL/min. In Mr. G's case, he was not yet motivated to reach abstinence, and, therefore, naltrexone was the best choice to help reduce his drinking, with the eventual goal of abstinence. The on-call clinician should apply brief alcohol counseling techniques (see Chap. 4), connect patients and families with community resources, such as Alcoholics Anonymous and Al-Anon, particularly groups oriented toward the older adults, or refer to formal treatment programs.

(b) Treatment for Non-alcohol Use Disorders While illicit substance use is less common in this population, persons aged 65 years or older consume more prescribed and over-the-counter medications than any other age group [46].

It is particularly risky for the geriatric patients to abuse *benzodiazepines*, as there is a positive correlation between the use of benzodiazepines and confusion, falls, and hip fractures [52]. Benzodiazepine withdrawal symptoms in geriatric patients are more likely to include confusion and disorientation and are less likely to include anxiety, insomnia, and perceptual changes [53]. Treatment of benzodiazepine dependence consists of a slow tapering of the medication. If the dependence is to a short-acting agent (e.g., alprazolam, triazolam, temazepam), conversion to an equivalent dose of a longer acting agent (e.g., lorazepam, clonazepam) may be done first, followed by slow tapering of this second medication.

The abuse of *opioids* is less common among geriatric patients, except if they have a history of abuse at a younger age or in the presence of comorbid alcohol abuse. Opioid detoxification of the geriatric patient often requires a medical setting because of the increased likelihood of comorbid medical illnesses. When on-call physicians assess patients seeking opioid pain medication, particularly in the ED settings, they should adhere to strict rules in order to minimize the risk of abuse and dependence. These include the following [54]:

- Document the encounter and have a progress note for every prescription written or telephoned to a pharmacy.

- Explain why a controlled drug is necessary, what alternatives have been considered, and document follow-up plans.
- Obtain an informed consent from the patient so there is no doubt about the treatment plan.
- Do not provide automatic refills.
- Assess all patients for past or present substance abuse and psychiatric illness.
- Lost, stolen, or misplaced medication should not be replaced; consideration of replacement should occur at a clinic visit with their PCP.
- Avoid "as-needed" or PRN medications.
- Do not prescribe long-acting or controlled release opioids (e.g., oxycontin, fentanyl patches, methadone) for acute pain.
- Opioids are generally contraindicated in patients currently addicted.
- Refer patients who are addicted to opioids to 12-step programs (e.g., Narcotics Anonymous, Pills Anonymous).

(c) Assess Whether There Are Concerns About Substance Use and Driving Physicians need to be familiar with the signs and symptoms that would raise concerns about drinking and driving. Screening, assessment, and appropriate referrals need to be considered, in addition to reporting patients to the government agency which licenses drivers, in accordance with applicable local legislation.

(d) Encourage Follow-Up with Members of the Patient's Caregiver Team Document care needs of geriatric patients with chronic pain who misuse opioids. Communicate your findings to the caregiver team, including the PCP.

10.2.8 The Insomnia Patient

Case Vignette Mr. H, a 71-year-old retired businessman, was recently admitted to a medical ward for uncontrolled hypertension, now under fairly good control with a diuretic. He had no history of substance misuse, was financially secure, exercised regularly, had an active social life, but had an unfulfilling relationship with his wife. He did not see divorce as an option. You were the on-call physician and asked to manage his chief complaint of insomnia. Selective review of the chart and examination of Mr. H revealed a long-standing, initial, and middle insomnia. He told you that insomnia was worse if he did not take lorazepam 0.5 mg at bedtime (prescribed for years by his PCP); trazodone 25 mg and mirtazapine 7.5 mg did not help. You noticed that lorazepam was not on his current medication list. You suspected underlying depression as a cause for his insomnia and joylessness, but there were no other symptoms or signs of major depression. Mr. H was not in any acute distress. You noticed the diuretic as a new factor for worsening his insomnia by increasing the rate of nocturnal voiding. Polysomnography study was not available. You elected to renew the medication order for lorazepam and asked the attending physician to review management of his insomnia the following day.

Sleep disturbance is a common complaint in geriatric hospitalized patients and is often secondary to existing medical and psychosocial morbidity. The principal psychiatric or physical illness, as well as medications (e.g., antidepressants, antihypertensives), can cause sleep disruption.

10.2.8.1 Assessment

The on-call physician should avoid prescribing sedating medications to geriatric patients with insomnia when requested by a staff member over the phone, without first assessing the situation.

(a) Before Seeing the Patient, Clarify with the Staff Clarify over the phone the following:

- Who requests help, the patient or the staff
- What the admission diagnosis is
- When the patient was admitted to the hospital
- Whether the patient had complaints of insomnia previous to this consult, and if so, what types of treatment were suggested, and whether they were beneficial
- If there has been any recent change in the patient's clinical status or medications
- If the patient has been anxious, agitated, or acting bizarrely, which may require a prompt evaluation (also refer to Section 10.2.2 on the violent patient)

(b) Conduct a Chart Review and History to Determine the Etiology of Insomnia Take a detailed history of insomnia, including the onset, duration, and nature of the patient's sleep complaint, severity, and impact on daytime function. Review factors that can be associated with insomnia, such as:

- Environmental (e.g., noisy or new environment for recently admitted patients, jet lag, situational anxiety, disturbed circadian rhythms because of daytime naps, nighttime disrupted sleep)
- Neuropsychiatric disorders (e.g., depressive, bipolar, anxiety, or psychotic disorders with intrusive hallucinations or paranoia, NCDs, Parkinson's disease)
- Systemic illness (e.g., pain, heart disease, thyroid disease)
- Medications (e.g., diuretics, antihypertensives, dopamine agonists, corticosteroids, cholinesterase inhibitors, antidepressants, psychostimulants); it is imperative to elicit recent changes in prescribed or over-the-counter medications and to recognize and avoid potentially inappropriate medications
- Substance use (e.g., caffeine, nicotine, cocaine)
- Substance withdrawal (e.g., alcohol, benzodiazepines, opioids)
- Other sleep-wake disorders associated with insomnia in geriatric patients (e.g., obstructive sleep apnea, advanced sleep phase syndrome, REM sleep behavior disorder, restless legs syndrome). (Also see Chap. 17 for section of disturbances of sleep and parasomnias.)

Be cognizant of the age-related physiological changes of sleep, which include:

- Longer duration to initiate sleep
- Decreased threshold of arousal, increased number of awakenings, and sleep experienced as interrupted and less restorative
- Decreased total sleep time
- Advanced sleep phase, experienced as difficulty in staying awake in the evening and waking earlier than the younger adults
- Earlier awakening (without a phase advance)
- Dream content may be distressing

Clinical Recommendation
The clinician's task is to distinguish symptoms of benign sleep difficulties from underlying conditions that require further evaluation and for which a sedative/hypnotic medication may be contraindicated (e.g., delirium other than alcohol related, sleep apnea, hepatic or respiratory failure, myasthenia gravis, or concurrent use of opioids due to potentiation effect).

10.2.8.2 Management

(a) Treat the Underlying Medical Problems When possible, select a medication for insomnia that also treats the underlying condition. As in Mr. H's case, the on-call physician can consider renewing the medication order for insomnia if the patient is not in acute distress and has a history of difficulty initiating or maintaining sleep that responded well to that medication in the past. If there is no daytime compromise in function, monitor the insomnia and defer treatment with hypnotics/benzodiazepines. If insomnia is debilitating, determine the need for a hypnotic/sedative medication in accordance with the metabolic profile for drugs and the patient's hepatic and renal function.

Clinical Recommendation
Once a hypnotic/sedative medication is selected during the on-call shift, start with a low dosage, limit the treatment period, and document the need for the attending physician to continue monitoring for improvement, watch for drug-related adverse effects (e.g., residual drowsiness, confusion), and address the risk of falls.

Figure 10.6 summarizes the on-call pharmacotherapy options for insomnia in this population [55–57].

(b) Recommend Non-pharmacological Approaches Always recommend non-pharmacological approaches to geriatric patients with chronic insomnia, tailored to the respective institutional setting (see Table 10.4) [58].

Recommend	Avoid
• *GABA-benzodiazepine receptor agonists used as hypnotics,* initial doses: eszopiclone 1 mg, zopiclone 3.75-5 mg, zaleplon 5 mg, zolpidem 5 mg. • Short-to-intermediate acting *benzodiazepines*, initial doses: triazolam 0.125 mg for sleep initiation, temazepam 7.5 mg for sleep maintenance. • Other options, initial doses: *melatonin-receptor agonist* (ramelteon 8 mg in adults, not studied in elderly), or *orexin-receptor antagonist* (suvorexant 10 mg in adults, not studied in elderly). • *Sedating TCAs*: these can moderately reduce sleep latency and increase total sleep time. *Nortriptyline* is preferred to amitriptyline due to fewer anticholinergic effects. *Doxepin,* initial dose: 3 mg, 30 minutes before bedtime, increase to 6 mg if indicated (effective for frequent or early morning awakenings and inability to return to sleep). • *Mirtazapine*, initial dose: 7.5-15 mg (especially if insomnia is due to depression). • *Trazodone*, initial dose: 25-50 mg (in patients with chronic "sundowning" - nighttime agitatation due to major neurocognitive disorder). • *Monitoring tips:* (a) Closely monitor patients with a history of substance abuse given benzodiazepines. (b) Use the lowest effective dose for the shortest duration possible. (c) Hypnotics should only be continued beyond 4 weeks when documented benefits clearly outweigh actual or potential harms and when other techniques (e.g., behavioral interventions) have not been effective. (d) For those on benzodiazepines for >1 year, it is prudent to taper dose by approx. 10 % every 2–4 weeks until discontinued. Peak-trough variability can be sufficient to cause withdrawal symptoms when tapering short acting benzodiazepines, and thus consider switching to an alternative with a longer half-life to prevent withdrawal.	• Avoid use of most *antipsychotics* and *antihistaminics* due to daytime sedation and other side effects. However, *quetiapine* 12.5-25 mg may be trialed if other options failed. • Avoid *amitriptyline* due to anticholinergic effects and possible confusion. • *Doxepin* ≥25 mg is nonselective and responsible for undesired anticholinergic, antiadrenergic, and cardiac conduction side effects. Doxepin is contraindicated in patients with severe urinary retention and narrow angle glaucoma. • Avoid *benzodiazepines* with *long half-lives* because of cumulative effect when given repeatedly, causing sedation with possible delayed in expression by days or weeks. • Avoid *beta-blockers*, especially lipophilic compounds (e.g., metoprolol, propranolol), which can cause difficulty falling asleep, increased awakenings, and vivid dreams. • Avoid *caffeine* before bedtime; the effect of caffeine can last up to 14 hours and may be more pronounced in elderly because of decreased caffeine clearance with decreased liver function. Note that caffeine is present in many over-the-counter analgesics, cold, and allergy remedies. • Avoid *nicotine,* a stimulant that affects sleep similar to caffeine (e.g., difficulty falling asleep, decreased sleep duration). • *Melatonin* has little to no effect, with the possible exception in patients with circadian rhythm disorders; use of controlled release melatonin may help facilitate discontinuation of benzodiazepines. • Some *herbals* may be effective, but evidence is poor and side effects may be of concern.

Fig. 10.6 On-call management considerations for bedtime treatment of insomnia in geriatric patients [55–57]. *AD* antidepressant, *CYP450* cytochrome P450, *ECG* electrocardiogram, *ECT* electroconvulsive treatment, *SIADH* syndrome of inappropriate antidiuretic hormone, *SNRIs* serotonin norepinephrine reuptake inhibitors, *SSRIs* selective serotonin reuptake inhibitors, *TCAs* tricyclic antidepressants

Table 10.4 Non-pharmacological approaches to insomnia [58]

Brief behavioral treatment approaches	A. Do not go to bed unless you are sleepy
	B. Do not stay in bed unless you are asleep
	C. Reduce your time in bed; if unable to fall asleep in 20 min (subjective sense, not clocked) get up and engage in a quiet activity (e.g., reading) until sleepy before attempting to sleep again; if unable to fall asleep in 20 min, repeat the process
	D. Get up at the same time every day of the week, no matter how much you slept the night before

(continued)

Table 10.4 (continued)

Elements of sleep hygiene	(a) Use a quiet, comfortable room environment
	(b) No visible time cues in room; always use an alarm clock
	(c) Reinforce waking hours with exposure to light early in the day and physical activity
	(d) Avoid stimulating activities 2 h before bedtime (including screen based activity)
	(e) Decrease daytime napping
	(f) Avoid caffeine, alcohol, and nicotine, particularly before bedtime
	(g) Promote relaxation, e.g., prepare for sleep with 30 min of breathing exercises, meditation, soft music
	(h) Avoid catastrophic thoughts, e.g., "I'll die if I have another night like the last one," or "If *X* happens, I won't sleep"
	(i) Insert positive thoughts
	(j) Address life stressors

Key Points

- Depressive disorders, anxiety disorders, and NCDs are common in the geriatric patients, and their symptoms are likely to comprise the majority of the on-call or crisis chief psychiatric complaints.
- Enhancing clinician's knowledge and skill in identifying geriatric psychiatric syndromes in those with medical comorbidities that can confuse the psychiatric diagnosis is crucial in the provision of the acute care.
- Common screening tools used specifically in the geriatric patients to identify various psychiatric syndromes are essential to know for the on-call practice.
- Always employ safe principles when implementing on-call pharmacological intervention.
- Physicians need to rigorously follow their local policy on several important matters, such as the use of mechanical restraint, duty to inform in case of patient's dangerousness, and duty to report patients whom they believe to be unfit to drive due to medical illness.

References

1. Tsoi KF, Chan JC, Hirai HW, Wong SS, Kwok TY. Cognitive tests to detect dementia: a systematic review and meta-analysis. JAMA Intern Med. 2015;175:1450–8. doi:10.1001/jamainternmed.2015.2152.
2. Carpenter CR, Bassett ER, Fischer GM, Shirshekan J, Galvin JE, Morris JC. Four sensitive screening tools to detect cognitive dysfunction in geriatric ED patients: brief Alzheimer's screen, short blessed test, Ottawa 3DY, and the caregiver-completed AD8. Acad Emerg Med. 2011;18(4):374–84.
3. Dubois B, Slachervsky A, Litvan I, Pillon B. The FAB: a frontal assessment battery at bedside. Neurology. 2000;55:1621.

4. Burnett J, Dyer CB, Naik AD. Convergent validation of the kohlman evaluation of living skills as a screening tool of older adults' ability to live safely and independently in the community. Arch Phys Med Rehabil. 2009;90(11):1948–52.
5. Holsinger T, Deveau J, Boustani M, et al. Does this patient have dementia? JAMA. 2007;297:2391–404.
6. CMA Driver's Guide. Determining medical fitness to operate motor vehicles. 8th ed. https://www.cma.ca/En/Pages/drivers-guide.aspx. Accessed 27 Aug 2015.
7. Sessums LL, Zembrzuska H, Jackson JL. Does this patient have medical decision-making capacity? JAMA. 2011;306(4):420–7.
8. Kroenke K, Spitzer RL, Williams JB. The PHQ-9: validity of a brief depression severity measure. J Gen Intern Med. 2001;16:606–13.
9. Kroenke K, Spitzer RL, Williams JB. The patient health questionnaire-2: validity of a two-item depression screen. Med Care. 2003;41:1284–92.
10. Hoyl MT, Alessi CA, Harker JO, et al. Development and testing of a five-item version of the geriatric depression scale. J Am Geriatr Soc. 1999;47:873–8.
11. Burke WJ, Roccaforte WH, Wengel SP. The short form of the geriatric depression scale: a comparison with the 30-item form. J Geriatr Psychiatry Neurol. 1991;4:173–8.
12. Adshead F, Cody DD, Pitt B. BASDEC: a novel screening instrument for depression in elderly medical inpatients. BMJ. 1992;305(6850):397.
13. Mayfield D, McLeod G, Hall P. The CAGE questionnaire: validation of a new alcoholism screening instrument. Am J Psychiatry. 1974;131(10):1121–3.
14. Conigliaro J, Kraemer K, McNeil M. Screening and identification of older adults with alcohol problems in primary care. J Geriatr Psychiatry Neurol. 2000;13(3):106–14.
15. Fink A, Morton SC, Beck JC, et al. The alcohol-related problems survey identifying hazardous and harmful drinking in older primary care patients. J Am Geriatr Soc. 2002;50(10):1717–22.
16. Weiner MF, Tractenberg RE, Jin S, Gamst A, Thomas RG, Koss E, Thal LJ. Assessing Alzheimer's disease patients with the Cohen-Mansfield Agitation Inventory: scoring and clinical implications. J Psychiatr Res. 2002;36(1):19–25.
17. Cummings JL, Mega M, Gray K, Rosenberg-Thompson S, Carusi DA, Gornbein J. The Neuropsychiatric Inventory: comprehensive assessment of psychopathology in dementia. Neurology. 1994;44(12):2308–14.
18. Inouye SK, van Dyck CH, Alessi CA, et al. Clarifying confusion: the confusion assessment method. A new method for detection of delirium. Ann Intern Med. 1990;11:941–8.
19. Inouye SK. Delirium in older persons. N Engl J Med. 2006;354(11):1157–65.
20. Bourgeois JA, Hategan A, Losier B. Delirium in the hospital setting: emphasis on geriatric patients. Curr Psychiatry. 2014;13(8):29. 36–42, A.
21. American Psychiatric Association. Diagnostic and statistical manual of mental disorders. 5th ed. Arlington: American Psychiatric Publishing; 2013.
22. Chan PKY. Clarifying the confusion about confusion: current practices in managing geriatric delirium. BCMJ. 2011;53(8):409–15.
23. CCSMH National Guidelines for Seniors' mental health: the assessment and treatment of delirium. http://www.ccsmh.ca/pdf/guidelines/NatlGuideline_Delirium.pdf. Accessed 14 Sep 2015.
24. Gage L, Hogan DB. CCSMH guideline update: the assessment and treatment of delirium. Toronto: Canadian Coalition for Seniors' Mental Health (CCSMH); 2014. www.ccsmh.ca.
25. Meyer-Massetti C, Cheng CM, Sharpe BA, Meier CR, Guglielmo BJ. The FDA extended warning for intravenous haloperidol and torsades de pointes: how should institutions respond? J Hosp Med. 2010;5(4):E8–16.
26. Alexopoulos GS, Streim J, Carpenter D, et al. Using antipsychotic agents in older patients. J Clin Psychiatry. 2004;65:5–99.
27. Canadian Coalition for Seniors Mental Health. National guidelines for seniors' mental health: the assessment and treatment of mental health issues in long-term care homes. http://www.ccsmh.ca/pdf/guidelines/NatlGuideline_LTC.pdf. Accessed 3 Oct 2015.

28. Chaimowitz GA, Glancy G. The duty to protect. Ottawa: Canadian Psychiatric Association; 2002. Position Paper 2002–42. Available at https://ww1.cpa-apc.org/Publications/Position_Papers/duty.asp.
29. Targum SD. Treating psychotic symptoms in elderly patients. Prim Care Companion J Clin Psychiatry. 2001;3(4):156–63.
30. Lacro JP, Jeste DV. Geriatric psychosis. Psychiatry Q. 1997;68(3):247–60.
31. Gugger JJ, Wagner ML. Rapid eye movement sleep behaviour disorder. Ann Pharmacother. 2007;41(11):1833–41.
32. Evers S, Ellger T. The clinical spectrum of musical hallucinations. J Neurol Sci. 2004;227(1):55–65.
33. Palmer BW, McClure FS, Jeste DV. Schizophrenia in late life: findings challenge traditional concepts. Harv Rev Psychiatry. 2001;9(2):51–8.
34. Chang B, Gitlin D, Patel R. The depressed patient and suicidal patient in the ED: evidence-based management and treatment strategies. Emerg Med Pract. 2011;13(9):1–23.
35. Canadian Coalition for Seniors Mental Health. National guidelines for seniors mental health: the assessment of suicide risk and prevention of suicide. 2006. http://www.ccsmh.ca/en/natlguidelines/suicide.cfm. Accessed 2 Oct 2015.
36. Mahgoub N, Klimstra S, Kotbi N, Docherty JP. Self-injurious behavior in the nursing home setting. Int J Geriatr Psychiatry. 2011;26(1):27–30.
37. Draper B, Brodaty H, Low LF, Richards V, Paton H, Lie D. Self-destructive behaviors in nursing home residents. J Am Geriatr Soc. 2002;50(2):354–8.
38. Hirschfeld RMA, Russell JM. Assessment and treatment of suicidal patients. N Engl J Med. 1997;337:910–5.
39. Heisel MJ, Duberstein PR, Talbot NL, King DA, Tu M. Adapting interpersonal psychotherapy for older adults at risk for suicide: preliminary findings. Prof Psychol Res Pr. 2009;40(2):156–64.
40. Unützer J, Tang L, Oishi S, Katon W, Williams J, Hunkeler E. The IMPACT investigators. Reducing suicidal ideation in depressed older primary care patients. J Am Geriatr Soc. 2006;54:1550–6.
41. Buchanan D, Tourigny-Rivard MF, Cappeliez P, et al. National guidelines for seniors' mental health: the assessment and treatment of depression. Can J Geriatr. 2006;9 Suppl 2:S52–8.
42. FDA. Drug Safety Communication: revised recommendations for Celexa (citalopram hydrobromide) related to a potential risk of abnormal heart rhythms with high doses. 28 Mar 2012. http://www.fda.gov/Drugs/DrugSafety/ucm297391.htm. Accessed 27 Aug 2015.
43. Menza MA, Liberatore BL. Psychiatry in the geriatric neurology practice. Neurol Clin. 1998;16(3):611–33.
44. Saltz BL, Robinson DG, Woerner MG. Recognizing and managing antipsychotic drug treatment side effects in the elderly. Prim Care Companion J Clin Psychiatry. 2004;6 suppl 2:14–9.
45. Blazer DG, Wu LT. Non-prescription use of pain relievers among middle aged and elderly community adults: national survey on drug use and health. J Am Geriatr Soc. 2009;57:1252–7.
46. Oslin DW. Evidence-based treatment of geriatric substance abuse. Psychiatr Clin North Am. 2005;28(4):897–911.
47. Mersy DJ. Recognition of alcohol and substance abuse. Am Fam Physician. 2003;67(7):1529–3152.
48. Akbik H, Butler SF, Budman SH, Fernandez K, Katz NP, Jamison RN. Validation and clinical application of the Screener and Opioid Assessment for Patients with Pain (SOAPP). J Pain Symptom Manage. 2006;32(3):287–93.
49. Butler SF, Budman SH, Fernandez KC, Houle B, Benoit C, Katz N, Jamison RN. Development and validation of the current opioid misuse measure. Pain. 2007;130(1–2):144–56.
50. Sullivan JT, Sykora K, Schneiderman J, et al. Assessment of alcohol withdrawal: the revised clinical institute withdrawal assessment for alcohol scale (CIWA-A). Br J Addict. 1989;84:1353–7.

51. Hecksel KA, Bostwick JM, Jaeger KM, et al. Inappropriate use of symptom-triggered therapy for alcohol withdrawal in the general hospital. Mayo Clin Proc. 2008;83:274–9.
52. Leipzig RM, Cumming RG, Tinetti ME. Drugs and falls in older people: a systematic review and meta-analysis: I. Psychotropic drugs. J Am Geriatr Soc. 1999;47(1):30–9.
53. Kruse WH. Problems and pitfalls in the use of benzodiazepines in the elderly. Drug Saf. 1990;5(5):328–44.
54. Lessenger JE, Feinberg SD. Abuse of prescription and over-the-counter medications. J Am Board Fam Med. 2008;21(1):45–54.
55. Hong IS, Bishop JR. Sedative-hypnotics for sleepless geriatric patients: choose wisely. Curr Psychiatry. 2014;13(10):36. -39, 46–50, 52.
56. Health Canada: Zopiclone. Drug product search. Modified 2014. Available at: http://webprod5.hc-sc.gc.ca/dpd-bdpp/info.do?code=43233&lang=eng. Accessed 3 Oct 2015.
57. Markov D, Doghramji K. Doxepin for insomnia. Curr Psychiatry. 2010;9(10):67. -68, 74, 76–77.
58. Becker PM. Put your patient to sleep: useful nondrug strategies for chronic insomnia. Curr Psychiatry. 2008;7(10):13–4. 17–20.

The Chief Physical Complaints

11

Calvin H. Hirsch and Tricia Woo

11.1 Background

The single greatest challenge for the on-call psychiatrist, who may be unfamiliar with an individual patient, is to correctly identify the severity of a symptom and the level of acuity in order to determine whether the patient can remain safely on the unit, should be transported to the emergency department (ED), or (if the psychiatric unit is located within a hospital) requires an urgent medical or surgical consultation. Key factors influencing this decision include the psychiatrist's own level of comfort with medical diagnosis and management, the availability and turnaround time of diagnostic modalities (laboratory tests, imaging studies), the availability of medical consultation, the ability of the unit's nurses to monitor the patient and carry out prescribed treatment, and patient/family preferences.

11.2 Management of Comorbid Conditions

The majority of geriatric patients admitted to psychiatric units and general hospitals have multiple medical comorbidities and are prescribed multiple medications. In an epidemiological sample, 80 % of US veterans with unplanned hospitalizations (mean age 76 years) were taking ≥ 5 medications at the time of admission [1]. Patients are usually continued on their prescribed outpatient medical regimen for "stable" chronic conditions not directly affected by the admitting diagnosis. However, these comorbidities often require active management.

C.H. Hirsch, MD (✉)
Department of Internal Medicine, Division of General Medicine, University of California Davis Medical Center, Sacramento, CA, USA
e-mail: chhirsch@ucdavis.edu

T. Woo, MD
Division of Geriatric Internal Medicine, McMaster University, Hamilton, ON, Canada

A. Hategan et al. (eds.), *On-Call Geriatric Psychiatry: Handbook of Principles and Practice*, DOI 10.1007/978-3-319-30346-8_11

- Comorbid conditions may not have been optimally managed as a result of disease progression, failure to follow up with the primary care physician, medication nonadherence, or poor self-care (e.g., dietary indiscretion in diabetes mellitus).
- Because diet and medication oversight are carefully controlled in the inpatient setting, medication doses adapted to the patient's outpatient lifestyle potentially may result in overtreatment. This is especially true of hypertension and diabetes mellitus, which often require adjustment of outpatient doses.

Clinical Recommendation
All newly admitted geriatric patients should have their blood pressure monitored at least daily (or more frequently, depending on institutional policy). Patients on antihypertensives should receive blood pressure checks every shift until stabilized, and then the monitoring frequency should be reassessed as appropriate.

Clinical Recommendation
Nearly 40 % of community-dwelling geriatric patients age 65 and older have orthostatic hypotension, which is often asymptomatic [2]. The autonomic dysfunction caused by prolonged bed rest and many medications has the potential to cause or exacerbate orthostasis. Orthostatic hypotension is an important risk factor for syncope and falls. Whenever possible, psychiatric patients should have an orthostatic blood pressure check at admission (holding the standing position for 3 min), which should be repeated every 3–4 days if the patient spends most of the time in bed. Significant orthostasis, especially if symptomatic, should prompt further work-up and treatment, starting with reduction in the doses of antihypertensive medication. Psychotropic medications with their own risk of orthostatic hypotension (e.g., tricyclic antidepressants, quetiapine, clozapine) require monitoring for orthostasis, especially as doses are escalated.

Clinical Pearl
The outpatient prescription of ≥ 3 antihypertensives should alert the clinician to possible medication nonadherence.

- Management of diabetes mellitus requires special vigilance. If a patient has a superimposed acute medical or surgical condition, metformin should not be prescribed because of the risk of lactic acidosis. Otherwise, outpatient hypoglycemic agents can be continued if the patient is eating normally. If intake is variable, the doses should empirically be reduced or the patient switched to a sliding-scale insulin regimen until it is safe to resume the previous hypoglycemic regimen.

Clinical Recommendation
Point-of-care (POC, "finger stick") blood glucose monitoring should be obtained fasting in the AM and just before lunch and dinner in all diabetics for at least the first 24 h; POC testing should be continued indefinitely if the patient is taking insulin.

Clinical Pearl
The psychiatrist should be aware that the addition or dose increase of a second-generation (atypical) antipsychotic may worsen glycemic control (see Chap. 12).

- Medications prescribed in the outpatient sector may not necessarily be the most appropriate, effective, or safest for the patient. In addition to a medication reconciliation *(what the patient is taking versus what the patient has been prescribed)*, a thorough medication review for appropriateness should be conducted (see Chap. 12). If perusal of the outpatient medical record does not elucidate the rationale for a medication that may be inappropriate, the primary care physician should be contacted.

11.3 Special Challenges with Geriatric Patients

Case Vignette 1 Mr. H was an 88-year-old man admitted to a psychiatric unit for passive wishes of death, poor sleep, tearfulness, and refusal to eat, drink, and get out of bed for 5 days shortly following the unexpected death of his wife during sleep. Nine days earlier, in late September, the couple had returned from the Middle East following a religious pilgrimage. On the return flight home, many passengers were coughing. His wife developed a fever and cough during a 12-h stopover and was given an antibiotic at the airport urgent care center, with resolution of symptoms within 2 days. At admission, he was tearful, uninterested in any activities, and demanded to be allowed to die so he could join his wife. Mr. H also had an intermittent dry cough and complained of being weak and uninterested in eating or drinking. He previously had been in fair health with well-compensated diastolic dysfunction, a history of atrial fibrillation treated by ablation and a pacemaker, and stage III chronic kidney disease. His physical exam was unremarkable except for a low-grade fever of 38.0 °C. His WBC count was 9.7 K/mm^3 and his chest X-ray showed no evidence of an infiltrate or heart failure. His chemistry panel was notable for a serum creatinine of 1.7 mg/dL (150.5 μmol/L), increased from a baseline of 1.5 mg/dL (132.6 μmol/L). Sertraline 25 mg q AM and methylphenidate 5 mg BID were started, and the patient was encouraged to eat and drink. Over the next 2 days, his dry cough worsened, with increased weakness and fever to 39.2 °C. On hospital day 3, the on-call psychiatric consultant prescribed azithromycin 500 mg PO X 1, followed by 250 mg PO daily for 4 days for a possible community-acquired pneumonia despite a normal repeat chest X-ray. On hospital day 8, the patient no longer could sit up without assistance, wheezes were now audible on lung exam, and he was transferred to the inpatient medical ward. His chest X-ray showed heart failure. An infectious disease consultation obtained a nasal swab that was positive for influenza A. Cardiac enzymes revealed a troponin I of 0.42 ng/mL (0.42 μg/L; normal<0.04 ng/mL/0.04 μg/L), consistent with demand ischemia attributable to influenza and decompensated heart failure, and the methylphenidate was stopped. He was placed on oseltamivir for the influenza A, given bumetanide 0.5 mg BID for the heart failure exacerbation, and started on a metoprolol succinate 25 mg daily and aspirin 81 mg daily. The Psychiatry Liaison Service provided ongoing psychiatric consultation during the remainder of the patient's hospital stay and effectively increased the sertraline to 100 mg q AM at the time of discharge to a skilled nursing facility on hospital day 17.

Case Analysis It is important to distinguish between symptoms resulting from systemic medical illness and neurovegetative symptoms of depression (loss of appetite, loss of energy). If the diagnosis is still in question, it is prudent to institute an antidepressant trial to see whether symptoms improve, while monitoring for potential medical illness. Mr. H's only symptoms of the "flu" were a low-grade fever and a dry cough. He did not have rhinorrhea, nasal stuffiness, or a sore throat. Oseltamivir would have been more effective in blunting the course of his influenza and possibly could have averted secondary heart failure had it been administered early in the course, but because of the atypical presentation, influenza was not suspected until he worsened despite antibiotics.

11.3.1 Atypical Presentation

Aging is associated with a greater likelihood of an *atypical* presentation of illness [3, 4], although the majority of patients still present with *typical* signs and symptoms. An atypical presentation may take several forms.

11.3.1.1 Failure to Manifest Many of the Usual and Expected Features of a Disease Process

Examples are lack of rhinorrhea, nasal stuffiness, and sore throat in a patient with acute influenza and absence of cough or leukocytosis in a patient with bacterial pneumonia. Using ambulatory electrocardiographic monitoring, asymptomatic ("silent") coronary ischemia can be detected in>30 % of geriatric patients with known coronary heart disease (CHD). The incidence of silent coronary ischemia is higher in geriatric diabetics with CHD [5].

11.3.1.2 Nonspecific Symptoms

These are symptoms that do not readily suggest a specific cause. Rather than presenting with crushing substernal chest pressure, an older patient with a myocardial infarction may complain of acute fatigue or nausea and vomiting. Instead of right lower quadrant pain suggestive of appendicitis, the patient initially may complain of generalized abdominal discomfort, nausea and vomiting, or just loss of appetite, as in the clinical vignette. A woman with a urinary tract infection may simply feel tired, rather than complaining of dysuria and frequency.

11.3.1.3 Symptoms Apparently Unrelated to the Involved Organ System

Acute illness in a frail, older patient can manifest as a disturbance in an organ system that is remote from the involved organ. For example, disturbances in the central nervous system (CNS) can be the only manifestation of an infection or other acute pathology, regardless of location, leading to delirium, gait disturbances, or loss of balance. A patient with pneumonia may present with mild confusion and new urinary incontinence. Physical signs and symptoms developing from pathology in a seemingly unrelated organ system are thought to arise from the inability of the patient, as an integrated organism, to respond to physiologic challenges to homeostasis due to reduced physiologic reserve and resilience. This state of impaired homeostatic function underlies the construct of frailty [6, 7]. A variation of this phenomenon is acute dysfunction in a diseased but compensated organ under severe physiologic stress. For example, a patient who has recovered from a stroke may again manifest symptoms of the previous stroke when septic. A patient with well-compensated heart failure may develop an exacerbation of heart failure because of a respiratory infection *(see case study above).*

11.3.1.4 Presentation of Symptoms Due to Failure to Mount an Appropriate Physiologic Response

Impaired function in one or more organ systems can lead to a failure to mount a compensatory response that would prevent or mitigate symptoms. For example, aging is associated with a blunting of the normal thirst response to volume depletion and a hyperosmolar state [8], making geriatric patients more susceptible to hypotension, light-headedness, and acute kidney injury from illnesses, like gastroenteritis, that cause volume loss or reduce oral intake. Roughly 30 % of the elderly have impaired vasoconstriction during assumption of an upright posture, leading to orthostatic hypotension [9], typically defined as a drop of 20 mmHg in systolic blood pressure or 10 mmHg of diastolic blood pressure. The result may be light-headedness or syncope. If the patient is allowed to maintain the upright posture for more than 3 min, the prevalence of orthostatic hypotension rises to as high as 40 % [10]. Orthostatic hypotension can be exacerbated by the heart's inability to increase the heart rate to maintain cardiac output, either through cardiac conduction-system abnormalities or autonomic dysfunction. These maladaptive age-related changes, while not reflecting normal aging, are common and can be worsened by comorbidities and medications that affect an organ's compensatory response (e.g., beta-blockers that prevent tachycardia).

11.3.2 The Older Psychiatric Patient as Poor Historian

In approximately 20 % of patients admitted to a medical inpatient service, the history alone is sufficient to arrive at an accurate diagnosis, and the history and physical examination lead to an accurate diagnosis in 80 % of cases [11]. Psychiatric conditions can impair history taking and thus the diagnostic process for all age groups, but the greater prevalence of neurocognitive disorders in the elderly adds an additional obstacle to accurate history taking. Among persons age 65+, mild cognitive impairment has a prevalence of 3.7 % or 7.9 %, using the DSM-5 or Petersen criteria, respectively [12]. Only 19 % of cases of delirium in hospitalized, non-demented patients 65 and older fully resolve by 24 weeks [13]. Delirium has been found in approximately 15 % of psychiatric inpatients, with the highest incidence among those with bipolar disorder; fewer than half of the cases of delirium were recognized at the time of occurrence [14]. Chronic diseases prevalent in the elderly, such as diabetes and end-stage chronic kidney disease (CKD-V), contribute to neurocognitive dysfunction [15], in part due to cerebral white matter disease. An atypical presentation or an inadequate history from the patient requires collateral information from family or health providers who have been closely involved with patient care during the period leading up to the current presentation.

Psychiatric patients may develop strong beliefs in the cause of symptoms, potentially misdirecting the work-up or causing the clinician to dismiss the symptoms as not being real.

Case Vignette 2 Mrs. M was a 74-year-old obese woman with obsessive-compulsive disorder, who was admitted for suicidal ideation with a clear plan. Her past medical history was notable for hypertension, hypercholesterolemia, osteoarthritis, and gastroesophageal reflux disease (GERD). Although taking a daily proton pump inhibitor, she intermittently complained of substernal chest pain. ("I know it's my heartburn, and it's getting worse! Please give me something for it!") The on-call psychiatrist acquiesced and prescribed 30 mL of aluminum hydroxide/magnesium carbonate antacid as needed, usually with relief of symptoms after 15–20 min. On hospital day 6, she was found unresponsive in bed at 6:00 AM. A "code blue" was called, but after 15 min of unsuccessful resuscitation efforts, she was declared dead. An autopsy revealed pathological features of acute and healing myocardial infarctions.

Case Analysis In retrospect, Mrs. M's frequent chest pain represented an angina equivalent. Because the patient had a history of GERD, the psychiatrist assumed the patient's belief that she had heartburn was accurate and did not take a careful history or perform an exam to rule out other causes of chest pain.

Case Vignette 3 Mr. K was an 89-year-old practicing businessman admitted with acute onset of hallucinations attributed to use of ropinirole for restless leg syndrome. He had stage III chronic kidney disease (CKD-III), knee osteoarthritis, mild cognitive impairment, and gout, for which he had been prescribed colchicine 0.6 mg BID as an outpatient. All of his outpatient prescriptions were stopped at admission.

His psychotic symptoms remitted. While an inpatient, he complained of nearly daily gouty attacks in his big toes and requested that the colchicine be resumed.

Case Analysis His complaints of gouty attacks led his primary care physician to prescribe colchicine despite his chronic kidney disease. On examination of his feet, he had no evidence of joint swelling, erythema, warmth, or tenderness to palpation. Roentgenograms of the feet revealed only osteoarthritic changes in the toes. The colchicine was not resumed, and he was given acetaminophen (paracetamol) 500 mg TID as needed for pain in the toes with good relief of symptoms.

In Ekbom's syndrome, or delusional infestation, psychiatric patients may attribute chronic pruritus to parasites or some other infestation, despite an underlying paresthesia caused by diabetes mellitus, hypo- or hyperthyroidism, lupus erythematosus, uremia, opioids, or other medications, as well as other chronic diseases [16]. Chronic dry skin (xerosis) affects more than 50 % of the elderly due to loss of the epidermal water barrier and is an important cause of chronic pruritus in this age group [17].

11.4 General Approach to Physical Complaints and Symptoms

Diagnosis and management of acute medical symptoms in the geriatric psychiatric patient require a fundamental understanding of disease processes and their treatment, but working through potentially atypical features and incomplete historical information can be facilitated by addressing the following questions, which may help to narrow the differential diagnosis:

- What are the symptoms and when did they begin (acute vs. gradual onset[1])?
- In what context did the present symptoms or behaviors begin? Are there any recent exposures that could explain the symptoms? (Example: 88-year-old bipolar man, stable on lithium treatment, presenting with nausea, and vomiting 4 days after exposure to his great-grandson, who had a diarrheal illness[2])
- Is there any relationship between the symptoms and the start or dose change of a medication? (Example: Inability to void in a 77-year-old patient with schizophrenia, 24 h after his dose of olanzapine was doubled to 10 mg qhs.[3])
- What are the patient's underlying medical problems, and could any of these symptoms be attributable to them or to the medications used to treat them?

[1] Conditions with acute onset can be divided into two types: those precipitated by a new intervention (e.g., medication or surgery) or those representing a potential medical emergency.

[2] The history of exposure and the patient's symptoms suggest transmission of a viral gastroenteritis, possibly complicated by lithium toxicity. Thus, serum lithium level and "watchful waiting" would be justified, provided the patient can receive adequate fluids by mouth or parenterally.

[3] Olanzapine's anticholinergic activity, in the setting of probable prostatic hypertrophy in this 77-year-old man, contributed to urinary retention.

(Examples: 66-year-old man with Parkinson's-related neurocognitive disorder admitted for severe psychosis, presenting with new hypoxemia on vital signs ($SaO_2 = 89$ %) after his dose of levodopa-carbidopa was reduced, with resulting worsening of parkinsonism.[4] A 77-year-old man 2 months status post non-ST-elevation myocardial infarction (NSTEMI) with placement of a drug-eluting stent, admitted for major depression and self-neglect, whose nurse reports that he appears exhausted walking from his bed to the bathroom.[5])

11.5 Approach to Specific Geriatric Conditions

11.5.1 Delirium

In geriatric orthopedic patients, hyperactive delirium is less common than the hypoactive type, but is associated with worse outcomes (death, nursing-home placement) [18–20]. However, hypoactive delirium is more likely to be missed, especially in patients whose somnolence may be attributed to psychotropic medication. Neither type of delirium is stable and fluctuations between the two types commonly occur [21]. Regardless of the severity or type, new-onset delirium should be regarded as a medical emergency, as it may represent potentially life-threatening organ system dysfunction (e.g., myocardial infarction), metabolic derangement, infection, or an adverse drug reaction/interaction. There is no "standard" work-up for acute delirium; prioritization of individual tests should be tailored to the individual's unique risk factors [22], bearing in mind that delirium often is multifactorial. Table 11.1 provides a systematic approach to delirium assessment. A default diagnosis of idiopathic delirium should not be made until treatable causes have been ruled out [23–25].

11.5.2 Falls

The US Centers for Medicare and Medicaid Services consider falls a quality indicator and does not reimburse hospitals for patient injuries resulting from nosocomial falls. Falls are associated with delirium and may be the result of lower extremity weakness, cerebellar or vestibular dysfunction, peripheral or autonomic neuropathy, neurodegenerative disorders (e.g., Parkinson's disease), visual impairment, orthostatic hypotension, prior stroke, cardiac arrhythmias, or the effects of medications (e.g., benzodiazepines). In many cases, there is more than one contributing factor. Patients who fall require an evaluation to assess for injury as well as the etiology.

---

[4] Worsened parkinsonism should alert the examiner to associated dysphagia and the risk of aspiration.

[5] Because of self-neglect, the patient may not have taken his aspirin or clopidogrel, resulting in stent occlusion and acute coronary ischemia or heart failure, manifested atypically by acute exhaustion without chest pain or shortness of breath.

- Although amnesia for the fall often limits the accuracy of the history [26], as much information as possible should be obtained from the patient and any witnesses in order to ascertain preceding symptoms like light-headedness and the exact circumstances surrounding the fall. Vital signs should be obtained immediately. Loss of consciousness (LOC), even if transient and not accompanied by injury, must be evaluated. Once the patient has been ruled out for injuries (see below), lying, seated, and standing blood pressures should be obtained to evaluate for orthostatic hypotension. An electrocardiogram with rhythm strip should be obtained; if an explanatory arrhythmia for LOC is not revealed, the patient will require telemetry and thus admission to a medical ward. The most common causes of syncope in geriatric patients include orthostatic hypotension, neurally mediated syncope ("vasovagal syndrome"), carotid sinus syndrome, and arrhythmias [26].

Table 11.1 A targeted stepwise approach to the differential diagnosis of acute delirium in geriatric patients

Step	Assessment	Comments
Assessment that should be performed in nearly all cases		
1	Obtain vital signs: Include oxygen saturation and core temperature. Pulse rate and type (regular vs. irregular) and respiratory rate should be accurately obtained by counting for at least 20 s.	A fever of $\geq$ 38 °C should be taken as a sign of infection until proven otherwise. True tachypnea (respiratory rate > 18) suggests an acute pulmonary process. A room-air SaO_2 < 92 % implies pulmonary compromise unless the patient has known underlying chronic lung disease. A heart rate $\geq$ 100 beats per min. suggests possible cardiopulmonary distress. Patients with prolonged bed rest are at risk for pulmonary embolism, for which an unexplained tachycardia is the most sensitive indicator
2	Medical history	Are there underlying medical conditions that increase the risk of metabolic compromise? Examples: Diabetes, especially if on glucose lowering medication Significant chronic lung disease that predisposes to hypoglycemia History of admissions for heart failure Chronic liver disease, with potential for hyperammonemia. Any history or suspicion of drug or alcohol withdrawal? If yes, the patient should empirically receive 100 mg of thiamine before receiving intravenous glucose to prevent Wernicke's syndrome *Any person suspected of diabetes should have a stat finger-stick glucose obtained*
3	Review medications	Any new medications (or dose changes in medications) with action on the CNS? Medications are the most common cause of delirium in the elderly. Patients recently started on valproic acid or on an increased dose should have a stat ammonia level obtained (see Chap. 12)

(continued)

Table 11.1 (continued)

Step	Assessment	Comments
4	*Targeted* stat/urgent laboratory testing, based on underlying conditions and the resulting probability of clinically significant abnormalities	A complete blood count (CBC) should be obtained in all patients A urinalysis usually should be obtained, especially in a patient with a current or recently discontinued bladder catheter, history of prostatic hypertrophy, or urinary retention. Available evidence supports an association between urinary tract infection and delirium [25]. Both men and women at prolonged bed rest have an increased risk for urinary retention An electrolyte panel (Na, K, BUN, creatinine) should be obtained in patients who could have a high serum sodium (from dehydration) or hyponatremia from diuretics or the inappropriate secretion of antidiuretic hormone (see Chap. 12) Additional electrolyte studies like calcium (looking for hypercalcemia) should be targeted toward patients whose past medical history suggests increased risk (e.g., hyperparathyroidism, excessive vitamin D or calcium ingestion) A cardiac troponin level should be obtained if coronary ischemia is suspected *Nonurgent* folate, B_{12} levels can be obtained if erythrocyte macrocytosis is seen or nutritional deficiencies suspected A magnesium level should be obtained in patients on chronic diuretics but is not a recognized cause of delirium
5	*Targeted* electrocardiogram (ECG)	An ECG is indicated when coronary ischemia or an arrhythmia is suspected based on known risk factors. Because coronary heart disease is prevalent in the elderly, and an atypical presentation of coronary ischemia is relatively common, an ECG is indicated in *most* cases (along with a troponin level), provided another explanation is not readily apparent
6	Poorly controlled pain	Inadequately controlled pain in patients unable to articulate their symptoms can present as delirium
Testing that should be performed only in specific circumstances		
7	*Targeted* imaging studies	Chest X-ray (CXR): If the patient has no respiratory symptoms, normal vital signs, and clear lungs on auscultation, and probable etiologic factors have been identified, a CXR is not required. However, one should be obtained if readily available, since delirium is associated with an increased risk of aspiration pneumonitis and pneumonia may present atypically Cranial imaging (computed tomography or magnetic resonance imaging): These have a low yield and should be limited to patients in whom a head injury is suspected, those taking anticoagulation in whom an intracranial hemorrhage is being considered, and those in whom new abnormal neurological findings raise suspicion of an acute stroke-like event [24]
8	*Targeted* electroencephalogram (EEG)	In delirium, the EEG generally displays nonspecific slowing with generalized theta or delta slow-wave activity [23] and has utility only in the rare circumstance when akinetic seizures are suspected – usually when delirium is sustained and no other cause can be identified
9	*Targeted* lumbar puncture (LP)	Rarely should an LP be performed in the evaluation of delirium. The exception is in patients with an acute or subacute neurocognitive decline unexplained by other causes and for which an encephalitis is suspected

Table 11.1 (continued)

Step	Assessment	Comments
Miscellaneous conditions associated with delirium that should be considered		
10	Fecal impaction	If the patient has not had a bowel movement recorded for days, a rectal examination and/or an abdominal X-ray should be obtained if no other causes of delirium have been identified
	Urinary retention	Similarly, urinary retention has been associated with delirium. A post-void residual by bladder ultrasound or in-and-out catheterization should be obtained if no other causes of delirium have been identified. Note that a fecal impaction can cause urinary retention

- For an unwitnessed fall, a careful neurological examination is mandatory, but is recommended for all fallers, looking for new, abnormal neurological signs and symptoms that may suggest stroke or intracranial bleed. As part of the motor exam, the patient also should be assessed for musculoskeletal injuries, and the ability to weight-bear and walk without new or worsened pain should be assessed.
- Because cervical spinal injury can occur without evidence of spinal cord injury, in an unwitnessed fall, the patient's neck should be immediately immobilized in a rigid collar pending cervical spinal X-rays. Following head trauma, intracranial bleeding can occur insidiously, delaying the development of neurological symptoms for hours to days. Computed tomography (CT) of the brain is therefore recommended – and must be obtained if the patient is taking an anticoagulant. If a head CT is not available, nurses should perform frequent neurological checks (evaluating level of consciousness and gross motor and cognitive function) for at least 48 h.
- Gait stability should be assessed following the fall to determine if a new walking aid or physical therapy should be prescribed.
  - Can the patient stand without pushing off with his/her hands? If not, the quadriceps muscles may be weak, constituting a risk factor for future falls.
  - With the patient one step in front of the chair (for safety if he/she falls backward), can the patient stand with feet together and eyes closed for 10 s without holding on for support? If no, proprioceptive, vestibular, or cerebellar function may be affected. Does the patient tend to fall backward when attempting to stand? If so, check for other signs of parkinsonism.
  - What is the gait like? Look for stride length and arm swing, posture (stooped vs. erect), ability to walk in a straight line (versus staggering), reaching out to touch walls or furniture for support (reflecting a fear of falling), and the stability of the 180° turn to come back.

11.6 Approach to Other Common Complaints

This section *does not* cover all common symptoms, but provides basic guidelines to prevent misdiagnosing potentially serious conditions in geriatric psychiatric patients.

11.6.1 Eyes

- Acute eye pain or changes in vision may represent acute glaucoma or other ocular emergencies. Immediate ophthalmologic evaluation is required.
- A *painless* spontaneous hemorrhage beneath the conjunctiva without associated changes in vision (Fig. 11.1) is benign, and the patient can be reassured that the blood will be reabsorbed within 2–4 weeks.

11.6.2 Headache

- Infrequent, minor headaches without neurological symptoms can be managed locally.
  - Any persistent or chronic daily headache or a new migraine-like headache in a patient without a history of migraine headaches should be referred for consultation. Any meningeal signs (e.g., nuchal rigidity) should prompt an acute ED visit or urgent neurology or medical consultation.

11.6.3 Upper Respiratory Infections and Cough

- Mild viral-like upper respiratory symptoms (stuffy nose, sore throat, nonproductive cough) should be monitored for progression and severity. An isolated cough requires a thorough history and exam. A dry cough can occur weeks to months after initiation of an angiotensin converting enzyme inhibitor for hypertension. If the patient complains of symptoms consistent with a postnasal drip (productive cough when supine, frequent tickle in the throat, with or without a "cobblestone" appearance and/or mucus in the nasopharynx), management of the postnasal drip with saline nasal rinses and a nasal steroid can be tried on the psychiatric unit.

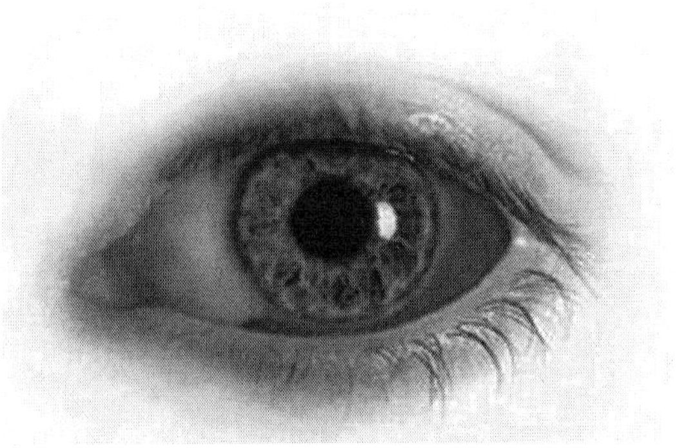

Fig. 11.1 Subconjunctival hemorrhage

11.6.4 Dyspnea

- Dyspnea is associated with many chronic and acute illnesses which may coexist in an older adult. It may be useful to determine whether the dyspnea is a new complaint or a worsening chronic complaint. Persisting dyspnea may be a result of advanced cardiopulmonary illness, such as advanced heart failure or chronic obstructive pulmonary disease (COPD). The presence of associated features such as cough, chest pain, or peripheral edema can be helpful in elucidating the underlying causative mechanism [27]. Symptoms of heart failure can include exertional shortness of breath, orthopnea, paroxysmal nocturnal dyspnea, and swelling of the lower limbs. Exertional symptoms are less prominent in older adults partially due to reduced physical activity, and patients may complain of nonspecific fatigue.
- As with many other infections, pneumonia in geriatric patients may present with atypical features such as fatigue, functional decline or loss of appetite. Up to one quarter of this population may not mount a fever.

Clinical Pearl
Dyspnea can represent a number of different sensations and some have been linked with specific pathology. For example, pulmonary edema is often described as "suffocation;" patients with cardiac deconditioning often complain of "heavy breathing;" and patients with COPD, asthma, or pulmonary fibrosis commonly describe an increased effort or harder work to breathe [28].

11.6.5 Chest Pain

- For patients over age 65, ischemic heart disease is a major cause of mortality and should be considered whenever the presenting complaint is chest pain. Other causes of chest pain can include noncardiac causes such as pulmonary embolism or esophageal reflux [29]. The National Registry of Myocardial Infarction (NRMI) reported that only 40 % of patients over age 65 presented with a chief complaint of chest pain. Other nonspecific symptoms such as abdominal pain, confusion, or dizziness may be present instead of chest pain [30]. Typical angina presents as a substernal chest pressure which may be provoked by exertion and improved with rest or nitroglycerin. If the chest pain radiates to the back, it may suggest aortic dissection or GERD. Associated features such as diaphoresis or dyspnea may be supportive of cardiac ischemia [31].

Clinical Pearl
If the patient has had a myocardial infarction in the past, asking if the current pain is similar to previously experienced pain can be an important clue.

11.6.6 Gastrointestinal (GI) Symptoms

- *Dyspepsia:* Occasional mild postprandial dyspepsia or substernal burning can be treated symptomatically with an antacid,[6] but the frequency and associated factors (e.g., exercise induced) should be closely monitored in case the symptoms represent an atypical presentation of heart disease, esophagitis, gastritis, peptic ulcer disease, cholecystitis, or another, potentially serious condition.
- *Abdominal pain:* Acute abdominal pain requires a thorough history and exam and usually requires urgent medical or surgical consultation. Absent or hypoactive bowel sounds suggest an ileus or partial ileus and can be confirmed by an abdominal X-ray ("kidney-ureter-bladder" series). In the elderly, pain from an acute abdominal process like diverticulitis, cholecystitis, pancreatitis, or appendicitis may not localize immediately. Localized pain may suggest the origin and help guide whether a surgical or medical consultation is called. Because valproic acid (VPA) can cause acute pancreatitis, epigastric pain in a patient on VPA should have blood drawn for a serum lipase. *Acute abdominal pain should not be managed on a psychiatric unit unless the patient is receiving terminal palliative care.*

Clinical Pearl

It is important to differentiate intra-abdominal from musculoskeletal abdominal pain, the latter most commonly resulting from abdominal wall hernias. Localized pain from abdominal wall hernias, such as spigelian hernias at the intersection of the medial and lateral rectus muscles, can be accentuated by asking the patient to sit up, which tenses the abdominal musculature and thus pinches the omentum or small bowel trapped inside. Large hernias are less likely to cause incarceration than smaller ones. Inability to reduce a hernia suggests incarceration and requires urgent surgical consultation. Persistent pain at the hernia site, even at rest, suggests possible strangulation and is an emergency, especially if associated with an ileus (suggesting infarcted bowel).

- *Nausea and vomiting:* In patients with nausea and vomiting, a history should explore associated factors, contacts with similar symptoms, and the severity and duration of symptoms. An isolated event associated with a foodstuff or new dose of a medication can be monitored; persistent nausea or vomiting, and all cases of hematemesis, should receive prompt medical consultation. Hematemesis is a medical emergency. Diabetics with nausea and vomiting require a stat POC blood sugar. Nausea and vomiting can be associated with fecal impaction (see below).

---

[6]The H_2 blockers, ranitidine and cimetidine, should be avoided because of their anticholinergic properties. Famotidine is safer. Proton pump inhibitors may take up to 24 h to provide symptomatic relief. Magnesium-containing liquid antacids should be avoided in patients with stage IV and V chronic kidney disease.

- *Constipation:* Constipation affects > 20 % of community-dwelling elderly and up to 75 % of institutionalized elderly [32]. The high frequency in older patients reflects the prevalence of contributing factors, such as the use of opioids and other constipating drugs, poor intake of dietary fiber, decreased mobility, dehydration, and age- and disease-associated autonomic dysfunction. Psychiatric medications with anticholinergic properties (e.g., tricyclic antidepressants, paroxetine, and clozapine) can contribute to constipation. Despite the popularity of docusate sodium for the treatment of constipation, there is little empiric evidence that demonstrates its efficacy, and it has been shown to be less effective than bulking agents like psyllium [33], which in turn are less effective than osmotic laxatives like polyethylene glycol (PEG), sorbitol, and lactulose [34]. Docusate sodium may help to maintain soft stool. Osmotic laxatives and sennosides are safe for everyday use in patients with chronic constipation, but studies suggest that PEG may be the most effective [32]. More potent stimulant laxatives like milk of magnesia and bisacodyl should be reserved for occasional constipation.

  When a patient complains of constipation, a history should be obtained about the frequency and consistency of bowel movements, as many North Americans define "constipation" as less than one bowel movement per day but have perfectly normal bowel function. Patients who feel the need to defecate but are unable to pass stool require a rectal examination. An over-distended rectum may lose its ability to contract properly. If the stool is soft, a local stimulatory laxative like a bisacodyl suppository may be sufficient to evacuate the rectum, but manual disimpaction still may be required. Because manual disimpaction of hard feces can be painful, the stool first should be softened with an oil-retention enema.

  Sustained constipation can result in a fecal impaction that can back up throughout the colon. In its most severe state, the patient can develop nausea, vomiting, and an ileus. An empty or nearly empty rectum does *not* rule out a fecal impaction.

Clinical Pearl
Fecal impaction should be considered in the differential diagnosis of loss of appetite, along with the side effects of medication, associated illness, and psychiatric disorders.

- *GI bleeding:* Black, tarry stools reported by the patient or nursing staff may reflect upper GI bleeding and should prompt immediate vital signs to screen for hypotension; if the patient is medically stable, a rectal examination should be performed looking for heme-positive stool to confirm GI bleeding, and blood work should be sent for a stat CBC and electrolyte panel to assess the presence and extent of anemia and volume depletion. Medical stability in the presence of GI bleeding is based on the stability of comorbid conditions, stable vital signs, and absence of brisk bleeding as defined by a hemoglobin > 10 mg/dL that has not dropped by > 2 mg/dL since admission. A proton pump inhibitor should be started immediately, preferably intravenously, if upper GI bleeding is suspected. Large-volume hematochezia is a medical-surgical emergency. However, small amounts of blood can color the toilet bowel red and appear more serious than it really is. All complaints of bright-red blood per rectum should prompt immediate vital signs to assess medical stability and an immediate rectal exam. If the amount of blood reported is small (e.g., blood on toilet paper) and external hemorrhoids are seen, the patient can be managed locally with a stool softener like docusate and an osmotic laxative like PEG to prevent straining at stool, along with application of hydrocortisone cream to the hemorrhoids. As selective serotonin reuptake inhibitors and serotonin-norepinephrine reuptake inhibitors can inhibit platelet aggregation, they should be held during acute GI bleeding. VPA can cause thrombocytopenia.

11.6.7 Edema

- Lower extremity edema is common in older patients and does not always signify poorly controlled heart failure. Table 11.2 lists common causes of peripheral edema. The clinician should exercise caution in treating non-heart-failure edema with diuretics, as they may cause excessive volume contraction and electrolyte abnormalities [35]. Diuretics should be reserved for patients in whom the edema cannot be controlled by leg elevation or compression stockings (the latter being contraindicated in significant peripheral vascular disease), and the edema threatens local cellulitis or skin breakdown. Venous stasis ulcers require specialized wound care best provided by a certified wound-care nurse. Hyperpigmentation that has accumulated around the ankles and shins suggests chronic venous stasis (CVS). Over time, CVS leads to dermal scarring, replacing pitting edema with firmer, darker tissue (so-called brawny edema), and eventually progresses to thickened, hardened skin with or without hard bumps (so-called woody edema).

Key Points

- Physical complaints may be more serious than they appear, and psychiatrists caring for geriatric inpatients are challenged by atypical presentations of acute illness and by inadequate or misleading medical histories.
- Every complaint should be assessed with a history from the patient and collateral sources, followed by a careful physical examination (see Chap. 2).
- Complaints arising from underlying chronic illnesses like chronic obstructive pulmonary disease and heart failure often require medical consultation for adjustment of medication.
- Medications for acute (and chronic) conditions should be carefully evaluated for potential side effects and drug-drug interactions (see Chap. 12).

Table 11.2 Common causes of lower extremity edema

Mechanism	Types	Comments
Increased plasma volume 2° salt and water retention	Congestive heart failure	Early heart failure may present with worsening lower extremity (LE) edema without dyspnea, especially if the patient is largely sedentary[a]
	Advanced kidney disease (CKD-III+)	Inability to excrete excess salt and water
Venous obstruction	Cor pulmonale	Seen in advanced primary and secondary pulmonary hypertension and right heart failure
	Unilateral: Acute venous thrombosis	Acute unilateral LE edema. *This is a medical emergency.* A stat Doppler ultrasound should be obtained for confirmation and urgent medical consultation obtained so that appropriate anticoagulation can be started. Low molecular weight heparin or oral anticoagulants can be used under close medical supervision. Patients receiving anticoagulation for proximal deep venous thrombosis usually can remain on the psychiatric unit
Venous insufficiency	Chronic venous stasis	Due to age-associated failure of venous valves. Also 2° increased venous pressure due to obesity
	Cirrhosis	Seen in advanced cirrhosis. Ascites usually accompanies peripheral edema, which also caused by hypoalbuminemia
	Unilateral: Post-thrombotic venous stasis	Chronic unilateral lower extremity edema following ipsilateral deep venous thrombosis. Often painful
	Status point unilateral saphenous venin harvesting for bypass grafting	May present with dependent edema on the side of the saphenous vein harvest. Usually mild and responds to leg elevation and compression stockings
	Varicose veins	LE varicosities can be present more on one leg than another. Edema usually mild and responds to leg elevation and compression stockings
Medications	Salt-retaining drugs	Examples include nonsteroidal anti-inflammatory drugs, glucocorticoids, fludrocortisone, thiazolidinediones ("glitazones" for diabetes mellitus), and dihydropyridine calcium channel blockers (amlodipine, nifedipine). Salt and water retention with these drugs often, but not always, occurs in the presence of heart failure or chronic kidney disease. Edema usually mild but can exacerbate edema from other causes
	Vasodilating drugs	Hydralazine, minoxidil, dihydropyridine calcium channel blockers. Edema usually mild but can exacerbate edema from other causes

[a]Except where noted, edema is usually bilateral. However, there may be asymmetry in the extent of the edema. An acute unilateral increase in edema should prompt concern for deep venous thrombosis

References

1. Marcum ZA, Amuan ME, Hanlon JT, et al. Prevalence of unplanned hospitalizations caused by adverse drug reactions in older veterans. J Am Geriatr Soc. 2012;60(1):34–41.
2. Cohen G, Zalomonson S, Press Y. Prevalence of orthostatic hypotension in the unselected ambulatory population of persons aged 65 years old and above. Blood Press. 2015;24(5):298–305.
3. Limpawattana P, Phungoen P, Mitsungnern T, Laosuangkoon W, Tansangworn N. Atypical presentations of older adults at the emergency department and associated factors. Arch Gerontol Geriatr. 2016;62:97–102.
4. Yahav D, Schlesinger A, Daitch V, et al. Presentation of infection in older patients – a prospective study. Ann Med. 2015;47(4):354–8.
5. Aronow WS, Mercando AD, Epstein S. Prevalence of silent myocardial ischemia detected by 24-hour ambulatory electrocardiography, and its association with new coronary events at 40-month follow-up in elderly diabetic and nondiabetic patients with coronary artery disease. Am J Cardiol. 1992;69(5):555–6.
6. Li Q, Wang S, Milot E, et al. Homeostatic dysregulation proceeds in parallel in multiple physiological systems. Aging Cell. 2015;14:1103–12.
7. Rodriguez-Manas L, Feart C, Mann G, et al. Searching for an operational definition of frailty: a Delphi method based consensus statement: the frailty operative definition-consensus conference project. J Gerontol A Biol Sci Med Sci. 2013;68(1):62–7.
8. Kenney WL, Chiu P. Influence of age on thirst and fluid intake. Med Sci Sports Exerc. 2001;33(9):1524–32.
9. Ricci F, De Caterina R, Fedorowski A. Orthostatic hypotension: epidemiology, prognosis, and treatment. J Am Coll Cardiol. 2015;66(7):848–60.
10. Campos AC, de Almeida NA, Ramos AL, Vasconcelos DF, Freitas MP, de V Toledo MA. Orthostatic hypotension at different times after standing erect in elderly adults. J Am Geriatr Soc. 2015;63(3):589–90.
11. Paley L, Zornitzki T, Cohen J, Friedman J, Kozak N, Schattner A. Utility of clinical examination in the diagnosis of emergency department patients admitted to the department of medicine of an academic hospital. Arch Intern Med. 2011;171(15):1394–6.
12. Lopez-Anton R, Santabarbara J, De-la-Camara C, et al. Mild cognitive impairment diagnosed with the new DSM-5 criteria: prevalence and associations with non-cognitive psychopathology. Acta Psychiatr Scand. 2015;131(1):29–39.
13. Cole MG, Bailey R, Bonnycastle M, et al. Partial and no recovery from delirium in older hospitalized adults: frequency and baseline risk factors. J Am Geriatr Soc. 2015;63:2340–8.
14. Ritchie J, Steiner W, Abrahamowicz M. Incidence of and risk factors for delirium among psychiatric inpatients. Psychiatr serv (Washington, DC). 1996;47(7):727–30.
15. Verdelho A, Madureira S, Moleiro C, et al. Depressive symptoms predict cognitive decline and dementia in older people independently of cerebral white matter changes: the LADIS study. J Neurol Neurosurg Psychiatry. 2013;84(11):1250–4.
16. Kimsey LS. Delusional infestation and chronic pruritus: a review. Acta Derm Venereol. 2015;96:298–302.
17. Berger TG, Shive M, Harper GM. Pruritus in the older patient: a clinical review. JAMA. 2013;310(22):2443–50.
18. Marcantonio E, Ta T, Duthie E, Resnick NM. Delirium severity and psychomotor types: their relationship with outcomes after hip fracture repair. J Am Geriatr Soc. 2002;50(5):850–7.
19. Meagher DJ, Leonard M, Donnelly S, Conroy M, Adamis D, Trzepacz PT. A longitudinal study of motor subtypes in delirium: relationship with other phenomenology, etiology, medication exposure and prognosis. J Psychosom Res. 2011;71(6):395–403.
20. Robinson TN, Raeburn CD, Tran ZV, Brenner LA, Moss M. Motor subtypes of postoperative delirium in older adults. Arch Surg. 2011;146(3):295–300.
21. Albrecht JS, Marcantonio ER, Roffey DM, et al. Stability of postoperative delirium psychomotor subtypes in individuals with hip fracture. J Am Geriatr Soc. 2015;63(5):970–6.

22. Inouye SK, Westendorp RG, Saczynski JS. Delirium in elderly people. Lancet (London, England). 2014;383(9920):911–22.
23. Jacobson S, Jerrier H. EEG in delirium. Semin Clin Neuropsychiatry. 2000;5(2):86–92.
24. Vijayakrishnan R, Ramasubramanian A, Dhand S. Utility of head CT scan for acute inpatient delirium. Hosp Top. 2015;93(1):9–12.
25. Balogun SA, Philbrick JT. Delirium, a symptom of UTI in the elderly: fact or fable? a systematic review. Can Geriatr J : CGJ. 2014;17(1):22–6.
26. Brignole M. Distinguishing syncopal from non-syncopal causes of fall in older people. Age Ageing. 2006;35 Suppl 2:ii46–50.
27. Mahler DA, Fierro-Carrion G, Baird JC. Evaluation of dyspnea in the elderly. Clin Geriatr Med. 2003;19(1):19–33. v.
28. Scano G, Stendardi L, Grazzini M. Understanding dyspnoea by its language. Eur Respir J. 2005;25(2):380–5.
29. Brieger D, Eagle KA, Goodman SG, et al. Acute coronary syndromes without chest pain, an underdiagnosed and undertreated high-risk group: insights from the Global Registry of Acute Coronary Events. Chest. 2004;126(2):461–9.
30. Alexander KP, Newby LK, Cannon CP, et al. Acute coronary care in the elderly, part I: non-ST-segment-elevation acute coronary syndromes: a scientific statement for healthcare professionals from the American Heart Association Council on Clinical Cardiology: in collaboration with the Society of Geriatric Cardiology. Circulation. 2007;115(19):2549–69.
31. Chun AA, McGee SR. Bedside diagnosis of coronary artery disease: a systematic review. Am J Med. 2004;117(5):334–43.
32. Vazquez Roque M, Bouras EP. Epidemiology and management of chronic constipation in elderly patients. Clin Interv Aging. 2015;10:919–30.
33. CADTH Rapid Response Reports. Dioctyl Sulfosuccinate or Docusate (Calcium or Sodium) for the prevention or management of constipation: a review of the clinical effectiveness. Ottawa: Canadian Agency for Drugs and Technologies in Health Copyright (c) 2014 Canadian Agency for Drugs and Technologies in Health; 2014.
34. Pare P, Fedorak RN. Systematic review of stimulant and nonstimulant laxatives for the treatment of functional constipation. Can J Gastroenterol Hepatol. 2014;28(10):549–57.
35. Wehling M. Morbus diureticus in the elderly: epidemic overuse of a widely applied group of drugs. J Am Med Dir Assoc. 2013;14(6):437–42.

12 The Chief Adverse Effects of Medications

Calvin H. Hirsch, Shyam Maharaj, and James A. Bourgeois

12.1 Background

12.1.1 Polypharmacy and Specific Drug Toxicity States with Psychotropic Medications

Polypharmacy (defined as five or more prescription drugs) is common in geriatric patients who have multiple comorbidities and increases the risk of adverse drug events (ADEs), which can result in significant morbidity and potentially avoidable emergency department (ED) and hospital admissions. Age-related changes in body composition and organ–system function affect the pharmacokinetics (metabolism) and pharmacodynamics (action) of many medications, often requiring lower dosing than recommended in the dosing guidelines developed by pharmaceutical companies. Polypharmacy and ADEs can be reduced by avoiding *potentially inappropriate medications* (PIMs), which are medications that pose disproportionately high risks compared to benefits in geriatric patients. Clinicians can use tools like the Beers Criteria and the START/STOPP Criteria to identify PIMs in order to inform their prescribing to their older patients.

Certain classes of medication pose a high risk to geriatric patients. Anticholinergic properties are found in numerous, commonly prescribed medications, including

C.H. Hirsch, MD (✉)
Department of Internal Medicine, Division of General Medicine, University of California Davis Medical Center, Sacramento, CA, USA
e-mail: chhirsch@ucdavis.edu

S. Maharaj, BSc. Pharm, PhD
Department of Psychiatry and Behavioural Neurosciences, McMaster University, Hamilton, ON, Canada

J.A. Bourgeois, OD, MD
Department of Psychiatry/Langley Porter Psychiatric Institute, University of California San Francisco, San Francisco, CA, USA

A. Hategan et al. (eds.), *On-Call Geriatric Psychiatry: Handbook of Principles and Practice*, DOI 10.1007/978-3-319-30346-8_12

first-generation antipsychotics, tricyclic antidepressants, the first-generation SSRI paroxetine, the atypical antipsychotic olanzapine, and first-generation antihistamines, and should be minimized because of their potential to affect cognitive function and precipitate delirium. Several antipsychotics may cause diabetes mellitus and the metabolic syndrome. Lithium (Li) has a low therapeutic index, especially in geriatric patients, in part caused by the co-prescription of medications such as diuretics, which increase the risk of Li toxicity by volume depletion.

Neuroleptic malignant syndrome (NMS) and serotonin syndrome (SS) are rare but potentially life-threatening dysautonomias that present with overlapping symptoms, including hypertension, tachycardia, hyperthermia, and muscle rigidity. NMS represents an idiosyncratic response to dopamine-blocking agents (most commonly antipsychotic medication). SS arises from direct toxicity from serotonergic agents. Multiple classes of medications in addition to antidepressants have serotonergic agonism, including several opioids. For both NMS and SS, management is largely supportive after discontinuation of the offending medication(s).

A variety of psychotropic medications increase secretion of the antidiuretic hormone vasopressin, contributing to the syndrome of inappropriate antidiuretic hormone (SIADH), to which geriatric patients are more susceptible than younger patients. SSRIs may inhibit platelet aggregation and have been associated with gastrointestinal bleeding and should be prescribed with caution to older patients at high risk for intracranial hemorrhage. Tricyclic antidepressants, certain SSRIs, and several atypical antipsychotics may prolong the electrocardiographic QTc interval, increasing the risk of a life-threatening form of ventricular tachycardia called torsades de pointes. A number of medications commonly prescribed to older patients also prolong the QTc, including macrolide antibiotics and the antiarrhythmic amiodarone, and may precipitate ventricular tachycardia when coadministered together or with QTc-prolonging psychotropics.

12.2 Epidemiology of Adverse Drug Events

In a study looking at men aged 70 and older, polypharmacy, defined as ≥5 prescription drugs, was associated with an increased risk of frailty, disability, mortality, and falls [1]. Polypharmacy contributes to significant drug–drug interactions (DDIs) and ADEs [2, 3]. Between 2003 and 2008, ADEs accounted for 0.75 % of ED visits by residents aged ≥66 in Ontario, Canada [4], and for an estimated 10 % of all admissions to US Veterans Administration Hospitals between 2003 and 2006. Ninety-three percent of the ADE-related admissions occurred in veterans taking five or more medications [5]. The number of prescribed medications rises with age due to an increasing number of comorbidities. Based on a random sample of 4,500 Australians ≥age 50 surveyed between 2009 and 2010, the Australian National Census of Medications found that fewer than 10 % of men and women aged 60–64 reported taking ten or more medications, but the proportions rose to nearly 30 % for women and 15 % for men after age 74 [6]. Not surprisingly, the potential for significant DDIs rises with the number of prescriptions. Retrospective screening of the prescriptions intended for use for at least 14 days among 81,650 outpatients at a Taiwanese medical center in 2004 identified an exponential risk of potential DDIs as the number of prescriptions rose, such that by five drugs, the average number of potential DDIs was two, and for 8–9 drugs was four [7]. Despite the associated risks, polypharmacy is an almost ineluctable consequence of the treatment of multiple comorbidities, some of which individually require more than one drug as standard of care. In 1999, 15 % of US seniors age 65–69 had four or more chronic conditions, compared to approximately 80 % of seniors over age 80 [8].

To complicate the challenge of prescribing for older adults, the metabolism of many medications (pharmacokinetics) changes with age due to physiologic changes and alterations in body composition, requiring awareness of a drug's distribution in the fat and water compartments, site(s) of metabolism, and modes of elimination (see Table 12.1). Age-related changes also modify the pharmacodynamics of certain medications, i.e., the type and extent of the pharmacologic actions of a given dose of drug (see Table 12.2). Standard dosing guidelines for many drugs, developed by pharmaceutical companies and approved by the US Food and Drug Administration, the Therapeutic Goods Administration of

Table 12.1 Summary of age-related changes that affect drug metabolism

Physiologic change	Pharmacokinetic consequence
Decreased serum albumin	Increased free fraction in plasma for highly protein-bound acidic drugs
Increased α-1-acid glycoprotein	Decreased free fraction of alkaline drugs
Decreased lean body mass Decreased total body water	Increased plasma concentrations of hydrophilic drugs
Increased body fat	Increased volume of distribution and $T_{1/2}$ of lipophilic drugs
Decreased hepatic blood flow	Potentially decreased first-pass metabolism
Decreased hepatic mass	Phase I metabolism (CYP oxidation, reduction, hydrolysis) slightly ↓ Phase II metabolism (glucuronidation, acetylation, sulfation) *preserved*
Decreased renal blood flow and GFR	Renal elimination ↓

Table 12.2 Examples of pharmacodynamic changes

Drug	Pharmacodynamic effect	Age-related change
Furosemide	Peak diuretic response	↓
Morphine	Analgesic effect	↑
Verapamil	Acute antihypertensive effect	↑
Scopolamine	Cognitive function	↓
Temazepam	Postural sway	↑
Diazepam	Sedation, postural sway	↑
Warfarin	Anticoagulant effect	↑

Australia, Health Canada, and other national regulatory agencies, are based on studies which only provide standard adult dosing without consideration of potentially clinically significant differences in the pharmacokinetics and pharmacodynamics of medications in older patients. The patients used in these studies are often not representative of the older population. To account for known limitations in prescribing to older individuals, a good rule of thumb is to select a dose at or below the standard starting dose for adults and then to titrate the dose upward as needed to achieve the desired outcome.

Polypharmacy and ADEs also result from inappropriate prescribing (see Table 12.3). An important principle of drug prescribing for the older adults entails avoidance, whenever possible, of PIMs. PIMs are defined as medications that pose more risks than benefits to geriatric patients, especially if there are safer alternatives. The use of PIMs has been associated with a 43 % greater risk of an ADE [9]. In the USA, PIMs are used by the Centers for Medicare and Medicare Services in

Table 12.3 Types and examples of high-risk prescribing in the elderly

Type	Examples
"Silo prescribing": Prescribing, by specialists who are not up-to-date with the management of diseases outside their specialty, without awareness of potential contraindications and DDIs (see PIMs below)	Oxybutynin prescribed by gynecologist for urinary urgency in patient with mild cognitive impairment Doxazosin prescribed by urologist for urinary hesitancy in patient with orthostatic lightheadedness Paroxetine prescribed by psychiatrist for depression in patient with glaucoma
Medication prescribed to treat unrecognized side effect of another medication	Haloperidol for new hallucinations in patient begun on ropinirole for restless leg syndrome Donepezil for "early dementia" in patient routinely taking amitriptyline, lorazepam, and hydrocodone/acetaminophen (paracetamol) Meclizine prescribed for "dizziness" in patient taking high-dose gabapentin
Using standard "adult" doses without accounting for altered drug metabolism and effects due to age-related physiologic changes	A given dose of fluoxetine may have higher serum levels and delayed elimination in older patients, especially women Age-related increase in sedation and postural sway with benzodiazepines, leading to increased risk of falls Prescription of morphine to elderly patients due to age-related reduction in renal function (reduced clearance of drug)
Use of potentially inappropriate medications (see text for discussion)	Bupropion to treat depression in a patient with history of seizures First-generation antihistamine (e.g., diphenhydramine) in older patient with allergic rhinitis Calcium channel blocker (e.g., amlodipine) for hypertension in older patient with constipation Amitriptyline for depression or neuropathic pain

developing guidelines for Part D formularies and by the National Committee for Quality Assurance and the Healthcare Effectiveness Data and Information Set as quality measures.

Because it is impossible to know all the harmful side effects and interactions of even commonly prescribed medications, PIM tools have been developed for clinicians. Two of the most widely used are the Beers Criteria [10] and the STOPP/START Criteria [11]. The Beers Criteria were originally developed in 1991 and revised in 1997, 2003, 2012, and 2015 to reflect the constantly evolving pharmacopeia, knowledge of drug interactions, and epidemiology of ADEs. The 2015 Beers Criteria were updated by a 13-member expert panel consisting of geriatricians, nurses, pharmacists, and experts in research and quality measures. Using standardized criteria, the Beers Criteria rate both the strength of their recommendations to avoid (strong, weak, insufficient) and the quality of the supporting evidence. New to the criteria are lists of select drugs that should be avoided or have their dose adjusted based on the individual's kidney function and select drug–drug interactions documented to be associated with harms in older adults.

The STOPP/START Criteria, developed in Ireland, stand for the "Screening Tool of Older People's Prescriptions" and the "Screening Tool to Alert to Right Treatment." STOPP consists of 65 prescribing situations organized by organ system and by clinical condition (including falls plus analgesic and duplicate drugs). Developed by a Delphi process, STOPP overlaps with but is not identical to the Beers Criteria. Although listing PIMs, STOPP does not provide the strength of supporting evidence or prescribing recommendations. To compare the sensitivity of the STOPP and Beers Criteria to identify drugs causing ADEs, an expert panel evaluated 600 consecutive patients aged 65 and older admitted to a university hospital. The researchers identified 329 ADEs in 158 patients. The Beers Criteria identified 20.4 % of the drugs responsible for the ADEs, compared to 51.7 % by the STOPP criteria. Of the 151 ADEs considered contributory to the admission and avoidable, PIMs based on the Beers Criteria detected 22.5 %, whereas the STOPP Criteria identified 62.3 % [12]. The Beers Criteria list a number of drugs not found in Europe, whereas STOPP/START targets drugs available in Europe. Some clinicians may disagree with the recommendations in the Beers Criteria, such as the categorical recommendation against the use of conventional and atypical antipsychotics as treatment for the behavioral problems of major neurocognitive disorder (NCDs) (formerly dementia) or the recommendation to avoid the antiarrhythmic amiodarone as first-line treatment for atrial fibrillation. PIMs ultimately are guides to prudent prescribing and are not meant to be prescriptive, but clinicians should become familiar with at least one tool and integrate it into their prescribing practice for geriatric patients. Which decisional support tool is selected should be based on its appropriateness for the setting, ease of use, and availability, whether as a pocket guide, software package accessible on a hospital information system, or an application on a PDA or smartphone. The Beers Criteria can be downloaded as part of the iGeriatrics Mobile App for Apple™ or Android™ [13].

12.3 Avoiding ADEs in Older Patients: Special Cases

12.3.1 Minimize Anticholinergic Burden

Case Vignette 1 Ms. G was an 82-year-old woman admitted to the Orthopedic Service following a fall resulting in a right intertrochanteric hip fracture. At baseline, she was independent in her activities of daily living, shopped for groceries with her daughter, and paid her own bills. Her active medical problems included heart failure with preserved ejection fraction (HFpEF), hypertension, osteoarthritis, osteoporosis, and mixed urinary incontinence. For these problems, she was prescribed with furosemide 20 mg daily, lisinopril 20 mg daily, oxybutynin 5 mg extended release daily, and acetaminophen (paracetamol) 500 mg as needed. In the hospital, her outpatient medications were continued, except that the lisinopril was held on the day of surgery and the acetaminophen (paracetamol) was scheduled four times daily. Anesthesiology provided a regional nerve block for control of her hip pain. On hospital day 2, after she underwent an uneventful open reduction and internal fixation, Ms. G was given hydrocodone/acetaminophen (paracetamol) 5 mg/325 mg every 6 h as needed for pain, with hydromorphone 0.4 mg IV every 4 h prescribed for severe breakthrough pain. She vomited after both hydrocodone and hydromorphone intake and was given prochlorperazine 25 mg rectal suppositories every 12 h as needed to control nausea.

In the evening of hospital day 3, the orthopedic surgeon requested an urgent psychiatric consultation for severe agitation after Ms. G pulled out her IV and bladder catheter, started screaming and slapping her nurse, and tried to get out of bed. On evaluation, she was unable to complete a cognitive assessment due to variable levels of consciousness, agitation, and distractibility. The on-call psychiatrist prescribed rapidly dissolving oral olanzapine 2.5 mg SL stat, to be repeated in 1 h if no effect, then subsequently ordered 2.5–5 mg at bedtime and up to every 6 h as needed to control agitation that jeopardized the health or safety of the patient.

In the AM of hospital day 4, the patient was difficult to arouse and her WBC rose to 14,500/mm^3. A chest roentgenogram revealed a right lower lobe infiltrate consistent with aspiration. For the next 3 days, the patient's level of alertness waxed and waned, ranging from somnolent, confused, but cooperative to hyperalert, easily agitated, requiring wrist restraints. Her cognitive status on formal testing fluctuated as well, with MoCA scores ranging for 0–14. The patient was uncooperative with physical therapy and was discharged to a skilled nursing facility on hospital day 8 and was alert but still very confused.

Over half of adults 65 and older take at least one anticholinergic medication [14], making anticholinergics one of the most common causes of ADEs in older patients. Numerous psychotropic medications have anticholinergic properties, and moderately to highly anticholinergic drugs are commonly prescribed to treat vertigo, urinary urgency, allergies, insomnia, nausea, diarrhea, and extrapyramidal symptoms (see Table 12.4). Since these conditions often co-occur, older inpatients can simultaneously receive multiple anticholinergic medications (e.g., olanzapine, paroxetine, chlorpromazine), leading to a cumulative risk of severe anticholinergic side effects.

Table 12.4 Examples of anticholinergic medications

Medication class	Medication name	Anticholinergic activity[a]	Examples of safer alternatives
Antipsychotic			
Atypical	Olanzapine	H	Aripiprazole
	Quetiapine	M	
	Risperidone	M	
	Ziprasidone	M	
Typical	Haloperidol	M	
	Trifluoperazine	H	
	Chlorpromazine	H	
Antidepressant			
SSRI	Paroxetine	M	Second-generation SSRIs
Tricyclic	Amitriptyline	H	
	Nortriptyline	H	
Antidiarrheal			
	Loperamide	M	
Antiemetic			
	Prochlorperazine	H	Ondansetron[b]
H2 blocker antacids			
	Ranitidine	M[c]	Proton pump inhibitors, H2 blocker: famotidine
	Cimetidine	M	
All first-generation antihistamines			
	Diphenhydramine[d]	H	Second-generation ("non-sedating") antihistamines: cetirizine, loratadine
	Chlorpheniramine	H	
	Clemastine	H	
	Hydroxyzine	H	
Anti-vertigo antihistamines			
	Meclizine	H	
	Dramamine	H	
Bladder antispasmodics			
	Trospium	H	Mirabegron (beta-3 agonist)
	Oxybutynin	H	Darifenacin, solifenacin[e]
	Tolterodine	H	
Antiparkinson medications			
	Benztropine	H	
	Amantadine	M	

Adapted from Ref. [15]

[a] *M* moderate, *H* high

[b] May cause QTc prolongation

[c] Considered low risk by one anticholinergic scale, but has been associated with delirium in the elderly in case reports

[d] Diphenhydramine is also found in over-the-counter (nonprescription) sleep aids

[e] M3 selective, not associated with cognitive impairment; may cause constipation and dry mouth

It has been known for some time that first-generation antihistamines (e.g., diphenhydramine), which cross the blood–brain barrier, bind to brain histamine receptors and, especially in geriatric patients, can cause a range of symptoms from sedation to impaired cognition and delirium. Validated scales quantifying the risk of anticholinergic side effects of medications have been developed. Using such a scale, investigators in Australia demonstrated a monotonic relationship between the number of moderate to strong anticholinergic medications and the risk of hospitalization for major NCDs or confusion. Compared to non-anticholinergic medications, the adjusted incident risk ratio went from 1.17 for one anticholinergic medication to 3.87 for three anticholinergic medications [16]. A dose-dependent association has been found between long-term, cumulative exposure to anticholinergic medications and the development of NCDs in general and Alzheimer disease in particular [17]. In addition to adverse central nervous system (CNS) side effects, anticholinergic medications contribute to constipation, urinary retention, dry mouth, dry eyes, provocation or exacerbation of narrow-angle glaucoma, and tachycardia, all in a dose-dependent fashion. Numerous drugs have mild anticholinergic activity that individually confers little risk of an ADE, but in combination can raise the total anticholinergic burden (see Table 12.5) [15].

Case Analysis 1 Ms. G was taking a potent anticholinergic medication (oxybutynin) plus a mild anticholinergic medication (furosemide). In addition to these, she was given the anticholinergic antiemetic prochlorperazine. When she became delirious, her agitation was managed with olanzapine, itself a strongly anticholinergic drug. For delirium patients, olanzapine is often chosen due to a lower likelihood of increased QTc interval when compared to other antipsychotics, but its anticholiner-

Table 12.5 Drugs with mild anticholinergic activity that can add to the total anticholinergic burden

Psychotropic drugs	Cardiac drugs (include diuretics)	Miscellaneous	(Indication)
Alprazolam	Atenolol	Codeine	(Pain)
Bupropion	Captopril	Colchicine	(Gout)
Clorazepate	Digoxin	Hydrocortisone	(Inflammation)
Diazepam	Chlorthalidone	Morphine[a]	(Pain)
Fluvoxamine	Dipyridamole	Timolol malleate	(Ocular topical for glaucoma – some systemic absorption)
Haloperidol	Furosemide	Theophylline[b]	(Bronchodilator)
Trazodone	Hydralazine	Warfarin	(Anticoagulant)
	Isosorbide		
	Metoprolol		
	Quinidine[b]		
	Triamterene		

Adapted from Ref. [15]

[a]Not recommended in elderly due to decreased renal clearance

[b]Rarely prescribed due to high potential for toxicity and drug interactions

gic burden (as illustrated in this case) can actually increase the risk of delirium. The opioids certainly added to the risk of delirium, but the quartet of anticholinergic medications contributed both to its onset and duration.

Clinical Recommendations
Be alert to the total anticholinergic burden and either discontinue nonessential anticholinergics or change to safer alternatives whenever possible. Among atypical antipsychotics commonly used for delirium, risperidone, quetiapine, ziprasidone, and aripiprazole have less anticholinergic effects and are often good alternatives to olanzapine, especially if the patient has been exposed to other anticholinergic medications. Consult with a pharmacist if unsure of a drug's anticholinergic properties.

12.3.2 Treatment-Induced Diabetes Mellitus and Metabolic Syndrome

Case Vignette 2 Mr. M was a 71-year-old mildly obese male (BMI 31 kg/m^2) with a long history of schizophrenia, who was switched from risperidone to olanzapine 5 mg at bedtime, after developing akathisia and mild gynecomastia which were attributed to risperidone. His past medical history was significant for hypertension and benign prostatic hypertrophy, but there was no history of diabetes mellitus. Initially, his psychotic illness was well controlled, but after 3 months, he developed recurrent auditory hallucinations directing him to harm himself, and he was brought to the ED by his son. After evaluation by the psychiatrist on duty, he was admitted to the acute inpatient unit on a psychiatric commitment order for danger to self. His olanzapine was increased to 10 mg at bedtime with an additional PRN dose of 2.5 mg PO q6h for psychosis. His random blood glucose in the ED was elevated at 142 mg/dL (7.89 mmol/L), but no insulin was administered.

After 5 days, Mr. M's hallucinations had improved significantly, but he developed polyuria, polydipsia, lethargy, and new confusion. Laboratory studies revealed normal electrolytes but a serum glucose of 300 mg/dL (16.67 mmol/L). Ten units of regular insulin were administered and he was placed on an insulin sliding scale. Diabetes mellitus associated with olanzapine was diagnosed. The olanzapine was immediately held and the patient's treatment was changed to aripiprazole 10 mg qAM and 5 mg PO q6h PRN for psychosis. His fasting blood glucose renormalized within 4 days and his psychotic symptoms continued to be well controlled. A hemoglobin A1C was obtained that showed chronic glucose intolerance (6.2 %).

Patients taking atypical antipsychotics have higher rates of metabolic syndrome, hyperlipidemia, and diabetes mellitus than those taking conventional antipsychotics or mood stabilizers. Using pharmacy and medical claims data for older patients residing in the western United States, Erickson et al. performed a cross-sectional, case–control study to ascertain whether atypical antipsychotics were associated with an increased odds ratio of having new treatment-dependent diabetes mellitus. After adjustment for confounders, exposure to atypical antipsychotics was associated with a 32 % greater odds ratio of diabetes mellitus, compared to individuals not taking these agents [18]. However, other pharmacoepidemiologic studies have provided conflicting information, possibly due to limitations in study design. Meta-analysis of these studies is made difficult by significant study heterogeneity. At present, the preponderance of evidence suggests that risperidone and quetiapine do not increase the risk of diabetes mellitus, compared to conventional antipsychotics, whereas clozapine and especially olanzapine do [19]. However, using conventional antipsychotics as the frame of reference may be misleading. Compared to remote users, geriatric patients currently taking an atypical antipsychotic had an adjusted odds ratio (aOR) of 1.44 for a hospital visit due to hyperglycemia. Geriatric patients using a typical (conventional) antipsychotic had an even greater, 2.86 aOR of a hospital visit for hyperglycemia [20]. The on-call psychiatrist should not assume that the risk of antipsychotic hyperglycemia requires chronic use and develops over time. In fact, significant hyperglycemia can develop in just days [21], especially in patients with obesity or a prior history of diabetes mellitus.

Case Analysis 2 Mr. M's new-onset hyperglycemia occurred within days of the dose increase of olanzapine. Risk factors for hyperglycemia included his borderline obesity and elevated random blood sugar. A routine fasting blood glucose daily or every other day might have detected his hyperglycemia before he became symptomatic. Obtaining a baseline hemoglobin A_1C at admission, once his risk factors for diabetes mellitus were known, would have reinforced the need for close glucose monitoring.

Clinical Recommendations
In the hospital setting, the blood glucose should be monitored before and after initiation of a routinely scheduled antipsychotic, especially clozapine and olanzapine. Patients taking antipsychotics should be screened for metabolic effects periodically as outpatients and always upon admission to the ED, hospital, or inpatient psychiatric unit.

12.3.3 The Hazards of Lithium in the Hospitalized Older Patient

Case Vignette 3 Ms. H, a 73-year-old obese woman with a 30-year history of bipolar disorder and chronic lithium (Li) use, was admitted to the ward medicine service for cellulitis of the right lower extremity due to poorly controlled chronic venous stasis. As an outpatient, she was prescribed levothyroxine 0.125 mg for hypothyroidism, ramipril 5 mg daily for hypertension, Li carbonate 300 mg bid, and hydrocodone 5 mg/acetaminophen (paracetamol) 325 mg three times daily as needed for pain. On admission, her serum sodium was 146 mEq/L (146 mmol/L), serum creatinine 1.3 mg/dL (113 μmol/L), and Li level 0.5 mEq/L (0.5 mmol/L); therapeutic range for general population was 0.5–1.2 mEq/L (0.5–1.2 mmol/L).

With the exception of the opioids, she was continued on her home medications. In addition, she was started on intravenous antibiotics and intravenous furosemide 20 mg daily to control the edema, along with a low-sodium diet and a 1.5 l/day fluid restriction.

In the hospital, she was restless, excessively talkative with loud, pressured speech, and got up to pace the halls frequently, despite instructions to keep her legs elevated. An urgent psychiatry consultation was requested, which recommended risperidone 2 mg at bedtime plus a change in her Li carbonate to 450 mg bid. The patient complained bitterly of chronic knee pain and refused plain acetaminophen (paracetamol), claiming it was ineffective. The admitting medical team was reluctant to prescribe opioids and ordered naproxen sodium 250 mg every 12 h PRN for osteoarthritis pain, adding a proton-pump inhibitor to prevent gastritis.

On hospital day 3, she was noted to be slurring her speech and spilling food from her fork at mealtime. On examination, she was confused, dysarthric, ataxic, and had a resting hand tremor. A follow-up chemistry panel was ordered, which revealed elevated levels for serum sodium of 151 mEq/L (151 mmol/L) and a creatinine of 2.6 mg/dL (230 μmol/L). Her Li level had risen to 1.8 mEq/L (1.8 mmol/L).

Case Analysis 3 Lithium (Li) remains a first-line mood stabilizer treatment for bipolar disorder, as well as an augmentation agent for treatment-resistant unipolar depression. Chronic use can lead to chronic renal insufficiency, polyuria, and nephrogenic diabetes insipidus with difficulty concentrating urine, hypothyroidism, and hyperparathyroidism (with elevated serum calcium concentrations) [22, 23]. Age-associated physiologic changes increase the risk of Li toxicity. The glomerular filtration rate declines with age but is balanced by decreasing muscle mass and reduced production of creatinine, which may result in a normal range serum creatinine. Therefore, clinicians should not rely upon the serum creatinine alone as an indicator of renal function and should calculate the creatinine clearance. In healthy younger adults, polyuria results in compensatory polydipsia, but in the older patient, the thirst response can be blunted, causing a net loss in intravascular volume that may result in prerenal azotemia (elevated BUN to creatinine ratio) and an increased risk of dehydration and Li toxicity. The signs and symptoms of Li toxicity can be attributed easily to age-associated conditions. Dry mouth from dehydration can be mistakenly attributed to anticholinergic medication or sicca syndrome, a slight tremor or unstable gait to age-associated neurological changes. Common comorbid conditions among the older patients or their treatment increase the risk of Li toxicity directly, as exemplified by polyuria caused by hyperglycemia, loop diuretics for heart failure, NSAIDs for pain, and angiotensin-converting enzyme (ACE) inhibitors or angiotensin receptor blockers for hypertension. Confusion may be attributed to underlying psychosis or severe depression rather than to hypernatremia, delaying the recognition of Li toxicity.

Chronic use of loop diuretics (e.g., furosemide, bumetanide, torsemide) and ACE inhibitors each has been associated with a ≥60 % relative risk increase of hospitalization for Li toxicity in older patients; this risk increases roughly sixfold when these drugs have been newly dispensed within the past month [24], underscoring the need to closely follow Li levels when they are prescribed.

12.3.4 Recognizing, Managing, and Avoiding Neuroleptic Malignant Syndrome and Serotonin Syndrome

Case Vignette 4 Mr. A was a 71-year-old veteran with a history of schizophrenia, for which he had been taking risperidone 0.5 mg twice daily with good results. Due to problems with housing and inadequate social support, he began to experience mood instability, for which he was started on Li carbonate 300 mg BID, resulting in a therapeutic Li level. Paranoid delusions redeveloped, and his risperidone was increased to 2 mg BID over the course of 1 week. After 3 days on 4 mg per day of risperidone, he presented to the ED with acute changes in mental status. On exam, he was febrile to 40.5 °C, hypertensive to 170/100 mmHg, tachycardic (115 BPM), diaphoretic, and had severe, "lead-pipe" rigidity of his muscles with decreased deep tendon reflexes. He was agitated and confused. His initial creatinine was 1.8 mg/dL (159 μmol/L), compared to a baseline of 1.1 mg/dL (97 μmol/L). A creatine phosphokinase (CPK) level was 3,500 U/L (high). A presumptive diagnosis of neuroleptic malignant syndrome (NMS) was made. Both the risperidone and Li were held. He was admitted to the ICU for aggressive supportive care, given lorazepam 1 mg IV as needed for agitation, dantrolene (4 mg/kg/day PO/NGT) for his hypertonicity, and aggressive IV fluids. After 4 days in the ICU, he was transferred to the medical ward for 3 more days, where he received lorazepam 1 mg PRN every 6 h for agitation. As he recovered from his delirium, he developed a recurrence of his psychotic symptoms and was then discharged to a psychiatric inpatient unit. After 2 weeks of CPK monitoring, during which his CPK remained in the normal range, he was started on quetiapine 50 mg in the AM and 150 mg at bedtime. His CPK continued to stay within normal limits.

Case Vignette 5 Ms. H was a 79-year-old woman with a long-standing history of anxiety and depression for which she had been on a stable dose of sertraline 200 mg daily. After her daughters encouraged her to move into an assisted living facility, her anxiety worsened and she complained of severe insomnia. Her primary care physician added buspirone 10 mg tid for the anxiety, along with trazodone 50 mg at bedtime for insomnia. Because of persistent insomnia, the dose of trazodone was increased to 100 mg and then to 150 mg at bedtime. After 1 week on this regimen, she presented to the ED with altered mental status. Vital signs revealed a temperature of 41.0 °C, blood pressure of 190/88 mmHg, and pulse of 110 BPM. Her neurological exam was nonfocal, but notable for tremors in both hands, increased motor tone, hyperreflexia, and bilateral ankle clonus. Laboratory exam revealed a creatine kinase of 1,055 U/L (17.6 μkat/L) and a serum sodium of 121 mEq/L (121 mmol/L) with increased urinary osmolality. She was diagnosed with serotonin syndrome (SS) and the syndrome of inappropriate antidiuretic hormone (SIADH) and admitted to the ICU. There, all serotonin agonists (sertraline, buspirone, and trazodone) were stopped, she was placed on a 1.0 L/day fluid restriction, and quetiapine 25 mg PO q6h PRN was administered as needed for agitation. Within 6 days, her serum sodium normalized and all symptoms of SS resolved. Quetiapine PRN was discontinued. After discharge, she was switched to mirtazapine 7.5 mg at bedtime with periodic monitoring of her serum sodium.

Neuroleptic malignant syndrome (NMS) and serotonin syndrome (SS) belong to a group of dysautonomias that are potentially life-threatening adverse drug reactions that can be mistaken for one another. NMS is regarded as an idiosyncratic illness due to the use of dopamine-blocking agents (most commonly antipsychotic medication) that may appear suddenly during the course of treatment, although change in antipsychotic agent, high doses, and the rapidity and magnitude of upward titration are considered to be risk factors [25]. The addition of a mood stabilizer such as Li may also increase the risk of NMS. SS represents direct toxicity from serotonergic agents. Both syndromes can present with mental status changes, autonomic dysfunction, hypertension, tachycardia, hyperthermia (>40 °C), and increased motor tone. For each illness, not all features need to be present for a clinical diagnosis. Principal characteristics showing the similarities and differences between NMS and SS are shown in Table 12.6. Due to similarities in presentation [26], differentiating the two requires a careful review of medication exposure (including over-the-counter and "street" drugs) and examination for key differentiating features. An important differentiating exam finding is hyperreflexia/clonus in SS (vs. typically decreased reflexes in NMS). In the psychiatric patient, coadministration of both an antipsychotic and a serotonergic antidepressant is common, so that the onset of symptoms relative to the initiation or dose increase of an antipsychotic or antidepressant can be helpful. However, this association only provides a clue and should not be considered definitive. Clinicians should avoid premature closure in making a diagnosis of NMS or SS and should carefully weigh all clinical evidence.

12.3.4.1 Neuroleptic Malignant Syndrome

NMS is believed to be precipitated by the unavailability/depletion of dopamine in the CNS or by the blockade of dopamine type 2 receptors (D_2). Central dopaminergic blockade has been advanced as the best possible explanation, as antipsychotic drugs block dopamine receptors in multiple regions of the CNS, including the

Table 12.6 Similarities and differences between the neuroleptic malignant and serotonin syndromes

Condition	Vital Signs	Skin	Pupils	Oral Mucosa	Bowel Sounds	Muscle Tone	Reflexes	Mental Status
Neuroleptic Malignant Syndrome	Hypertension Tachycardia Tachypnea Hyperthermia (T° > 40° C)	Diaphoresis Pallor	Mydriasis	Sialorrhea	Normal or decreased	Marked rigidity in all muscle groups	Slow, depressed	Alert to stupor and coma Delirium
Serotonin Syndrome	Hypertension Tachycardia Tachypnea Hyperthermia (T° > 40° C)	Diaphoresis	Mydriasis	Sialorrhea	Hyperactive	Increased, primarily in lower extremities	Hyperreflexia Clonus	Coma Delirium (usually agitated)

Adapted from Ref. [27]

The shaded columns represent findings that predictably differentiate the two hypothalamus, corpus striatum, the basal ganglia, and spinal areas. All antipsychotics, not just high-affinity D_2 receptor drugs, have been associated with NMS, including clozapine, quetiapine, aripiprazole, and olanzapine. High-dose antipsychotics and a rapid rate of upward dose titration increase the risk of NMS. More than half of reported cases have involved the coadministration of two or more psychotropics [25], but it is unclear whether this association represents potentiation or simply reflects the severity of psychiatric illness. NMS, or an NMS-like syndrome, has been seen after the abrupt withdrawal of dopaminergic drugs for Parkinson's disease.

12.3.4.2 Serotonin Syndrome

Because SS is both rare and underdiagnosed, reliable data on its incidence are lacking. However, the widespread use of SSRI and SNRI antidepressants, together with the frequent administration of drugs which are serotonin agonists or which interfere with the metabolism of SSRIs, SNRIs, or MAO inhibitors, suggests that the risk of SS is rising. Although the majority of cases of SS result from increased CNS serotonin levels from the addition of a second (or subsequent) serotonin agonist, roughly 40 % of cases arise from a single agent [28]. Table 12.7 lists medications which can increase brain serotonin levels. In patients receiving a serotonergic psychotropic agent, non-phenanthrene opioids should be avoided or discontinued whenever possible, including tramadol, methadone, propoxyphene, meperidine, and fentanyl. The phenanthrene opioids, such as hydrocodone, morphine, and codeine, can be used safely with serotonin antidepressants [29]. Serotonergic pain medications (especially tramadol) by themselves have been associated with SS [28]. Dextromethorphan (a cough suppressant found in many over-the-counter cold remedies) also can precipitate SS. The anticonvulsant carbamazepine and the antibiotic erythromycin (but not azithromycin) inhibit the metabolism of SSRIs. The oxazolidinone class of antibiotics (linezolid, tedizolid phosphate) are weak MAO-B inhibitors, with the potential to induce SS in patients receiving a serotonin-enhancing antidepressant [30].

SS can present insidiously across a continuum of severity with only one or a few of the characteristics. Mild, subacute cases can be missed, the symptoms being attributed to common morbidities in the older patients (e.g., hypertension, infection) or to the underlying psychiatric disorder in the case of akathisia and anxiety. In more severe cases, tremor can be suppressed by hypertonicity (see Fig. 12.1) [27].

12.3.4.3 Basic Principles of Treatment

Patients with NMS and severe cases of SS require close medical and nursing management and should be transferred to the ED or to the intensive care unit.

Care for NMS is supportive and requires discontinuation of the antipsychotic. Because 30–50 % of NMS patients who are later re-challenged with an antipsychotic will experience recurrence of NMS [25], simple dose reduction is not recommended as part of initial treatment. In NMS, the dopamine agonists bromocriptine or amantadine can help to counteract the D_2 blockade, but bromocriptine increases the risk of SS and may worsen psychosis. Amantadine may precipitate delirium in

Table 12.7 Medications that may contribute to serotonin syndrome

Drug class	Drugs
Antidepressants	SSRIs
	SNRIs
	Trazodone
	Tricyclic antidepressants
	MAOIs
	St. John's wort (*Hypericum perforatum*)
Anxiolytics	Buspirone
Mood stabilizers	Lithium
	Valproic acid
	Carbamazepine
Amphetamines and derivatives	Dextroamphetamine
	Methylphenidate
	Sibutramine (Meridia, withdrawn in the USA)
	3,4-Methylenedioxymethamphetamine (Ecstasy)
	Methamphetamine
Analgesics	Fentanyl
	Meperidine
	Tramadol
Muscle relaxants	Cyclobenzaprine
Antiemetics	Ondansetron
	Metoclopramide
Anti-migraine drugs	Triptans
	Ergot alkaloids
Miscellaneous	Cocaine
	Linezolid
	Tedizolid
	5-Hydroxytryptophan
	Tryptophan

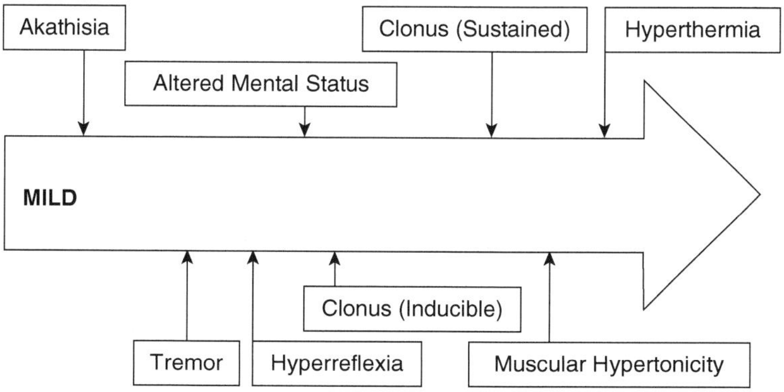

Fig. 12.1 Spectrum of severity of serotonin syndrome (Adapted from Ref. [27])

older patients and thus may cloud evaluation of the mental status. For severe agitation, intermediate-acting benzodiazepines may be necessary, despite the risk of exacerbating or prolonging confusion.

For SS, the first step in treatment is discontinuing or reducing the doses of the offending drugs. Even when the precipitating agent appears to have been identified (e.g., the recent start of tramadol for pain in a patient on a stable dose of citalopram), the antidepressant also should be stopped or its dose reduced to hasten recovery, despite the risk of serotonin withdrawal. Case reports have suggested that the serotonin and histamine antagonist, cyproheptadine, which is used in carcinoid syndrome, can be helpful if the patient can take per os. Atypical antipsychotics can be used to block the effect of excess serotonin at the postsynaptic 5HT2 receptor.

In both NMS and SS, vital signs should be monitored frequently. Severe hyperpyrexia (>40 °C) can lead to seizures and irreversible brain damage and requires aggressive external cooling with a cooling blanket or ice packed around the patient. Severe muscle rigidity induced by involuntary isotonic muscle contractions can lead to rhabdomyolysis, especially in NMS, so muscle relaxants are often indicated. Dantrolene is more effective than benzodiazepines and is associated with relatively lower risk of inducing delirium. Serum electrolytes and a complete blood count should be obtained in all patients and serially monitored. A creatine kinase level (CK) should be obtained. Elevated CK (>1,000 U/L/16.7 μkat/L) reflects significant muscle injury, which releases myoglobin that is filtered by the kidney. The toxicity of high levels of myoglobin to the renal tubules can precipitate acute renal failure, especially in older patients with chronic kidney disease. Rhabdomyolysis requires close medical management involving intravenous fluids and diuresis, alkalinization of the urine in severe cases, and monitoring for heart failure.

Case Analysis 4 Mr. A's NMS likely resulted from the rapid increase in risperidone; the addition of Li may have contributed to the NMS, although its role has been disputed [25]. He had significant muscle rigidity causing rhabdomyolysis and hyporeflexia, the latter feature distinguishing NMS from SS. Dantrolene helped the muscle rigidity and its consequences (rhabdomyolysis and hyperpyrexia).

Case Analysis 5 Ms. H experienced classic SS due to three concurrent serotonergic drugs (sertraline, buspirone, and trazodone). Of note, she also experienced clinically significant SIADH, to which both the SSRI and trazodone likely contributed. The degree of hyponatremia was sufficient to have independently caused delirium.

12.3.5 Important Comments About SIADH

A rapid lowering of the serum sodium into the 120 s (mEq/L/mmol/L), or a serum sodium of ≤120 mEq/L (120 mmol/L), may precipitate delirium and/or seizures due to brain swelling. Hyponatremic seizures represent a medical emergency and require transfer to the ED or medical ICU. In the presence of symptomatic low serum sodium, urine and serum electrolytes and urine and serum osmolality should be obtained stat. An inappropriately high urine osmolality (usually much higher than serum osmolality) is consistent with SIADH. Diuretics, especially loop diuretics like furosemide, can cause hyponatremia but do not increase the urine osmolality.

12.3.5.1 Treatment of SIADH

In patients with hyponatremia-associated seizures, the sodium concentration should be increased rapidly by 4–6 mEq/L over 4–6 h, but then not more than 9 mEq/L = mmol/L over 24 h and 18 mEq/48 h. Initially, 100 ml of 3 % hypertonic saline can be given over 1 h in severe cases, pending transfer to the ED or ICU. Serum electrolytes should be obtained every 2 h initially, then every 4–6 h until the serum sodium is >125 mEq/L, since a rate of rise in the serum sodium faster than the above parameters can lead to myelinolysis. Asymptomatic or mildly symptomatic hyponatremia (e.g., lethargy, confusion) can be treated with aggressive fluid restriction pending an internal medicine consultation (800 ml fluids per 24 h). Drugs contributing to hyponatremia should be stopped or at least reduced as much as safely possible. Salt tablets can be combined with fluid restriction. However, in SIADH, physiologic sodium handling is not affected. Patients susceptible to heart failure should not receive supplemental salt tablets, and intravenous 3 % saline should be administered only under close medical supervision on a medical unit.

12.3.6 Miscellaneous Adverse Reactions to Psychotropic Medications

12.3.6.1 SSRIs and Gastrointestinal Bleeding

Serotonin plays an important role in platelet aggregation, and serotonin reuptake inhibitors can reduce platelet serotonin by up to 90 % [26]. Therefore, it follows that when SSRIs are taken in a patient predisposed to gastritis or peptic ulcer disease, for example, through the ingestion of nonsteroidal anti-inflammatory drugs, or when taken together with an antiplatelet agent like aspirin, the risk of gastrointestinal bleeding rises [31]. SSRIs have also been associated with an increased risk of stroke from subarachnoid hemorrhage [32].

12.3.6.2 QTc Prolongation and Ventricular Arrhythmias

Case Vignette 6 Ms. R was a 68-year-old woman with a history of paroxysmal atrial fibrillation, diabetes mellitus with neuropathy, and major depression. Her medications included metoprolol succinate 25 mg daily, amiodarone 200 mg daily, warfarin 2.5 mg daily, metformin 500 mg twice daily, and amitriptyline 50 mg at bedtime. Her psychiatrist recently increased her fluoxetine from 20 to 40 mg daily. After a witnessed fall with loss of consciousness, she was admitted through the ED to a telemetry bed for a work-up of syncope. Her serum electrolytes and magnesium were within normal limits and her INR was 1.8 (subtherapeutic). An ECG showed atrial fibrillation at a rate of 80 BPM with frequent premature atrial contractions and a QTc of 520 ms. During the first 24 h of telemetry, her heart rate consistently was below 100 BPM, but she showed frequent premature ventricular contractions (PVCs) and one asymptomatic six-beat run of ventricular tachycardia. An urgent psychiatry consultation was requested to review her psychotropic medications.

A prolonged corrected QT interval (QTc) on the electrocardiogram (>450 ms in men, >470 ms in women) increases the risk of a potentially life-threatening ventricular tachycardia known as torsades de pointes (TdP). In addition to congenital QTc prolongation, the QT interval can be prolonged from bradycardia, hypocalcemia, hypokalemia, and hypomagnesemia, the latter two frequently seen as a complication of loop diuretics. Age itself has been associated with prolongation of the QTc. Although case reports suggest an association between QTc prolongation and phenothiazines, haloperidol (and its cousin, droperidol), and the second-generation antipsychotics (risperidone, quetiapine, ziprasidone, and clozapine, less so olanzapine and aripiprazole), epidemiologic evidence has not shown a consistent, predictable class effect with these drugs [33]. Moreover, the incidence of associated TdP or sudden death is very low. Tricyclic antidepressants have been linked to QTc prolongation [34], as has fluoxetine and citalopram (leading to a lowering of the maximum dose of citalopram to 20 mg in older patients). Escitalopram has not been clearly linked to QTc prolongation, but because it is the s-enantiomer of citalopram, Health Canada advises caution when used in older patients. Sertraline and paroxetine are associated with a lower degree of risk.

The risk of TdP and sudden cardiac death may be increased by the coadministration of common medications known to prolong the QTc interval. Of importance are the macrolide antibiotics (erythromycin, clarithromycin, and azithromycin), chloroquine (an anti-malarial commonly used as an immunomodulator), the antihistamine astemizole, methadone, the antiemetic ondansetron, and multiple antiarrhythmics (amiodarone, dronedarone, sotalol, procainamide, quinidine, disopyramide). There are case reports of galantamine and donepezil causing QTc prolongation, but the association is not definitive.

Case Analysis 6 Ms. R was taking three QTc-prolonging medications, amiodarone, amitriptyline, and fluoxetine, resulting in a QTc of 520 ms. The etiology of her syncope could have been due to atrial fibrillation with unrecognized rapid ventricular response, but the prolonged QTc and ventricular tachycardia suggest that she had experienced non-sustained TdP. Given that she was in atrial fibrillation despite amiodarone, the psychiatrist could have questioned the rationale for continuing the amiodarone. An additional concern is the coadministration (in any patient) of fluoxetine, paroxetine, or fluvoxamine and any tricyclic antidepressant. Due to DDIs, these three SSRIs can increase TCA levels, leading to TCA-referable side effects. As such, if patients are to continue to receive TCA at any dose and for any indication, any of these three SSRIs should be stopped and an alternative SSRI (e.g., sertraline) substituted. The amitriptyline and fluoxetine were stopped. After 3 days, her QTc had improved to 480 ms and fewer PVCs were seen on telemetry. She was discharged home with plans to visit her psychiatrist in 2 weeks for consideration of a replacement SSRI.

Psychiatrists should follow the following guidelines when considering a QTc-prolonging medication:

Clinical Recommendations

- Before prescribing a QTc-prolonging drug, obtain a baseline ECG.
- Reevaluate the need for the medication if the QTc is lengthened; select a safer alternative whenever possible.
- Avoid concurrent use of more than one QTc-prolonging medication by stopping nonessential QTc-prolonging drugs whenever possible.
- Monitor the QTc closely after starting the medication and after dose increases.

Key Points

- Table 12.8 provides a summary of key points to remember regarding psychotropic medications for the older patients.
- Prescribing psychotropic medication to older patients represents a major challenge due to the prevalence of polypharmacy, the potential for adverse drug events due to age-associated changes in pharmacokinetics and pharmacodynamics, and complex drug–drug interactions.
- Adverse events like torsades de pointes, neuroleptic malignant syndrome, and serotonin syndrome can be directly life-threatening, while complications like syncope and falls can lead to injuries resulting in disability, death, and impaired quality of life.
- All older patients seen in psychiatric consultation require a careful review of their medications and assessment of the risk for drug interactions and side effects before prescribing.
- Prudent prescribing is essential, which includes minimization of inappropriate medications based on accepted criteria (e.g., the Beers Criteria).

Table 12.8 Summary of common adverse drug events by class of psychotropic medication

Drug class	Examples	Notes		
		Side effect concerns	Conditions with increased risk for adverse events	Drug combinations with risk for serious drug interactions
Antipsychotics	Phenothiazines Haloperidol Atypical antipsychotics	EPS (especially dystonia and akathisia), orthostatic hypotension, sedation, anticholinergic effects, diabetes mellitus, QTc prolongation, hyperprolactinemia	Parkinsonism, epilepsy, long QTc	Multiple antipsychotics (initiate therapy ¼–½ usual starting dose and titrate gradually) Anticholinergic agents Serotonergic agents
Antidepressants	Tricyclics (e.g., amitriptyline)	Anticholinergic effects, increased fall risk	Glaucoma, urinary retention, delirium, SIADH	Serotonergic agents
	Bupropion	Lowers seizure threshold	Active seizure disorder	Other drugs which lower seizure threshold, serotonergic agents
	SNRI (e.g., venlafaxine)	Akathisia, torsades de pointes, mild anticholinergic effects with full dose of venlafaxine SIADH Bleeding (do not use post-hemorrhagic CVA, with thrombocytopenia. Use with caution with aspirin or nonsteroidal anti-inflammatory drugs) Hepatotoxicity with duloxetine Do not use duloxetine in renal or hepatic failure	QT prolongation, hyponatremia, SIADH from other causes	Antipsychotics, serotonergic agents
	SSRI (paroxetine)	Cause/worsen delirium (due to anticholinergic effect; other SSRIs not anticholinergic) SIADH Bleeding (do not use in post-hemorrhagic CVA, with thrombocytopenia. Use with caution with aspirin or nonsteroidal anti-inflammatory drugs)	Cognitive impairment, hyponatremia/SIADH from other causes	Other drugs with strong anticholinergic effects, serotonergic agents, fluoxetine has very long duration, coadministered TCAs (primarily an issue with paroxetine, fluoxetine, fluvoxamine), SSRI can lead to elevated TCA levels and thus TCA side effects

Anxiolytics	Benzodiazepines	Dizziness, sedation, falls, fractures, confusion, and disorientation	Unsteady gait, history of falls Pre-existing cognitive impairment	Cumulative effect with other CNS depressants; caution with long-acting drugs
Sedative hypnotic	"Z drugs," i.e., zopiclone, zolpidem	Daytime sedation	Chronic use should be avoided in elderly (see Beers Criteria)	Cumulative effect with other CNS depressants
Mood stabilizers	Carbamazepine	Sedation, fatigue, ataxia, tremor, blurred vision	Liver impairment, hyponatremia, narrow therapeutic index; therapeutic levels may be increased by CYP3A4 inhibitors	Cumulative effect with other drugs which cause confusion, anticholinergic agents
	Valproic acid	Hepatotoxicity, hyperammonemia, thrombocytopenia, pancreatitis	Liver disease, urea cycle enzyme deficiencies, history of pancreatitis, thrombocytopenia	Interaction with carbamazepine
Cholinesterase inhibitors	Donepezil, rivastigmine, galantamine	Gastrointestinal intolerance (anorexia, nausea, diarrhea), syncope, fatigue, vivid nightmares	Bradycardia (heart rate < 60) or drugs which slow heart rate (digoxin, beta-blockers, verapamil) Epilepsy	Other drugs with CNS depressant activity

References

1. Gnjidic D, Hilmer SN, Blyth FM, et al. Polypharmacy cutoff and outcomes: five or more medicines were used to identify community-dwelling older men at risk of different adverse outcomes. J Clin Epidemiol. 2012;65(9):989–95.
2. Hanlon JT, Pieper CF, Hajjar ER, et al. Incidence and predictors of all and preventable adverse drug reactions in frail elderly persons after hospital stay. J Gerontol A Biol Sci Med Sci. 2006;61(5):511–5.
3. Obreli Neto PR, Nobili A, de Lyra Jr DP, et al. Incidence and predictors of adverse drug reactions caused by drug-drug interactions in elderly outpatients: a prospective cohort study. J Pharm Pharm Sci. 2012;15(2):332–43.
4. Wu C, Bell CM, Wodchis WP. Incidence and economic burden of adverse drug reactions among elderly patients in Ontario emergency departments: a retrospective study. Drug Saf. 2012;35(9):769–81.
5. Marcum ZA, Amuan ME, Hanlon JT, et al. Prevalence of unplanned hospitalizations caused by adverse drug reactions in older veterans. J Am Geriatr Soc. 2012;60(1):34–41.
6. Morgan TK, Williamson M, Pirotta M, Stewart K, Myers SP, Barnes J. A national census of medicines use: a 24-hour snapshot of Australians aged 50 years and older. Med J Aust. 2012;196(1):50–3.
7. Lin CF, Wang CY, Bai CH. Polypharmacy, aging and potential drug-drug interactions in outpatients in Taiwan: a retrospective computerized screening study. Drugs Aging. 2011;28(3):219–25.
8. Wolff JL, Starfield B, Anderson G. Prevalence, expenditures, and complications of multiple chronic conditions in the elderly. Arch Intern Med. 2002;162(20):2269–76.
9. Lund BC, Carnahan RM, Egge JA, Chrischilles EA, Kaboli PJ. Inappropriate prescribing predicts adverse drug events in older adults. Ann Pharmacother. 2010;44(6):957–63.
10. By the American Geriatrics Society Beers Criteria Update Expert P. American Geriatrics Society 2015 updated beers criteria for potentially inappropriate medication use in older adults. J Am Geriatr Soc. 2015;63(11):2227–2246.
11. O'Mahony D, O'Sullivan D, Byrne S, O'Connor MN, Ryan C, Gallagher P. STOPP/START criteria for potentially inappropriate prescribing in older people: version 2. Age Ageing. 2015;44(2):213–8.
12. Hamilton H, Gallagher P, Ryan C, Byrne S, O'Mahony D. Potentially inappropriate medications defined by STOPP criteria and the risk of adverse drug events in older hospitalized patients. Arch Intern Med. 2011;171(11):1013–9.
13. GeriatricsCareOnline.org. iGeriatrics-Mobile App. 2015. http://geriatricscareonline.org/ProductAbstract/igeriatrics-mobile-app/B019/?param2=search. Accessed 6 Oct 2015.
14. Mulsant BH, Pollock BG, Kirshner M, Shen C, Dodge H, Ganguli M. Serum anticholinergic activity in a community-based sample of older adults: relationship with cognitive performance. Arch Gen Psychiatry. 2003;60(2):198–203.
15. Carnahan RM, Lund BC, Perry PJ, Pollock BG, Culp KR. The Anticholinergic Drug Scale as a measure of drug-related anticholinergic burden: associations with serum anticholinergic activity. J Clin Pharmacol. 2006;46(12):1481–6.
16. Kalisch Ellett LM, Pratt NL, Ramsay EN, Barratt JD, Roughead EE. Multiple anticholinergic medication use and risk of hospital admission for confusion or dementia. J Am Geriatr Soc. 2014;62(10):1916–22.
17. Gray SL, Anderson ML, Dublin S, et al. Cumulative use of strong anticholinergics and incident dementia: a prospective cohort study. JAMA Intern Med. 2015;175(3):401–7.
18. Erickson SC, Le L, Zakharyan A, et al. New-onset treatment-dependent diabetes mellitus and hyperlipidemia associated with atypical antipsychotic use in older adults without schizophrenia or bipolar disorder. J Am Geriatr Soc. 2012;60(3):474–9.
19. Ramaswamy K, Masand PS, Nasrallah HA. Do certain atypical antipsychotics increase the risk of diabetes? A critical review of 17 pharmacoepidemiologic studies. Ann Clin Psychiatry. 2006;18(3):183–94.

20. Lipscombe LL, Levesque LE, Gruneir A, et al. Antipsychotic drugs and the risk of hyperglycemia in older adults without diabetes: a population-based observational study. Am J Geriatr Psychiatry. 2011;19(12):1026–33.
21. Bishara A, Phan SV, Young HN, Liao TV. Glucose disturbances and atypical antipsychotic use in the intensive care unit. J Pharm Pract. May 6;2015.
22. Rej S, Herrmann N, Shulman K. The effects of lithium on renal function in older adults – a systematic review. J Geriatr Psychiatry Neurol. 2012;25(1):51–61.
23. Shine B, McKnight RF, Leaver L, Geddes JR. Long-term effects of lithium on renal, thyroid, and parathyroid function: a retrospective analysis of laboratory data. Lancet. 2015;386(9992):461–8.
24. Juurlink DN, Mamdani MM, Kopp A, Rochon PA, Shulman KI, Redelmeier DA. Drug-induced lithium toxicity in the elderly: a population-based study. J Am Geriatr Soc. 2004;52(5):794–8.
25. Perry PJ, Wilborn CA. Serotonin syndrome vs neuroleptic malignant syndrome: a contrast of causes, diagnoses, and management. Ann Clin Psychiatry. 2012;24(2):155–62.
26. de Abajo FJ. Effects of selective serotonin reuptake inhibitors on platelet function: mechanisms, clinical outcomes and implications for use in elderly patients. Drugs Aging. 2011;28(5):345–67.
27. Boyer EW, Shannon M. The serotonin syndrome. N Engl J Med. 2005;352(11):1112–20.
28. Abadie D, Rousseau V, Logerot S, Cottin J, Montastruc JL, Montastruc F. Serotonin syndrome: analysis of cases registered in the French pharmacovigilance database. J Clin Psychopharmacol. 2015;35(4):382–8.
29. Jhun P, Bright A, Herbert M. Serotonin syndrome and opioids – what's the deal? Ann Emerg Med. 2015;65(4):434–5.
30. Douros A, Grabowksi K, Stahlmann R. Drug-drug interactions and safety of linezolid, tedizolid, and other oxazolidinones. Expert Opin Drug Metab Toxicol. 2015;1–11.
31. Jiang HY, Chen HZ, Hu XJ, et al. Use of selective serotonin reuptake inhibitors and risk of upper gastrointestinal bleeding: a systematic review and meta-analysis. Clin Gastroenterol Hepatol. 2015;13(1):42–50.e43.
32. Shin D, Oh YH, Eom CS, Park SM. Use of selective serotonin reuptake inhibitors and risk of stroke: a systematic review and meta-analysis. J Neurol. 2014;261(4):686–95.
33. Takeuchi H, Suzuki T, Remington G, Uchida H. Antipsychotic polypharmacy and corrected QT interval: a systematic review. Can J Psychiatry. 2015;60(5):215–22.
34. Vieweg WV, Wood MA, Fernandez A, Beatty-Brooks M, Hasnain M, Pandurangi AK. Proarrhythmic risk with antipsychotic and antidepressant drugs: implications in the elderly. Drugs Aging. 2009;26(12):997–1012.

13 The Physical and Behavioral Indicators of Elder Mistreatment and Neglect

Calvin H. Hirsch, Deborah C. Francis, and James A. Bourgeois

13.1 Background

The on-call psychiatrist may encounter victims of elder mistreatment in all medical settings as part of the consultation process, psychotherapy, and evaluation of the psychiatric patient's acute medical complaints. Elder mistreatment may take the form of psychological abuse, physical abuse, neglect, financial exploitation, or combinations of abuse. Many authorities consider self-neglect, the inability to provide for one's basic needs because of physical and/or mental disability, as a form of elder mistreatment. Physical abuse includes hitting, scratching, or biting; unwanted sexual contact; and inappropriate restraint, either mechanical or through sedating medication. Psychological abuse involves the infliction of emotional harm through insults, threats, or isolation. Neglect refers to the inadvertent or intentional failure of the primary caregiver to adequately meet the care needs of a dependent adult. Financial exploitation involves the misappropriation of an elder's money or property through theft, fraud, or embezzlement. Elder mistreatment can lead to significant psychiatric pathology, cause acute physical harm, contribute to the exacerbation of chronic illnesses, is associated with an increased risk of hospitalization, and can result in premature mortality [1, 2].

C.H. Hirsch, MD (✉)
Department of Internal Medicine, Division of General Medicine, University of California Davis Medical Center, Sacramento, CA, USA
e-mail: chhirsch@ucdavis.edu

D.C. Francis, RN, MSN, GCNS-BC
Geriatric Clinical Nurse Specialist Co-Chair Bioethics Committee,
Kaiser Permanente South Sacramento Medical Center, Sacramento, USA

J.A. Bourgeois, OD, MD
Department of Psychiatry/Langley Porter Psychiatric Institute,
University of California San Francisco, San Francisco, CA, USA

A. Hategan et al. (eds.), *On-Call Geriatric Psychiatry: Handbook of Principles and Practice*, DOI 10.1007/978-3-319-30346-8_13

The prevalence of elder mistreatment varies considerably, depending upon the population surveyed, the survey instrument used, and the definitions given to the types of abuse. The 2008 National Elder Mistreatment Study estimated that approximately 10 % of cognitively intact US older adults aged 60 and older experienced various forms of mistreatment in the previous year, the most common being financial abuse (5.2 %), followed by neglect (5.1 %), psychological abuse (4.6 %), and physical abuse, including sexual mistreatment (2.2 %) [3] . Based on population studies, the prevalence of elder mistreatment ranges from 3.2 to 27.5 %. A systematic review of the epidemiology of elder abuse found that almost 25 % of respondents to elder-abuse surveys reported having experienced neglect, and approximately 20 % responded that they had been psychologically abused [4]. The prevalence of abuse in cognitively impaired older adults is believed to be much higher. Approximately one-third of US physicians detect elder abuse in a given year, but only half report the abuse to the local health authority [5]. Victims of elder mistreatment are common in the psychiatric setting; among 126 geriatric patients assessed for decisional capacity by a hospital geriatric psychiatry service covering both outpatients and inpatients, 16 % had suspected or confirmed abuse [6].

Consistent characteristics of victims of mistreatment include older age, nonwhite race, lower level of completed formal education, low household income, major neurocognitive disorders (NCDs) (formerly dementia), depression, functional impairment, demanding personality, and low social support [7, 8]. Caregiver dependence on the patient, inadequate housing, history of substance abuse, and stress also contribute to the risk of elder mistreatment [8]. In a New England (USA) cohort study of older adults, the development of cognitive impairment was associated with a fivefold increased risk of abuse, compared to cognitively intact participants, after adjustment for age, sex, race, and income [9]. Some of this abuse is provoked by the patient. Coyne et al. found that one-third of patients with a NCD threaten or engage in assaultive behavior against their caregivers, with the potential of inciting reciprocal rage and aggression [10]. In this setting, 12 % of these caregivers commit acts of physical violence toward the patient [10].

13.2 Screening for Elder Mistreatment

With dependent geriatric patients, elder abuse or self-neglect should be considered during the evaluation of depression, new behavioral disturbances in patients with a NCD, exacerbations of chronic illness, and acute physical injury. Table 13.1 provides clues to the possibility of elder mistreatment which should heighten suspicion. The presence of pressure ulcers at the time of admission always should raise the question of neglect or self-neglect, even if the patient was transferred from another healthcare facility.

Once the possibility of elder mistreatment has been entertained, the psychiatrist should ask the patient questions to confirm and clarify the type(s) of abuse. The conflict tactics scale has been widely applied in elder-abuse research as a general screening tool [13, 14], but pertains to family violence generally rather than being specific to elder abuse. The relatively brief Hwalek-Sengstock Elder Abuse Screening Test [15] also is a general screening tool that is suitable for clinical settings, includes

Table 13.1 Clues for possible elder mistreatment

General	Failure of caregiver to visit patient in hospital
	Patient and/or caregiver reluctance to answer questions about a suspicious physical finding or illness
	Implausible, vague, or inconsistent explanations for injuries given by caregiver or patient
	Tension or indifference between caregiver and patient
Suspicious physical signs	Multiple bruises or bruises at different stages of healing
	Bruises in unusual locations, such as the inner aspects of the thighs or chest wall
	Pattern injuries (injuries in the shape of the object used to inflict them, such as bite marks, cigarette burns)
	Unusual configuration of the bruise, such as a circumferential bruise around the arm from forceful grabbing
	Evidence of old injuries not previously documented
	Broken nose, teeth
	Radiographic evidence of old, misaligned fractures Subtherapeutic levels of drugs
	Patient lacking his or her eyeglasses, dentures, and/or hearing aids
Caregiver	Poor knowledge of patient's medical problems
	Excessive concern about costs
	Attempts to dominate medical interview
	Verbal abuse or hostility toward elder during encounter
	Hostility toward healthcare providers
	Evidence of substance abuse or irritable behavior
The victim	Fearfulness toward caregiver (e.g., flinching when caregiver comes close) Reluctance to make eye contact
	Diagnosis of a neurocognitive disorder (NCD) with history of disruptive behavior
	In a patient with NCD, unexplained resistance to, or fear of, physical touch, removing clothes, toileting, bathing of private parts
	Depression, anxiety, insomnia

Adapted from Refs. [11] and [12]
For additional clues related to physical and sexual abuse, see Table 14.1

questions about risk factors as well as actual abuse, and can be administered by any health professional. However, when a specific type of mistreatment is suspected, more focused questions are desirable (see Table 13.2). The psychiatrist should exercise caution when asking screening questions when the patient has a major NCD, as the responses could reflect misperceptions of reality or delusional thinking.

13.3 Interventions for Elder Mistreatment

Most US states have mandatory reporting requirements for suspected elder abuse. In Canada, reporting laws for suspected elder abuse vary by province and territory, with most provinces limiting reporting to health professionals [16]. However,

Table 13.2 Examples of questions to elicit information about specific forms of mistreatment

General lead-in questions about the safety of the home environment and who provides help	Do you feel safe where you live?
	Who helps you with the things that you have trouble doing yourself?
	Who handles your checkbook and pays the bills?
Questions concerning physical abuse	Are you afraid of anyone at home?
	Have you ever been slapped, punched, or kicked?
	Have you ever been tied down or locked inside your room or house against your will?
Questions about neglect	Are you made to wait a long time for food or medicine?
	Have you been left alone for long periods?
	When you need assistance, do you have trouble getting someone to help you?
Questions about psychological abuse	Are you yelled at?
	Have you been threatened with punishment or placement in a nursing home?
	Are you kept isolated from friends or other relatives?
	Do you get the "silent treatment" at home?
	Do you have frequent disagreements with your (principal caregiver)?
	When you disagree with caretakers what happens?

Adapted from Refs. [11] and [12]
For additional questions pertinent to suspected physical and sexual abuse, see Table 14.2

screening and reporting bring with them a challenging ethical dilemma. On the one hand, reports of suspected elder abuse can initiate interventions that can end the abuse and improve the victim's quality of life. On the other hand, an investigation into alleged abuse that does not lead to a satisfactory resolution for the patient may *increase* the risk of future abuse and lead the caregiver to isolate the patient or not seek appropriate healthcare after discharge. Adult Protective Services (APS) in the USA has been described as a "beleaguered resource" that is often underfunded and understaffed [17], and the lack of community resources to address the underlying causes of elder mistreatment, such as poverty, substance abuse, and the inavailability of in-home support, undermines the ability to prevent future abuse.

Reporting of suspected abuse is an insufficient response by itself and represents one facet of a broader, multidisciplinary strategy to assist the victim. Because of their training in interviewing, psychiatrists are uniquely positioned to take a leading role in the development of interventions while the patient is hospitalized. A social worker and discharge planner (if not the same individual) should be part of this team. The psychiatrist can assess for posttraumatic psychiatric illness and initiate psychotherapy for the older adult victim when appropriate (refer to Chap. 4 for on-call psychotherapy principles and Chap. 14 for trauma-informed care). For patients admitted from home, the family caregiver's perspective should be solicited in a non-accusatory manner in most cases involving suspected neglect and psychological abuse, as the reasons for the abuse may stem from caregiver ignorance, inadequate training, lack of resources, or excessive stress, all of which may be remediable through education and counseling without removing the patient from the home. By interviewing the caregiver, traits that suggest risk of future abuse also can be identified, such as a personality disorder, other psychiatric illness, and signs of substance abuse.

In planning for the hospital discharge of an elder-abuse victim, the patient's safety is paramount. Whenever possible (based on eligibility criteria imposed by health insurance), home health services should be ordered, which can provide an assessment of the home environment, help instruct the caregiver, and monitor for signs of abuse. Primary-care providers, who may have been unaware of the abuse, should be informed by the inpatient team so that they can be alert to signs of future abuse and reinforce patient and caregiver counseling.[1] The social worker should provide the family with information about community resources, such as specialized day programs for older adults which can offer the caregiver respite and provide socialization for the patient. The patient's insurance status, and thus eligibility for government-subsidized in-home support services, should be known at admission. Eligible patients and families without such support may not know how to apply or have not done so due to language barriers, lack of transportation, low literacy, and/or cultural barriers. It is incumbent on the social worker/discharge planner to identify these barriers and to try to develop individualized solutions (e.g., interpreter services).

In cases of potentially criminal physical abuse (e.g., bruises suggesting inflicted blunt trauma, signs of sexual assault), the police should be notified immediately and the patient should be examined by a trained forensic examiner. The psychiatrist and social worker should defer interviewing caregivers suspected of potentially criminal neglect (e.g., allegedly locking the dependent elder in a room for the entire day without access to food or water) until the case has been discussed with APS and/or the police.

Caregivers suspected of financial abuse should be interviewed regarding the patient's health-related concerns, but reference to the financial abuse should be avoided and its investigation left to the appropriate public authority. Suspected financial abuse does not preclude discharge home unless the abuse is responsible for the patient's present condition (e.g., suicidal ideation).

13.4 Case Vignettes

Case Vignette 1 – Neglect The on-call psychiatrist was asked to assess the decisional capacity of Ms. R, a 78-year-old woman admitted 3 days earlier following recurrent falls, rule out syncope. This was her third fall-related emergency

[1] For victims of abuse and neglect who are seen as outpatients, candid responses to questions that may reflect ongoing abuse or caregiver stress can best be obtained by interviewing the patient and caregiver separately.

department (ED) visit in the past 2 months. Per the patient and niece, she lost her balance trying to open the passenger door of her niece's car, falling backward and striking her head against the side walk. In the ED, she was alert and "oriented in four spheres (person, place, time, situation);" non-contrast computerized tomography of her head showed age-consistent atrophy but no evidence of intracranial bleeding or stroke. Her electrolytes and complete blood count were within normal limits except for a blood urea nitrogen of 26 mg/dL (9.3 mmol/L) and a creatinine of 1.3 mg/dL (114.9 μmol/L). Her electrocardiogram showed nonspecific ST-T wave changes. Per chart notes, on the admission physical examination, she appeared "well developed and well nourished," but had greasy, unkempt hair, dirt-encrusted skin on her back and abdomen, and an "unwashed" body odor. She wore loose-fitting upper dentures and had poor lower dentition. She required one-person assistance to stand and was very unstable on her feet, with decreased vibratory sensation to the knees but normal proprioception. Several mycotic toenails were several centimeters long. Her B_{12} level was 550 pg/mL (400 pmol/L) and her serum albumin was 3.8 g/dL (38 g/L), both within normal limits. After 2 days of physical therapy, Ms. R was able to transfer and ambulate safely with a front-wheeled walker, but was caught several times by nurses ambulating to the bathroom without it. Telemetry demonstrated normal sinus rhythm with infrequent, short runs of supraventricular tachycardia. The primary medical team believed she was medically stable for discharge, but because of concern about self-neglect and a possible underlying NCD, wanted a formal determination of decisional capacity for self-management in the community. The patient did not want to leave her house of 40 years and lose her independence and refused placement in a board and care facility, where she feared she would lose her privacy. She indicated that her son, who lived on her "sun porch," would take care of her. She did not know her son's cell phone number. According to the discharge social worker, APS had opened and closed a case on her within the past year because of the son's history of drug abuse, concluding that she was receiving adequate support.

On mental status evaluation, Ms. R scored 28/30 on the MoCA, missing the date and generating nine words in 1 min for the verbal fluency task (normal ≥11 words). Her clock draw was systematically and accurately executed, although the lines were shaky. When asked why she didn't bathe, she replied that the bathroom sink was broken, and she was afraid to take a shower out of fear of falling. She planned to call a plumber when she returned home. She acknowledged that her son was unreliable and sometimes used drugs but that he needed a place to stay. She stated that her niece was good at taking her shopping whenever she needed to go and would cook for her on occasion. When the psychiatrist asked if he could talk to the niece, she refused. "She's nice to me, but I don't trust her. She recently got divorced, and she needs money. She would say anything to get me conserved and use my money for herself." Ms. R was unwilling to consider a chore worker because of the cost and her mistrust of strangers coming into the home, stating, "I used to have a housekeeper, but she stole from me." The patient was receptive to a wireless lifeline device to summon help in an emergency, calling it a "good idea" because of her fall risk.

The psychiatrist concluded that the patient did not have a NCD and demonstrated logical reasoning and fair insight, although she did demonstrate possible paranoid ideation. Moreover, her home situation had been "vetted" by APS. Ethically and legally, the psychiatrist believed that the team did not have the right to violate the patient's wish for them not to contact the niece. Ms. R was discharged home the next day with an order for home health supports, along with a new referral to APS for neglect. The patient repeatedly did not answer the telephone when the home health support worker called to schedule a visit. Three weeks later the patient was readmitted for a hip fracture associated with hypotension and dehydration and later was discharged to a skilled nursing facility. APS had not reopened her case since discharge.

Case 1 Analysis Ms. R suffered from self-neglect, needing help with basic activities of daily living (ADLs) like bathing and grooming, as well as with instrumental activities of daily living (IADLs) like shopping. Her ability to manage finances, do laundry, and prepare food was not assessed. Without further investigation, the validity of her claims about her niece's intentions could not be determined. As a result of the decisional capacity assessment, the primary team took the patient's word that she had adequate home resources, despite physical evidence to the contrary, in part because of the difficulty obtaining further information. In addition, as in most acute care hospitals, there was pressure to discharge the patient as soon as possible, and pursuing conservatorship would have prolonged her hospitalization. The team may have given too much weight to APS' earlier investigation. The son, by virtue of living with his mother, should have recognized her self-care needs and in most US states would be held accountable for not providing for them, a prosecutable criminal offense in many jurisdictions. The quality and timeliness of investigation and extent of intervention for elder abuse vary widely by APS district, even within the same state [18], related in part to training and number of field investigators, case load, and budgetary constraints. APS agencies generally prefer letting families shoulder the responsibility for obtaining conservatorship. Failure to use standardized criteria to guide questioning, such as the MacArthur Competence Assessment Tool-Treatment (MacCAT-T), can affect the accuracy of the assessment, as measured by the percent agreement among providers [19]. From an ethical standpoint, it could be argued in this case that concern for patient safety ("beneficence") trumped respect for autonomy and would have justified contacting the niece, despite the patient's wishes to the contrary. Most elder-abuse laws are paternalistic and structured around the primacy of beneficence in the context of presumed vulnerability. The evaluation of decisional capacity should incorporate many sources of data to gain as complete an assessment as possible of the patient's functional abilities and the ability of family to address functional dependence [20]. Ideally, decisional capacity assessments for "self-determination" to live in the community, in addition to assessment of mental status (including cognitive assessment), should include in vivo assessment of skills at various "real-life" ADLs. A Kohlman Evaluation of Living Skills (KELS) assessment is a common assessment done by occupational therapy to address this area. Discharge should have been delayed until the plan for follow-up had been coordinated with all concerned parties (niece, APS, home health, and possibly the son).

Case Vignette 2 – Psychological and Financial Abuse
Mr. C was an 81-year-old man admitted to the inpatient psychiatry unit from the outpatient clinic for major depression with active suicidal ideation. On admission, he was wheelchair bound, thin, frail, malnourished (serum albumin 2.6 g/dL (26 g/L)), and smelled of urine. Sertraline 25 mg q AM was started, along with daily supportive psychotherapy sessions led by the psychiatrist. In the evening of day 6, the on-call psychiatrist was summoned to evaluate the patient, who was found screaming and ramming his wheelchair repeatedly into the wall in an attempt to hurt himself. When asked why he was doing this, the patient admitted that he was ashamed and humiliated by his life and wanted to die. The psychiatrist considered elder abuse as a contributor to the patient's psychiatric condition and asked open-ended questions, such as "Do you think you're getting enough help at home?" The psychiatrist learned that the grandson was using the patient's credit cards for online purchases and selling the patient's belongings, using the proceeds to buy expensive items like a new watch and leather jacket. In addition, the grandson repeatedly cursed and belittled him, especially when the patient needed a diaper change or help going to the toilet. The psychiatrist recommended adjustment of psychotherapy to focus on empowering the patient to take more control of his life and on providing him with viable alternatives to returning home. APS was contacted and initiated an investigation. With the help of social services, the patient's nephew, whom the patient trusted, agreed to be granted power of attorney over finances and arranged for the patient to be discharged to an assisted living facility, to which the patient agreed to go after much encouragement.

Case 2 Analysis Chronic psychological and financial abuse can lead to depression and suicidal ideation in vulnerable geriatric patients [21]. Fear of abandonment and institutional placement, embarrassment, and shame about their plight or fear of retribution from the caregiver inhibit many elderly victims from admitting their mistreatment and seeking help. Healthcare encounters may be the only opportunity to identify this abuse. An emphasis on history taking, psychotherapy, and counseling gives psychiatry an advantage among the health professions in detecting elder mistreatment – provided it is considered.

Case Vignette 3 – Physical Abuse
Mr. H was an 87-year-old resident of a memory-care unit within a skilled nursing facility (SNF) and carried a diagnosis of advanced Alzheimer's disease. He was brought to the ED and admitted to the ward medicine service because of recurrent assaultive behavior against his nursing assistants. At baseline, he was dependent in all ADLs, incontinent, and largely bedbound. On admission, he was inconsistently able to follow simple commands and made nonsensical vocalizations. On hospital day 1, he attempted to hit and kick his nurse, and the primary team wrote orders for wrist restraints and olanzapine 5 mg every 6 h as needed for violent or agitated

behavior. In addition, they requested psychiatric consultation for behavior management. The consultant psychiatrist asked the nurse to describe the patient's assaultive behavior and what seemed to trigger it. The nurse stated that Mr. H was generally pleasant and cooperative with feeding and grooming, although he tended to suck on his toothbrush. He also readily smiled when smiled at. However, every time she attempted to check or change his diaper, he would yell and withdraw and then strike out with his fists if she continued. The psychiatrist wondered if this was a reaction to a female nurse approaching his genitals and asked a male nurse to check the diaper. The same reaction occurred. The psychiatrist hypothesized that the cowering and striking out represented a fear response, possibly triggered by physically or verbally abusive behavior from caregivers that occurred in association with his incontinence.

The consulting psychiatrist conferred with the hospital's geriatric clinical nurse specialist (GCNS) to devise a behavior-modifying routine to associate diaper changes and perineal care with pleasant rather than unpleasant experiences. The GCNS encouraged the nurses to frequently touch the patient's shoulders and hold his hand to accustom him to gentle touch. She trained two nurses on each shift how to perform perineal care in a slow, gentle manner while talking in soothing voices and smiling frequently at the patient. She brought in an iPod™ so that relaxing music could be played into the patient's ears prior to and during perineal care. The psychiatrist recommended discontinuation of the restraints and reserving the olanzapine for dangerous behavior unresponsive to verbal calming interventions. Diapers were replaced by an absorbent waterproof pad placed beneath the patient. In anticipation of the first perineal cleansing after switching to the bed pad, the patient was introduced to a therapy dog and allowed to pet him for 10 min. For the next 2 days, Mr. H's nurses practiced the routine of relaxing music before and during perineal care while they carried on a soothing banter with the patient. Each time a clean diaper was laid over the patient's genitals but not attached. On hospital day 4, the patient allowed the diaper to be affixed and remained cooperative during subsequent diaper changes and perineal care. The discharge social worker was able to find a new SNF to which the patient was discharged on hospital day 9, with detailed instructions for continuing the current touch-talk-music intervention for perineal care. The psychiatrist and social worker wrote a formal letter to the ombudsman's office describing Mr. H's behavior and their suspicion of elder mistreatment at his former SNF.

Case 3 Analysis Elder mistreatment can be difficult to detect, especially when the victim cannot communicate reliably. Understanding risk factors can increase sensitivity to clues, like Mr. H's selective resistance to diaper changes. In patients with advanced, major NCD, other clues to abuse include withdrawal, refusal to eat, and other signs of superimposed depression. Regression, the unexplained acute or subacute progression of the major NCD, may occur as a result of any form of elder mistreatment. During the physical exam, the psychiatrist should be alert for bruises in unusual locations, such as a circumferential bruise on the wrist or arm from being tightly grabbed. In this case, the inventive behavioral modification plan underscores the potential effectiveness of non-pharmacological interventions and enabled the patient to be discharged without an antipsychotic.

Key Points

Victims of elder mistreatment are commonly found in the ED, hospital wards, and psychiatric units. The on-call psychiatrist should become familiar with risk factors and clues for elder mistreatment in the history, hints of its occurrence in the behavior of the patient and caregiver during the interview, and findings suspicious for abuse during the physical exam. Once suspected, additional screening is necessary, starting with non-threatening, open-ended questions. The medical team has a responsibility to develop a multidisciplinary, individualized plan to address the abuse prior to discharge by:

- Determining the victim's decisional capacity for returning home
- Determining the best discharge destination to ensure the patient's safety
- Determining contributors to abuse that may be remedied through education and counseling and initiating both before discharge
- Determining resources and community services that may alleviate caregiver stress and prevent further abuse
- Ensuring continuity of education, counseling, and monitoring after discharge by engaging home health and informing the patient's primary-care provider
- Engaging agencies that can monitor the patient's safety, in particular Adult Protective Services (where available) and ombudsman services

References

1. Dong X, Simon MA. Elder abuse as a risk factor for hospitalization in older persons. JAMA Intern Med. 2013;173(10):911–7.
2. Lachs MS, Williams CS, O'Brien S, Pillemer KA, Charlson ME. The mortality of elder mistreatment. JAMA. 1998;280(5):428–32.
3. Acierno R, Hernandez MA, Amstadter AB, et al. Prevalence and correlates of emotional, physical, sexual, and financial abuse and potential neglect in the United States: the National Elder Mistreatment Study. Am J Public Health. 2010;100(2):292–7.
4. Cooper C, Selwood A, Livingston G. The prevalence of elder abuse and neglect: a systematic review. Age Ageing. 2008;37(2):151–60.
5. Cooper C, Selwood A, Livingston G. Knowledge, detection, and reporting of abuse by health and social care professionals: a systematic review. Am J Geriatr Psychiatry. 2009;17(10):826–38.
6. Vida S, Monks RC, Des Rosiers P. Prevalence and correlates of elder abuse and neglect in a geriatric psychiatry service. Can J Psychiatry. 2002;47(5):459–67.
7. Dong XQ. Elder Abuse: Systematic Review and Implications for Practice. J Am Geriatr Soc. 2015;63(6):1214–38.
8. Jones JS, Holstege C, Holstege H. Elder abuse and neglect: understanding the causes and potential risk factors. Am J Emerg Med. 1997;15(6):579–83.

9. Lachs MS, Williams C, O'Brien S, Hurst L, Horwitz R. Risk factors for reported elder abuse and neglect: a nine-year observational cohort study. Gerontologist. 1997;37(4):469–74.
10. Coyne AC, Reichman WE, Berbig LJ. The relationship between dementia and elder abuse. Am J Psychiatry. 1993;150(4):643–6.
11. Kleinschmidt KC. Elder abuse: a review. Ann Emerg Med. 1997;30(4):463–72.
12. Lachs MS, Pillemer K. Abuse and neglect of elderly persons. N Engl J Med. 1995;332(7):437–43.
13. Cooper C, Maxmin K, Selwood A, Blanchard M, Livingston G. The sensitivity and specificity of the Modified Conflict Tactics Scale for detecting clinically significant elder abuse. Int Psychogeriatr. 2009;21(4):774–8.
14. Straus MA, Douglas EM. A short form of the Revised Conflict Tactics Scales, and typologies for severity and mutuality. Violence Vict. 2004;19(5):507–20.
15. Neale A, Hwalek M, Scott R, Sengstock M, Stahl C. Validation of the Hwalek-Sengstock Elder Abuse Screening Test. J Appl Gerontol. 1991;10(4):406–18.
16. Wang XM, Brisbin S, Loo T, Straus S. Elder abuse: an approach to identification, assessment and intervention. CMAJ. 2015;187(8):575–81.
17. O'Brien JG. Screening for Elder Abuse and Neglect. J Am Geriatr Soc. 2015;63(8):1689–91.
18. Mosqueda L, Wiglesworth A, Moore AA, Nguyen A, Gironda M, Gibbs L. Variability in Findings From Adult Protective Services Investigations of Elder Abuse in California. J Evid Inf Soc Work. 2015;1–11.
19. Guzman-Clark JRS, Reinhardt AK, Wilkins SS, Castle S. Decision-making capacity and conservatorship in older adults. Ann Longterm Care. 2012;20(9).
20. Falk E, Hoffman N. The role of capacity assessments in elder abuse investigations and guardianships. Clin Geriatr Med. 2014;30(4):851–68.
21. Wu L, Shen M, Chen H, et al. The relationship between elder mistreatment and suicidal ideation in rural older adults in China. Am J Geriatr Psychiatry. 2013;21(10):1020–8.

14 The Complaints of Physical and Sexual Trauma: A Trauma-Informed Approach

Caroline Giroux, Albina Veltman, Lisebeth Gatkowski, and Kolja Paech

14.1 Background

Given the increasing population of older adults, there are also a growing number of older adults reporting that they are the victims of abuse. Evidence shows that perpetrators of violence against seniors are most often adult children and current or former spouses, which may explain the reluctance of many older people to report the abuse for fear of retaliation. Research indicates that patients with major neurocognitive disorders (NCDs) (formerly dementia) are at greater risk of elder abuse than those without significant cognitive deficits. A decline in the older adult's physical and/or cognitive ability and/or a lack of training by healthcare professionals to properly assess and recognize signs of abuse can result in the underreporting of abuse. In addition to stress-related disorders, other

C. Giroux, MD (✉)
Department of Psychiatry and Behavioral Sciences, APSS Stockton Clinic,
University of California, Davis Health System, Sacramento, CA, USA
e-mail: cgiroux@ucdavis.edu

A. Veltman, MD
Department of Psychiatry and Behavioural Neurosciences, McMaster University,
Hamilton, ON, Canada
e-mail: veltmaa@mcmaster.ca

L. Gatkowski, RN, BScN
St. Joseph' Healthcare Hamilton, Faculty Mohawk College of Applied Arts and Technology,
Institute for Applied Health Sciences at McMaster, Hamilton, ON, Canada
e-mail: info@lisebethgatkowsi.ca

K. Paech, MD
Kaiser Permanente, Roseville, CA, USA
e-mail: koljapaech@hotmail.com

A. Hategan et al. (eds.), *On-Call Geriatric Psychiatry: Handbook of Principles and Practice*, DOI 10.1007/978-3-319-30346-8_14

consequences of abuse can involve increased healthcare issues, including bone or joint problems, digestive problems, chronic pain, hypertension and other cardiac conditions, depression, and anxiety.

Elder mistreatment worsens the quality of life of many older adults and indeed also reduces the lifespan of the victims considerably [1], with a risk of death three times higher than among those who do not experience mistreatment [2]. The identification of elder abuse is difficult in part because medical conditions and physiological characteristics of older adults may mask markers of abuse [3]. Since the vast majority of elder abuse is perpetrated by spouses and adult children [3] and can be experienced as particularly traumatic due to the power differential and underlying vulnerability that often accompanies advanced age, it is especially important to use a trauma-informed approach when providing care to this population.

Due to a variety of factors, including underreporting, the prevalence of abuse and neglect of older adults is unclear. In the community, the incidence is estimated at about 15 % (corresponding to a prevalence ranging from 3.2 to 27.5 %) [4]. In institutional settings, the extent of abuse and neglect of older adults remains largely unknown [5]; however, studies suggest it may be a common occurrence [6].

14.2 Definition, Assessment, and Management

14.2.1 Definition

Elder mistreatment is a single or repeated act or lack of appropriate action, occurring within any relationship where there is an expectation of trust which causes harm or distress to an older person [7]. Whereas a review of all types of abuse is presented elsewhere in the book (see Chap. 13), this chapter addresses the following chief complaints of alleged abuse, which the clinician could encounter during the on-call shift:

- *Physical abuse*: direct attacks against a person's body with or without a weapon (e.g., slapping, pushing, inappropriate use of restraints).
- *Sexual abuse*: any unwanted sexual experience or act.

Some overlap exists between categories (there is often an emotional component associated with other forms of abuse). Sexual abuse is the least acknowledged and reported type of elder abuse [8]. Due to ageism, older persons may be seen as asexual, and therefore, the risk of sexual abuse may not be taken seriously [8].

Case Vignette 1 You were the on-call physician and a nurse from an acute psychiatric unit called you with concerns about Ms. F, a patient with sudden change in behavior: "Doctor, I am calling about Ms. F, a 76-year-old woman with a prior diagnosis of major depression with psychotic features (persecutory delusions), a history of alcohol and cocaine use in the distant past, and a recent diagnosis of major NCD with Lewy bodies. Generally, she is mild-mannered and does not mingle with other patients. She was given a weekend pass, accompanied by her son who wanted to take her to a family function. She had returned to the unit accompanied in a disheveled condition, with soiled clothing, blood in her underwear and a strong smell of urine. She became agitated, crying, hypervigilant, pacing and muttering to herself, and stated that her son beat her up because she is *queer*." While over the phone with you, Ms. F was overheard yelling, allegedly at her son who was not there, and threatening retaliation for plotting to have her murdered. Then you heard that she threw a chair against the wall, thinking he was next to her. On your arrival to the unit, further report indicated that when staff tried to intervene, she spat and accused staff of being part of the "assassination plan." She also seemed confused, no longer immediately recognizing staff. Physical assessment included a strong odor of alcohol and poor motor coordination. Her blood pressure was 124/68 mmHg, pulse 110 BPM, and respiratory rate 26/ min. Her mouth appeared dry. Blood glucose was 223 mg/dl (12.4 mmol/L) and pupils at pinpoint. There were no visible wounds and no bruises, scratches, or reddened areas. Ms. F's medical history included type 2 diabetes mellitus, hypertension, and chronic anemia. The chart indicated that Ms. F had had a surrogate decision-maker for 4 years due to progressively decreasing decision-making capacity. You had not finished making your recommendations and you were paged to do a consultation in the emergency department (ED).

Case Vignette 2 Mr. S was a 68-year-old biracial (Caucasian and African-American) veteran and divorced man who was brought to the ED by law enforcement after being found in the streets shouting he had been "seriously molested, like in the army." You immediately noticed a black eye and a heavy smell of alcohol. He clung to a big garbage bag of dirty clothes and rotten food. He was supposed to be on "tons of medications" (which were not among his personal belongings) but did not remember for what exactly since he had not seen his primary care physician "in ages." He had a prior history of major depression with serious suicide attempts. He had been homeless for most of the past decade, but his son recently reconnected with him. Mr. S had not been sleeping much because of nightmares and vague pain in various locations. Upon examination, he appeared frightened and scanned the room. He had temporal muscle atrophy. He limped when he walked and seemed to be in pain, refusing to sit. His hygiene was poor and he was malodorous. His conjunctivae and face were pale. You noticed bruises of various stages on his extremities and on his torso. Hair was missing in some areas of his scalp. Some dots of burnt skin appeared on his buttocks and behind his ears. He was minimally cooperative but finally agreed to have you take pictures of his injuries. He startled upon hearing the click of your camera. He did not know the date and was surprised upon hearing what date it was. Otherwise, he scored 25 out of 30 on his MoCA (grade 12 education). In the interim, his son showed up, irate about his father having been seen without his presence. During the brief moment Mr. S and his son were in the same room, the nurse observed that Mr. S looked shaky and "nervous." He started pacing and speaking loudly to himself and eventually escalated to the point that you considered asking the nurse to put him under physical restraints to prevent harm to self and others.

As illustrated in both vignettes, a few common biopsychosocial "red flags" for complaints of alleged physical or sexual trauma are presented in Table 14.1 [9, 10].

14.2.2 Assessment

(a) *Rule out features for delirium.* Recognizing high-risk factors for delirium is essential. A full medical evaluation of the patient at the time of presentation to the ED is urgently needed in such cases. If a speculum or rectal exam is recommended, have a support person (female or male staff, depending on patient's preference) present while the trained clinician (e.g., emergency physician) explain all the steps to the patient to facilitate informed consent.
(b) *Identify medical conditions and iatrogenesis*; for instance, bruises could be caused by anticoagulants.
(c) *Consider underlying social problems along with chronic medical conditions* (e.g., neglect, physical abuse, sexual abuse, inappropriate medication administration, including poor adherence). Identify risk factors for elder

Table 14.1 Biopsychosocial "red flags" as indicators[a] for possible physical or sexual trauma

Patient	Caregiver
Injuries inconsistent with history provided (e.g., inadequately explained burns) Conflicting reports from patient and caregiver Fractures that are inconsistent with patient's mobility Sexually transmitted infections Pressure ulcers Difficulty walking or sitting Oversedation Malnutrition and dehydration Poor hygiene Inappropriate clothing Fear of caregiver Post-traumatic stress disorder symptoms (e.g., re-experiencing, avoidance, or hyperarousal) Depression Reluctance to answer questions Indifference or hostility Established problems that have not been properly addressed Delay in seeking care for injury Unusually frequent healthcare visits Physician or hospital shopping Frequently missed medical appointments	Poor knowledge of the patient's medical conditions Conflicting reports from patient and caregiver Failure by the caregiver to administer prescribed medications Repeated preventable injuries due to poor supervision Excessive concern with medical care costs Reluctance to leave patient alone with the healthcare provider Poor self-control (e.g., defensiveness, denial) Depression Implausible or vague explanations for injuries Reluctance to answer questions Indifference or hostility

Adapted from Refs. [9] and [10]
For additional clues to elder mistreatment in general, see Table 13.1
[a]For legal indicators and for additional physical and behavioral indicators of abuse, please refer to Chap. 13

mistreatment, but risk factors do not prove abuse. In some situations, the likelihood of mistreatment is high enough to take action based on a single encounter. These situations include extreme neglect that leads to physical and/or psychological abuse, objective evidence of medication misadministration, or injuries that cannot be self-induced or accidental. However, without abuse on the differential diagnosis, abuse will be missed, especially given the confounders of more prevalent explanations for many symptoms. For instance, rectal bleeding in the geriatric patients may be due to a diverticulosis, an arteriovascular abnormality, or neoplasm, but sexual abuse, although uncommon, is still possible. There is evidence that victims may benefit from referrals for trauma treatment services in an ED care setting, even if they are not seeking care for an acute trauma-related injury [11].

(d) *Consider exacerbation of underlying psychiatric illness*, such as psychotic disorder, major NCD (Ms. F's case), or reactivation of post-traumatic stress disorder (PTSD) (Mr. S's case). PTSD can sometimes manifest itself for the first time in old age [12]. A psychiatric history ruling out sexual abuse for older veterans while in the army should be offered and conducted when the patient feels ready. Not only military sexual trauma may be a risk factor for homelessness, it has also been found to be a stronger predictor of PTSD compared to civilian sexual assault [13]. The three most common psychiatric disorders among people who had a history of military sexual trauma were depressive disorders, PTSD, and substance-related disorders [13]. In cases of substance intoxication, a full psychiatric assessment should be performed once the patient is no longer intoxicated.

(e) *Assess for safety regarding suicidal/homicidal ideation or plan.* (See Chap. 10, Sect. 10.2.4 The Suicidal Patient.)

Case Analysis Both Ms. F and Mr. S presented with possible indicators of physical and sexual abuse. In Ms. F's case, the fact that she left for a short period of time and returned soiled and intoxicated were objective indicators that required further action and sexual abuse needed to be ruled out. Any history that Ms. F gave was likely unreliable due to her alcohol intoxication and major NCD. She was, however, thoroughly interviewed. In all cases of suspected or alleged mistreatment, the patient should first be interviewed alone. It is important to normalize this step, for instance, by saying "I always ask family to step out for part of my medical evaluation." Even though one might suspect delirium in this case, it is still important that the patient be informed about the upcoming evaluation, especially invasive procedures such as venipuncture, so that the patient knows what to expect. It is equally important to establish a calm and reassuring atmosphere, not to pressure the patient, and to give the patient the opportunity to ask questions or voice concerns. Some helpful sample questions for a clinician to adopt can be found in Table 14.2 [9, 14, 15]. No one should be coerced to participate in a trauma assessment unless they feel ready. In some situations, it is preferable to defer to another day and rather focus on the patient's physical and emotional safety and comfort in the on-call setting. At the same time, it is imperative to differentiate between a patient who

Table 14.2 Screening clinical questions for abuse

Routine screening for all geriatric patients	Prior to the trauma screen: use a framing statement, such as "Because traumatic events are so common and because they have direct, long-lasting effects on general health, I find it important to ask all patients about stressful or difficult experiences they may have had." "Many of the patients I see are dealing with abuse in their relationships. Some are too afraid or uncomfortable to bring it up themselves, so I ask about it routinely."
Physical abuse questions	"We know that violence is a problem for many older individuals in their lives. Is this a problem for you in any way?"; "Do you feel safe at home?" or "Are you afraid of anyone living in your home?"; "Sometimes patients tell me they have been hurt by someone close to them. Could this be happening to you?"; "Has anyone ever hurt, scolded, threatened, or made you feel bad at home?"; "Are you frequently by yourself?"; "Has anyone hurt you? If yes, how? What part of your body was hurt?"
Sexual abuse	"Has anyone made lewd or offensive comments to you?"; "Has anyone touched you sexually without your consent?"
Proceed with gradually more specific questions	*Open-ended questions:* "What happened?"; "What do you remember about how this injury occurred?" *Close-ended questions:* "Have you been struck, slapped, or kicked?"; "Does your son or daughter ever hit you when you two have a disagreement?"; "Do you have to wait a long time for your food or medicine?"; "Have you been tied down or locked in a room?"; "Have you ever been emotionally, physically, or sexually abused by your partner or someone important to you?"; "The injuries you have are like bruises and lacerations people get when someone hits them. Did someone hit you? Are you afraid?"; "Do you ever feel alone?"; "Have you been threatened with punishment, deprivation, or institutionalization?"; "Have you received 'the silent treatment'?"; "Have you been force-fed?"; "Has anyone touched you without permission?"
Caregiver questions	An opening, nonjudgmental statement can be: "You've been carrying a heavy responsibility for some time now and it's alright to feel burdened at times." "What are the challenges that you are experiencing from caring for your elderly relative?"; "How do you cope with feeling overwhelmed or with increased demands?"; "How do you express irritation or frustration?"; "Are you getting enough sleep?"; "What do you do to maintain a balanced lifestyle?"; "Are you struggling financially?"; "Do you have concerns or worries?"

Adapted from Refs. [9], [14], and [15]
For additional screening questions about elder mistreatment in general, see Table 13.3

clearly has decision-making capacity and one who is severely impaired. If a severely impaired patient disagrees with a medical evaluation, patient's preference and comfort is more a secondary consideration.

14.2.3 Management

(a) *Establish patient's safety first and intervene to stop the mistreatment if mistreatment is confirmed or highly suspected.* In the case example of Ms. F, she should not be allowed to leave her facility to spend time with her son if it is confirmed that he abused her. In other cases, removing a patient from their current living situation may be necessary. Hospitalization may be indicated for Mr. S, if no other immediate option such as a shelter is available. If there appears to be an immediate ongoing threat, law enforcement should be involved (refer to Chap. 13). In any case of alleged or suspected mistreatment, health professionals should contact Adult Protective Services in their jurisdiction or the Elder Care Locator in the USA (Toll-free: 800-677-1116), or any provincial and territorial resources on elder mistreatment in Canada (e.g., Victim Support Line in Ontario, Toll-free: 888-579-2888), or call the police. If mistreatment is suspected at the time of the evaluation in the ED or any medical setting but there is no confirmatory evidence, arrange for frequent follow-up home visits by a home health agency worker to gather more information once discharged home to their environment [9, 10]. The patients should be asked if they wish for a support person, nurse examiner, or social worker to attend during the on-call medical assessment. Identify if there is a power of attorney (POA) document for the patient. If there is a concern that the POA person is not acting in the patient's best interest or that the POA person is the abuser, consider involving other family members. Provide education, both to the patient and to the suspected abuser.

(b) *Address any underlying psychiatric condition and offer biopsychosocial treatments*. Oral medications are preferable as injection could be perceived as intrusive and re-traumatizing. Selective serotonin reuptake inhibitors (such as sertraline) and prazosin are good choices for trauma-based reactions. Benzodiazepines should be avoided since they can further impair cognitive functioning and should be used with caution, in small doses, very short term, and only when there is extreme agitation. In general, adding psychotropic medications should be avoided, especially highly sedating medications, benzodiazepines, or anticholinergic medications [12]. Antipsychotics should also be used with caution in geriatric patients, weighing risks and benefits, involving the patient or the POA person in this decision. If the patient has a major NCD, the emphasis should be to find a stable and expectable environment, preferably with familiar people to the patient.

14.3 The Experience of Trauma

Situations of physical and/or sexual trauma are overwhelming, threaten physical and emotional integrity, and can put persons at risk of developing trauma-related stress disorders such as acute stress disorder. Panic disorder, agoraphobia, PTSD, substance-related disorders, resistant depression, and borderline personality disorder can also develop, or be reactivated, as a result of traumatic experiences. Trauma affects the whole person and can become the organizing principle of the person's life. It can have a profound impact on identity and self-esteem. Advanced age is an especially critical period since disability, dependence, and other conditions that increase the person's vulnerability are common.

Acute stress in geriatric patients may be expressed in a more somatic way (e.g., pain, palpitations, digestive complaints). Additionally, mild reversible memory impairment after trauma has been unrecognized [12]. Therefore, making a diagnosis of major NCD might be premature in the immediate phase of a trauma, and it is preferable to obtain collateral information and repeat the cognitive assessment once the patient is ready.

14.3.1 Trauma-Informed Care

Trauma-informed care (TIC) involves providing services that are welcoming and appropriate to the special needs of those patients affected by trauma, and this framework for practice should be applied in all settings, including during brief encounters such as on-call consultations. TIC is a shift in attitude towards "patients first" language. Core principles of TIC include acknowledgement, safety, trust, choice and control (on the principle that the individual is an expert on his/her own life), compassion, and collaboration (or advocacy). The goal is to achieve a therapeutic relationship that offers *r*espect, *i*nformation, *c*onnection, and *h*ope (RICH) and to promote relationships that are consistent, predictable, nonviolent, non-shaming, and non-blaming [14].

First, it is essential to recognize the pervasiveness of traumatic or adverse life experiences and of trauma-based reactions. In order to be fully informed about a patient's condition, the clinician should review the chart carefully to find out about trauma history. Second, a trauma-sensitive approach is important. Trauma sensitivity can be expressed in many forms, such as (i) assisting in understanding the correlation between past traumatic experiences and current symptoms (i.e., physical, psychological, and/or behavioral), (ii) helping to identify triggers (e.g., sights, sounds, situations, smells, feelings) that could potentially remind the individual of traumatic events [14], and (iii) acknowledging that what happened to the patient was bad, but that the patient is not a bad person. In this spirit, interaction approaches that can be helpful include:

- Explaining each step of the assessment
- Screening for trauma history
- Empowering the patients by allowing them to set the pace of the interventions
- Minimizing re-traumatization, by including psychoeducational framing, using a cultural safety lens, de-escalation strategies, grounding, and emotional modulation techniques
- Using shared decision-making

Re-traumatization can occur in certain medical situations, including invasive procedures without proper explanation, physical restraints (which also tend to increase agitation [15]), or simply being left in an exam room without a sense of what is going on. Doing a proper closure by thanking the patient for sharing a difficult story can help to strengthen the alliance. Explain to the patient that what happened to them is not their fault.

The clinician's reaction to a disclosure of trauma is important. Key components include (i) accepting the information, (ii) expressing empathy and caring, (iii) re-emphasizing confidentiality, (iv) normalizing the experience, and (v) validating the disclosure. It may also be helpful to ask whether this is the first disclosure, discuss time limitations, collaborate with the person who has experienced trauma to develop an immediate plan of self-care, and recognize that action is not always required. For continued care, the clinician should discuss the implications of abuse history for future healthcare and interactions with other clinicians who are involved in the care of the patient and inquire about the patient's social supports [16]. For more information of ethical and legal considerations regarding reporting of suspected abuse, please see Chap. 13.

A few concepts of a safety plan and resources that a clinician can provide to patients who experienced trauma are presented in Table 14.3 [7, 16].

Table 14.3 Safety plan and resources for patients who experienced trauma [7, 16]

Safety plan	Resources (phone numbers, websites)
Should include: Safe places to go Strategies to reduce harm if ongoing contact with abuser Checklist of essential items; e.g., clothes, money, picture ID, prescribed medications to keep in a safe place Special considerations; e.g., arrangements for transportation needs Follow-up appointment with primary care physician or referral to other services Telephone numbers of family, friends, community organizations, and emergency service providers	www.trauma-informed.ca Local police, 9-1-1 *USA* National Domestic Violence Hotline **1-800-799-SAFE (7233)** National Sexual Assault Hotline **1-800-656-HOPE (4673)** National Clearinghouse on Abuse Later Life http://ncall.us/ *Canada* Provincial and territorial resources on elder abuse, available at: http://www.seniors.gc.ca/eng/pie/eaa/help.shtml www.advocacycentreelderly.org
Other characteristics: Individualized Options written down Stored in a safe place Reviewed regularly by the physician, the patient and a trusted friend or family member	Provide local resources [16]: Day programs Home care Respite care Legal services Shelters Elder abuse consultants

Key Points

- The complaints of alleged or suspected physical or sexual abuse by the patient or concerned clinicians are often challenging to distinguish from disease and normal aging in the elderly.
- Physical abuse does not necessarily cause visible injury (like pushing), but the psychological consequences should not be underestimated and need to be addressed by clinicians.

- Clinicians should be alert about the red flags of abuse, for example, the abusers often accompany the victimized patient and are reluctant the leave the abused person alone.
- Vulnerable populations (such as the older adults) can experience mistreatment as traumatic. The stress from abuse can be expressed via somatic complaints or transient memory impairment in geriatric patients.
- All levels of medical assessment and interventions should be trauma informed in order to avoid re-traumatization.
- The process of mandatory reporting of suspected abuse is jurisdiction specific; however, the patient with intact decision-making capacity has the right to refuse intervention.

References

1. Sandmoe A, Kirkevold M. Identifying and handling abused older clients in community care: the perspectives of nurse managers. Int J Older People Nurs. 2011;8:83–92.
2. Danesh MJ, Chang AL. The role of the dermatologist in detecting elder abuse and neglect. J Am Acad Dermatol. 2015;73:285–93.
3. Desmarais SL, Reeves KA. Gray, black and blue: the state of research and intervention for intimate partner abuse among elders. Behav Sci Law. 2007;25:377–91.
4. Cooper C, Selwood A, Livingston G. The prevalence of elder abuse and neglect: a systematic review. Age Ageing. 2008;37(2):151–60.
5. McDonald L. Elder abuse and neglect in Canada: the glass is still half full. Can J Aging. 2011;30(3):437–65.
6. McDonald L, Beaulieu M, Harbison J, Hirst S, Lowenstein A, Podnieks E, et al. Institutional abuse of older adults: what we know, what we need to know. J Elder Abuse Negl. 2012;24(2):138–60.
7. Wang XM, Brisbin S, Loo T, Straus S. Elder abuse: an approach to identification. Assessment and intervention. CMAJ. 2015;187(8):575–80.
8. Malmedal W, Iversen MH, Kilvik A. Sexual abuse of older nursing home residents: a literature review. Nurs Res Pract. 2015;1–7.
9. Allison EJ, Ellis PC, Wilson SE. Elder abuse and neglect: the emergency medicine perspective. Eur J Emerg Med. 1998;5:355–63.
10. Ahmad M, Lachs MS. Elder abuse and neglect: what physicians can and should do. Cleve Clin J Med. 2002;69:801–8.
11. Raja S, Hasnain M, Hoersch M, Gove-Yin S, Rajagopalam C. Trauma informed care in medicine – current knowledge and future research directions. Fam Community Health. 2015;38:216–26.
12. Sakauye K. Geriatric psychiatric interventions. In: Stoddard FJ, Pandya A, Katz CL, editors. Disaster psychiatry – readiness, evaluation, and treatment. Washington, DC: American Psychiatric Publishing, Inc.; 2011.
13. Pavao J, Turchik JA, Hyun JK, Karpenko J, Saweikis M, McCutcheon S, Kane V, Kimerling R. Military sexual trauma among homeless veterans. J Gen Intern Med. 2013;28 Suppl 2:S536–41.
14. Schachter C, Stalker C, Teram E, Lasiuk G, Danilkewich A. Handbook on sensitive practice for health care practitioners: lessons learned from adult survivors of childhood sexual abuse. Ottawa: Public Health Agency of Canada; 2008. http://www.integration.samhsa.gov/clinical-practice/handbook-sensitivve-practices4healthcare.pdf. Accessed 8 Dec 2015.

15. Kingston P, Penhale B. Elder abuse and neglect: issues in the accident and emergency department. Accid Emerg Nurs. 1995;3:122–8.
16. The Jean Tweed Centre for Women and their Families. Trauma matters – guidelines for trauma-informed practices in women's substance use services. 2013. http://jeantweed.com/wp-content/themes/JTC/pdfs/Trauma%20Matters%20online%20version%20August%202013.pdf. Accessed 8 Dec 2015.

Additional Resources

Bolton MJ, et al (Klinic Community Health Center, Winnipeg, Manitoba). Trauma-informed – the trauma toolkit. A resource for service organizations and providers to deliver services that are trauma-informed. 2nd ed. Winnipeg, MB 2013.

Buzgova R, Ivanova K. Elder abuse and mistreatment in residential settings. Nurs Ethics. 2009;16(1):110–26.

Cohen M, Halevy-Levin S, Gagin R, Prilutzky D, Friedman G. Elder abuse in long-term care residences and the risk indicators. Ageing Soc. 2010;30(6):1027–40.

Dong XQ. Elder abuse: systematic review and implications for practice. Am Geriatr Soc. 2015;63:1214–38.

Du Mont J, Macdonald S, Kosa D, Elliot S, Spencer C, Yaffe M. Development of a comprehensive hospital-based elder abuse intervention: an initial systematic scoping review. PLoS One. 2015;21:1–21.

Haviland S, O'Brien J. Physical abuse and neglect of the elderly: assessment and intervention. Orthop Nurs. 1989;8:11–8.

Hoover R, Polson M. Detecting elder abuse and neglect: assessment and intervention. Am Acad Fam Phys. 2014;89:453–60.

Lachs MS, Pillemer K. Elder abuse. Lancet. 2004;364(9441):1263–72.

Lindbloom EJ, Brandt J, Hough LD, Meadows SE. Elder mistreatment in the nursing home: a systematic review. J Am Med Dir Assoc. 2007;8(9):610–6.

Long-Term Care Task Force On Resident Care and Safety. Progress report: Long-Term Care Task Force on Resident Care and Safety. 2013. http://www.oanhss.org/oanhssdocs/Media_Centre/MediaReleases/Progress_Report_Final_January30_2013_English.pdf. Accessed 28 Sept 2015.

The Sexual Consent and Patients with Major Neurocognitive Disorders

15

Daniel L. Ambrosini, Ana Hategan, and James A. Bourgeois

15.1 Background

Because human sexuality is an important component of life regardless of age, the majority of geriatric persons report moderate or high levels of sexual interest well into their late life, and thus, documenting a sexual history taken during admission to an institution (e.g., hospital, long-term care home) needs to be part of a patient's medical evaluation and should easily be accessible to the on-call clinician [1].

The risks and benefits for patients with major neurocognitive disorders (NCDs) to provide their consent to participate in sexual activity has become an issue of increasing concern for clinicians, including geriatric psychiatrists [2, 3]. The tension lies in balancing protection of vulnerable patients from potential abuse while advocating for patient autonomy and freedom of sexual expression [4, 5]. Whether someone is capable to consent to sexual activity affects others including sexual partners, physicians, family members (who may be substitute decision-makers

D.L. Ambrosini, LLB/BCL, MSc, PhD (✉)
Legal Counsel, St. Joseph's Healthcare Hamilton, Hamilton, ON, Canada

Department of Psychiatry and Behavioural Neurosciences, Forensic Psychiatry Program, McMaster University, West 5th Campus, 3rd Floor, D328, 100 West 5th, Box 585, Hamilton, ON L8N 3K7, Canada
e-mail: dambro@mcmaster.ca

A. Hategan, MD
Department of Psychiatry and Behavioural Neurosciences, Division of Geriatric Psychiatry, Michael G. DeGroote School of Medicine, Faculty of Health Sciences, McMaster University, Hamilton, ON, Canada

J.A. Bourgeois, OD, MD
Department of Psychiatry/Langley Porter Psychiatric Institute, University of California San Francisco, San Francisco, CA, USA

Consultation-Liaison Service, University of California San Francisco Medical Center, San Francisco, CA, USA

A. Hategan et al. (eds.), *On-Call Geriatric Psychiatry: Handbook of Principles and Practice*, DOI 10.1007/978-3-319-30346-8_15

when patients have been found to have diminished decisional capacity), nursing staff, administration (hospitals and long-term care homes), courts, and ethicists. Sexual consent and capacity to consent to sexual activity are not always the same. Both should raise issues for clinicians about unwanted sexual advances, unwanted pregnancies, unsafe sexual practices, and management of relationships [6]. In this chapter, we explore some of the issues as they surface in on-call clinical practice for physicians and hospitals in managing the care of patients with major NCDs.

Case Vignette Mr. J was a 73-year-old man, with chronic schizophrenia and admitted to a psychiatric hospital for 4 months. Mr. J also showed early signs of Alzheimer's disease based on clinical examination and supportive neurocognitive tests; his attention, memory, and social cognition had become increasingly compromised. He had three adult children who visited him regularly in the hospital; his eldest daughter had assumed the role of substitute decision-maker as he had been declared by a court to be of diminished decisional capacity for medical treatment decisions. One night, Mr. J's nurse informed the on-call psychiatrist that she saw Mr. J having sexual intercourse with a 33-year-old female patient who was experiencing a manic episode. The nurse told the psychiatrist that she approached Mr. J about the incident and he replied that it was his "own business." The psychiatrist raised several questions including: *Does the hospital have a policy on sexual activity and conjugal visits? Should the family be informed, and if so, who? Was there consent to engage in sexual activity between Mr. J and the co-patient, or was it coercive behavior?* Several members of the team raised concerns about their role in reporting these incidents to their own managers, the hospital, and legal authorities, along with how to protect and educate patients with NCDs who engage in sexual activity.

The vignette above raises a host of clinical, ethical, legal, and even moral issues, not uncommonly found in the law, whereby individuals are expected to understand the local cultural, social mores governing sexual behavior in order to be considered capable to consent to sexual activity [7]. The vignette raises questions such as: *What constitutes "sexual" activity? What is the legal test to determine whether someone is able to consent to sexual activity?* We cover some of these clinical, ethical, and legal issues, noting that there is often overlap among them.

15.2 Clinical Issues

Sexual consent is the ability to freely give verbal or nonverbal communication of a feeling or willingness to engage in sexual activity [8]. Despite this definition, there is often little consensus on what constitutes "sexual activity" [9] and exactly how is it to be determined whether a patient has the requisite mental capacity to consent to sexual activity [10]. Patients with major NCDs pose unique challenges in providing sexual consent due to a typically progressive and gradual decline in their mental status. Of course, the severity of the illness is critical in appreciating the extent in which the patient is aware of his or her behavior.

Three clinical and legal criteria used by physicians and psychologists to assess sexual consent capacity are rationality, knowledge, and voluntariness [11]. A full medical evaluation will be required, along with testing and treatment in advance for sexually transmitted diseases. In cases where there is risk of sexual trauma, psychological support may need to be provided. (See Chap. 14.) Some cases will require close monitoring and educating patients about the relationship between sexual activity and pregnancy specifically the limits of sexual consent, what constitutes safe sexual practices, the use of contraception, and strategies for preventing the spread of sexually transmitted diseases [2, 3, 6, 9, 12]. Staff at the hospital and nursing homes will also need education about how to handle situations with both sensitivity and clinical skill [2, 5, 13].

Clinicians working within hospital settings are increasingly grappling with the status of institutional policies for conjugal visits [3, 14]. In a 1981 survey among 70 psychiatric units across the province of Ontario in Canada, for example, not a single unit had a written policy on how to manage sexual relationships between patients, and most respondents felt it was impossible to have a policy to include all emerging variables [14]. In the UK, the Royal College of Psychiatrists has recommended that all psychiatric facilities develop policies around sexual behavior for patients [15]. One UK study found that psychiatric institutions are inconsistent in their policies; most institutions prohibited or actively discouraged sexual activity [15]. This raises an issue for hospital and other healthcare facility administration on how to deal with sexual behavior of patients on a case-by-case basis, while still implementing a policy or guideline. There are at least four possible stances hospitals could take: (i) forbid all forms of sexual activity; (ii) forbid certain types of sexual activity and allow others, such as autoerotic practices; (iii) allow all forms of sexual activity; or (iv) allow all forms of sexual activity, but with certain safeguards (e.g., written guidelines, sex education) [3]. Other questions arise: *How long should a patient be in hospital before being able to obtain the "privilege" of sexual activity? Should sexual activity be treated as a "privilege" or as a "right"? Should it be permitted to occur on or off the unit* [11]*? How will clinicians safely facilitate, or in some cases even promote, safe sexual activity in a dignified manner?*

Lyden suggests determining sexual consent capacity involves three general methods: (i) review relevant medical records; (ii) hold discussions with others who know the patient; and (iii) conduct a face-to-face interview with the patient about their knowledge and voluntariness [11].

Clinical Recommendations

The severity of the illness is critical in appreciating the extent in which the patient with major NCD is capable of sexual consent for his or her sexual behavior. Clinical and legal criteria used by clinicians to assess sexual consent capacity are rationality, knowledge, and voluntariness.

15.3 Ethical Issues

Ethical and moral theoretical frameworks relating to sexual consent by patients with major NCDs should be addressed. The outcome of one's reasoning may differ from an "ethics of care" versus a "rights" perspective [3]. Although all humans have a fundamental right to autonomy, a patient's mental capacity can be diminished to the point that the patient may not be able to evaluate the foreseeable harms and consequences from any behavior.

Independent of patients' own views toward sexual behavior, there are various external ethical, moral, and religious beliefs that others hold about sexual behavior. These external perceptions of sexual behavior relate to fundamental values and beliefs that individuals may have of geriatric persons as a vulnerable group. One possibility is to adopt a supported "committee approach" in making a final decision of a patient's ability to consent to sexual activity that incorporates various perspectives that equally balance autonomy, dignity, and right to sexual expression [11].

Ethical Recommendations

Clinicians must not only ensure that geriatric patients are not unnecessarily exposed to harm or risks but also that the ethical and moral considerations around sexual behavior have been fully contemplated.

15.4 Legal Issues

Clinicians should also be aware of the various laws and regulations surrounding sexual consent among psychiatric patients, but note that the law is still evolving in this area. The *UN Convention on Rights of Persons with Disabilities* provides that State parties adopt awareness raising in terms of combating stereotypes, prejudices, and harmful practices relating to persons with disabilities (Article 8(1)(b)) [6, 16, 17]. It also states that persons with disabilities receive the same range, quality, and standard of free or affordable health programs as provided to other persons "including in the area of sexual and reproductive health" (Article 25(a)) [16]. Although most countries protect one's legal right to sexual privacy and the freedom of sexual expression, within the bounds of reasonable expectations, such rights may be curtailed where they infringe the rights of others or if they create an undue risk.

There has been a paucity of law in the USA addressing decisional capacity to provide sexual consent for patient with psychiatric disorders [18]; legal criteria adopted will vary depending on jurisdiction [2, 7, 19]. Most USA states have adopted a test that incorporates whether the individual has (i) knowledge of the relevant facts of the decision; (ii) the mental capacity and intelligence to rationally understand the risks and benefits; and (iii) voluntariness to engage in sexual activity without sexual coercion [2]. Yet, one may find varying thresholds across states.

In the UK, courts have in recent years heard several cases around the issue of sexual consent capacity that has led to commentary on what the legal standards should look like [19–21]. Herring and Wall propose a dichotomy of the legal test used by courts, as either *issue specific* (whether the individual understood the sexual act in the abstract, the physical nature of the act, medical risks, and/or risk of pregnancy) or *situation specific* (assess the individual in the context of a particular sexual act, facts about the other party, relational context) [21]. One of the issues courts struggle with is finding a "workable" test that can dovetail the general law of mental capacity with other closely related areas such as capacity to marry [19].

Clinicians working in hospitals and nursing homes may need to become familiar with tools and processes to assess mental capacity and sexual consent [7, 13]. In one survey conducted among 305 psychologists, researchers found that there are five factors in establishing criteria around sexual consent capacity: (i) knowledge of consequences of sexual activity; (ii) essential sexual knowledge; (iii) unessential sexual knowledge; (iv) knowledge of safety for self and others; and (v) basic safety skills [22]. Individuals at any age can become mentally incapable and may require additional protection; caution is warranted against developing potentially "ageist" views regarding geriatric sexuality. Some have advocated for the use of a sexual power of attorney as a specialized form of advance directive to keep others actively involved in the decision-making process [5].

While patients with psychiatric disorders are not anymore violent than the general public, unique risks may be present with forensic psychiatric patients regarding sexual consent and sexual decisional capacity [18]. There is the possibility for psychological violence or harm in the form of threatening behavior, coercion, or undue influence either by or toward the patient. There are also legal risks that need to be managed to minimize the risk that sexually transmitted diseases are contracted, certainly not knowingly, but also recklessly or negligently. The clinician must be concerned with not only the potential for psychological harm but also physical dangerousness, which may warrant conducting a clinical risk assessment to engage in sexual activity.

Hospitals, nursing homes, and other healthcare institutions will want to ensure that they are managing any potential risk for civil liability for failing in a duty to protect if they have not turned their attention to potential policies [3]. Hospitals have undertaken an obligation to protect all patients and to provide a safe and secure residence – *to what extent are they able to achieve this while still optimizing autonomy, choice, and freedom for sexual expression?* One example where these legal obligations may arise for hospitals is with Internet use by geriatric psychiatric patients who wish to engage in online dating for the purposes of seeking sexual intimacy [23]. Certain hospitals may also have their own moral or religious values that impact how clinicians deal with patients on issues of sexual consent or sexual issues with LGBT (lesbian, gay, bisexual, and transgender) patients. In those cases where a hospital may agree to establish a conjugal visit policy, they will need to consider how they balance the right to privacy and other important priorities.

Legal Recommendations

Clinicians should (i) be aware of the legal issues and facts that can arise with each patient who wishes to engage in sexual activity; (ii) determine whether the patient has the mental capacity and intelligence to rationally understand the risks and benefits; and (iii) evaluate whether there is a degree of voluntariness for the patient to engage in sexual activity without sexual coercion.

Key Points

- Sexual consent is the ability to freely give verbal or nonverbal communication of a feeling or willingness to engage in sexual activity.
- Patients will be required to understand the social mores of sexual behavior in order to be considered mentally capable to consent to sexual activity.
- Clinicians working in hospitals and nursing homes may need to become familiar with tools and processes to assess mental capacity and sexual consent.
- Clinicians must be concerned with the potential for dangerousness, which may warrant conducting a clinical risk assessment for patients admitted to an institutional setting and wish to engage in sexual activity.
- Patients with major NCDs pose unique challenges in providing sexual consent due to a progressive and gradual decline in their mental status.

References

1. Chow ES, Hategan A, Bourgeois JA. When it's time for 'the talk': sexuality and your geriatric patient. Curr Psychiatry. 2015;14(5):13, 14, 16–19, 29, 30.
2. Tang SL. When "yes" might mean "no": standardizing state criteria to evaluate the capacity to consent to sexual activity for elderly with neurocognitive disorders. Elder Law J. 2015;22(2):450–90.
3. McSherry B, Somerville MA. Sexual activity among institutionalized persons in need of special care. Windsor Yearbook Access Justice. 1998;16:90–131.
4. Breland L. Lost libido, or just forgotten? The legal and social influences on sexual activity in long-term care. Law Psychol Rev. 2014;38:177–92.
5. Hill E. We'll always have shady pines: surrogate decision-making tools for preserving sexual autonomy in elderly nursing home residents. William Mary J Women Law. 2014;20:469–90.
6. Dein K, Williams PS. Relationships between residents in secure psychiatric units: are safety and sensitivity really incompatible? Pyschiatry Bull. 2008;32:284–7.
7. Kennedy CH. Legal and psychological implications in the assessment of sexual consent in the cognitively impaired population. Assessment. 2003;10(4):352–8.
8. Humphreys TP, Brousseau MM. The sexual consent scale-revised: development, reliability, and preliminary validity. J Sex Res. 2010;47(5):420–8.
9. Perlin M, Lynch AJ. "All his sexless patients": persons with mental disabilities and the competence to have sex. Wash Law Rev. 2014;89:257–300.
10. Murphy GH, O'Callaghan A. Capacity of adults with intellectual disabilities to consent to sexual relationships. Psychol Med. 2004;34(7):1347–57.

11. Lyden M. Assessment of sexual consent capacity. Sex Disabil. 2007;25(1):3–20.
12. Spady A. The sexual freedom of eve: a recommendation for contraceptive sterilization legislation in the Canadian post Re Eve context. Windsor Rev Legal Soc Issues. 2008;25:33–67.
13. Lindsay JR. The need for more specific legislation in sexual consent capacity assessments for nursing home residents. J Leg Med. 2010;31(3):303–23.
14. Keitner G, Grof P. Sexual and emotional intimacy between psychiatric inpatients: formulating a policy. Hosp Community Psychiatry. 1981;32(3):188–93.
15. Bartlett P, Mantovani N, Cratsley K, Dillon C, Eastman N. 'You may kiss the bride, but you may not open your mouth when you do so': policies concerning sex, marriage and relationships in English forensic psychiatric facilities. Liverpool Law Rev. 2010;31:155–76.
16. UN convention on human rights for persons with disabilities. http://www.un.org/disabilities/convention/conventionfull.shtml. Accessed 21 Feb 2016.
17. Macgregor-Morris R, Ewbank J, Birmingham L. Potential impact of the Human Rights Act on psychiatric practice: the best of British values? BMJ. 2001;322(7290):848–50.
18. Perlin M. "Everybody is making love/or else expecting rain": considering the sexual autonomy rights of persons institutionalized because of mental disability in forensic hospitals and in Asia. Wash Law Rev. 2008;83:481–512.
19. Mackenzie R, Watts J. Capacity to consent to sex reframed: IM, TZ (no 2), the need for an evidence-based model of sexual decision-making and socio-sexual competence. Int J Law Psychiatry. 2015;40:50–9.
20. Curtice M, Mayo J, Crocombe J. Consent and sex in vulnerable adults: a review of case law. Br J Learn Disabil. 2012;41:280–7.
21. Herring J, Wall J. Capacity to consent to sex. Med Law Rev. 2014;22(4):620–30.
22. Kennedy CH, Niederbuhl J. Establishing criteria for sexual consent capacity. Am J Ment Retard. 2001;106(6):503–10.
23. Hategan A, Bougeois JA, Parthasarathi U, Ambrosini DL. Counseling geriatric patients about opportunity and risk when "digital dating". Curr Psychiatry. 2016 (in press).

Part III

On-Call Geriatric Psychiatry in Specific Medical Settings

16 Emergency Medicine Settings

Katren Tyler, Calvin H. Hirsch, Lorin M. Scher, and Dane E. Stevenson

16.1 Background

When called to the emergency department (ED) for a psychiatric issue in an older patient, the psychiatric consultant must understand the nature of the ED environment and the challenges it poses for diagnosis and management. Many emergency conditions are characterized by having to act with minimal background information. This is compounded in older patients by cognitive disorders or other underlying psychiatric illnesses, which may limit the ability to provide a clear history. Additionally, emergencies of any type, be they primarily systemic medical or psychiatric, or a combination of both, are commonly assessed initially in the fast-paced setting of a busy ED, with its emphasis on triage, stabilization, and rapid turnaround of patients. EDs are problematic for older patients because they are crowded and noisy; staff can be distracted by the spectacular medical emergencies and by disruptive or demanding patients. Often, privacy is minimal,

K. Tyler, MD (✉)
Geriatric Emergency Medicine Fellowship Director, Department of Emergency Medicine, University of California, Davis, Sacramento, CA, USA
e-mail: krtyler@ucdavis.edu

C.H. Hirsch, MD
Department of Internal Medicine, Division of General Medicine, University of California Davis Medical Center, Sacramento, CA, USA

L.M. Scher, MD • D.E. Stevenson, MD, MS
Department of Psychiatry, University of California, Davis, Davis, CA, USA

A. Hategan et al. (eds.), *On-Call Geriatric Psychiatry: Handbook of Principles and Practice*, DOI 10.1007/978-3-319-30346-8_16

lights are on continuously, and orienting stimuli like clocks and windows are out of sight [1, 2]. The ED environment can provoke anxiety, delirium, and agitation in vulnerable older patients, especially those with underlying psychiatric illness including neurocognitive disorders (NCDs). Once medically stabilized and awaiting admission, geriatric patients may not receive optimal monitoring and frequent orientation to prevent or manage delirium [1]. Those with psychiatric illness including NCDs may not be able to effectively communicate their physical and psychological distress. As a result, pain, a need to void, or feeling cold, hungry, thirsty, or frightened may go unrecognized or become channeled into undifferentiated agitation, for which staff may not have the time to perform a thorough assessment and instead will treat the *behavior*, rather than the *underlying cause*. Most hypoactive delirium is not identified by ED physicians, and delirium that is missed in the ED is nearly always missed by hospital physicians at the time of admission [3].

Although the emphasis of the ED is rapid stabilization and disposition (either back to the community or through hospital admission), disposition can be held up, sometimes for days, when no suitable discharge destination can be found. Busy EDs may experience delays moving a patient from the ED to a hospital bed (known as exit block or ED boarding). A study of ED boarding of patients age 65 or older in a large Eastern Canadian academic health facility found, after adjustment for age, sex, acuity, and comorbidity, that each hour in the ED was associated with a 3 % increase in the risk of an adverse event, with an adverse event approximately doubling the hospital length of stay [3]. The geriatric patient with complex systemic medical or psychiatric conditions may be stable and hospital admission unjustified (or not reimbursable by an insurer), but a long-term care facility willing to accept the patient may be difficult to find. For geriatric patients with comorbid medical illness presenting with a psychiatric emergency, transfer to a psychiatric facility without on-site primary care medical consultation may be similarly difficult. Such unintended prolonged stays in the ED while awaiting psychiatric placement, also referred to as "psychiatric boarding" [4], present the psychiatric consultant with the challenge of treating a psychiatric condition in a suboptimal environment that *itself* may be exacerbating the psychiatric condition.

16.2 Approach to the Geriatric Patient in the ED

There is a reciprocal relationship between systemic medical and psychiatric illness, particularly in older patients. Psychiatric illness is common in older patients presenting to the ED, and medical illness is common in older psychiatric patients. Data from the Canadian Study of Health and Aging showed a strong correlation between the number of frailty-defining factors and prevalent psychiatric illness (mostly depressive disorders) in community-dwelling persons age 65 or older without major NCDs (dementia). Over 30 % of the most severely frail had psychiatric illness [5]. In patients who are confused, the duration of the cognitive impairment initially may not be clear during the presentation; having collateral history is critical. It can be

Table 16.1 Differential diagnosis of confusion in the geriatric emergency department patient and a comparison of clinical features

	Delirium	Major neurocognitive disorder (NCD)	Major depressive disorder	Psychotic disorder
Onset	Sudden	Gradual	Variable	Variable, from early adulthood to late onset
Duration	Days to months	Lifelong once established	Months	Long term
Course	Fluctuating over hours to days	Months to years	Weeks to months to years	Weeks to months to years
Risk factors	Hospitalization Serious medical illness Preexisting cognitive impairment, especially major NCD Hip fractures Polypharmacy Withdrawal syndromes	Family history Vascular disease Comorbidities	Bereavement Sleep disturbance Disability Female sex	Complex
Attention	Fluctuating	Stable with gradual decline	Preserved	Preserved
Level of consciousness	Varies between somnolent and combative (RASS, −3 to +4)	Intact until advanced stages	Intact	Intact
Orientation	Disrupted	Disrupted in advanced stages	Intact	Intact
Psychotic features	Common	Uncommon until advanced stages	Variable	Common
Neuropsychiatric symptoms (NPS) of NCDs	Acute delirium may be easily confused with NPS	Common with disease progression	No	No
Treatment	Directed at underlying cause and management of agitation	Few effective treatments	Antidepressants usually effective Psycho-behavioral treatments	Antipsychotics
Outcome	Long-term increased mortality risk and increased cognitive impairment. Short-term fall risk as inpatient	Loss of higher cortical functions and progressive dependence	Older patients are high risk of completed suicide if depression is unrecognized or untreated	Long-standing functional decline and social isolation

nearly impossible to assess for fluctuating level of consciousness during a brief ED assessment as the fluctuations may require many hours of sustained observation to quantitate. Table 16.1 provides a summary of the differential diagnosis of confusion in the geriatric patient presenting to the ED and a comparison of the underlying clinical features.

Case Vignette 1 Ms. A was an 86-year-old woman brought to the ED after a ground-level fall in her residential skilled nursing facility. Past medical history included major NCD, hypertension, and type 2 diabetes mellitus. She had been increasingly agitated for 3 days prior to the fall and had received several doses of lorazepam in the previous 48 h. Vital signs in the ED revealed a blood pressure of 132/85 mmHg, heart rate of 113 BPM, temperature of 37.8 °C, respiratory rate of 18/min, and an oxygen saturation of 97 %.

Ms. A was disorientated, not following commands, but did not show any focal neurological deficits. She was agitated and verbally abusive to ED staff, occasionally striking out at them. The left lower extremity was shortened and externally rotated. Laboratory testing revealed a urinalysis consistent with a urinary tract infection (UTI), hemoglobin of 12.2 mg/dL (122 g/L), and normal serum electrolytes. A mildly displaced intertrochanteric fracture of the left femoral neck was visible on pelvic and femur roentgenograms.

Case Analysis This discussion focuses specifically on the ED geriatric patient with hyperactive delirium who is at risk of injury to themselves or others. It assumes that acute conditions such as hypoglycemia have already been reversed. (For additional discussion of causes, diagnosis, and management of delirium, see Chaps. 10, 11, and 18.) Ms. A had a preexisting delirium most likely precipitated by a UTI and, in an attempt to control agitated behavior at her residential facility, received several small doses of a benzodiazepine, which may have further contributed to the delirium.

16.2.1 Delirium and Agitation in the Geriatric Patient in the ED

16.2.1.1 Prevention of Delirium and the Limitations of Non-pharmacological Management

Prevention of delirium is critical for vulnerable, older patients in the ED. Patients who are particularly likely to develop delirium during their ED stay include patients who spend many hours in the ED, first waiting to be seen and then waiting for a hospital bed or transfer to another facility. Patients with preexisting cognitive impairment, severe pain, severe acute illness, and hip fractures are at high risk of developing delirium [6, 7]. A multimodal pain strategy is now the standard of care for hip (neck of femur) fragility fractures and includes intravenous opioids, regular acetaminophen (paracetamol), regional anesthesia ideally within the ED, and early operative fixation [7–9].

Non-pharmacological approaches (day-night appropriate lighting, a calm environment, frequent reorientation, early mobilization out of bed, and appropriate nutrition) often help to prevent and manage delirium in the inpatient setting [10, 11] and should be implemented whenever possible in the ED. (See Chap. 18, Table 18.1, for non-pharmacological delirium management.) However, in the ED, urgent stabilization and management of acute medical illness and/or injury drive clinical care, and medication management for severe agitation during hyperactive delirium is often unavoidable. Severe agitation is a serious risk for both significant patient injuries and injuries to health-care providers [12]. In this setting, non-pharmacological approaches may be too time-consuming, necessitating rapidly active sedation despite a desire to minimize the negative effects of medications [11]. Even the fastest intravenous medication will still take 5–10 min to take full effect. Use of the lowest possible dose of psychoactive medication for the shortest possible time should always be a goal, but the time course in the ED is often very different from the clinic or the medical ward. The geriatric axiom of "starting low and going slow" should still be attempted, but immediate control of behavioral symptoms may require more frequent dosing than is typically utilized in calmer circumstances.

16.2.1.2 Use of Restraints for the Agitated Geriatric Patient

Restraints provide a double bind in the acutely agitated patient. In the immediate short term, they may provide some protection against self-harm, but in the medium and long term, they may contribute to the development of delirium and may exacerbate agitation. If the psychiatric consultant discovers restraints being used on a geriatric patient, or recommends restraints, there should be a discussion with the ED physician and nurses regarding the most appropriate and least restrictive type. For confused patients who may reach for intravenous and catheter tubing or electrocardiogram leads, hand mitts may suffice. Patients who are striking out or physically resisting care may require wrist restraints. If attempting to get off the gurney (trolley), the patient may require a lap belt. The traditional vest restraint prevents the patient from turning from side to side or sitting up and may endanger older patients who cannot defend their airway from vomitus, contributing to pressure ulcers. Bilateral wrist restraints also prevent the patient from changing position and similarly contribute to the risk of pressure ulcers from the hard gurney. More modern vest restraints enable side-to-side shifts in position while preventing the patient from sitting up. In the USA and Canada, at least, behavioral restraint orders must be frequently reordered. Restrained patients need constant one-on-one observation (see Chap. 7). For the confused patient, medical devices such as oxygen tubing, intravenous lines, cardiac monitoring and urinary catheters may be experienced as a restraint.

16.2.1.3 When to Use Opioids for Hyperactive Delirium

In patients with a condition known to be painful, such as a hip fracture, control of pain should be the first step in the management of hyperactive delirium. All opioids can make delirium worse through direct effects on cognition. Morphine and meperidine are strongly associated with delirium in geriatric patients and should be avoided. Both have active metabolites that are renally cleared and thus have a relatively longer half-life in older patients, increasing the potential for toxicity. Hydromorphone has fewer active metabolites and is preferred in patients with renal impairment [13, 14]. If there is known or suspected pre-ED opioid use plus a constellation of symptoms that includes several common autonomic reactions seen in

Table 16.2 Nonpsychiatric symptoms of opioid withdrawal

Early symptoms (first 24 h)	Late symptoms (after 24 h)
Muscle aches	Diarrhea
Lacrimation	Abdominal cramps
Runny nose	Dilated pupils
Frequent yawning	Tachycardia
	Hypertension
	Cutis anserina ("goose bumps")

opioid withdrawal (see Table 16.2), then a small test dose of a short-acting opioid can be tried. Caution must be exercised in determining the effectiveness of the test dose. The clinical symptoms of opioid withdrawal are nonspecific and may be misinterpreted. In the absence of withdrawal, an opioid may lessen agitation because of sedation and may improve hypertension because of its vasodilatory effect. Therefore, effectiveness in *opioid withdrawal* should be determined based on improvement of multiple autonomic signs.

Prescription drug monitoring programs, where available (e.g., in California, USA), have proven useful in identifying patients of all ages who have multiple prescriptions for controlled substances. Obtaining prescriptions from multiple providers is a significant risk for opioid complications [15, 16] (see Chap. 10, Sect. 10.2.7.2 for opioid prescribing rules in the ED settings).

If providing analgesia does not adequately control agitated behavior in the patient with a clinical condition associated with severe pain, a decision has to be made about the use of psychoactive agents.

16.2.1.4 Selection of Psychoactive Medication for Agitation in the Geriatric ED Patient

When a psychoactive medication is required, the goal is to administer a dose sufficient to manage the behavior while avoiding excessive sedation. Antipsychotics remain the drug class of choice, with the initial and repeat doses titrated to the severity of the agitation and observed peak effect. (For details of antipsychotic selection and dosing for agitation in the geriatric patient, see Chap. 10, Sect. 10.2.1.2 "Management of Delirium.") In general, benzodiazepines should be reserved for delirium in four clinical situations: (1) when the patient requires immediate sedation, as, for example, when a bedside procedure must be performed or to prevent imminent self-injury; (2) to control agitation during withdrawal from alcohol, benzodiazepines, or barbiturates; (3) to control severe agitation in a substance-induced psychosis; and (4) for management in rare delirium syndromes where antipsychotics are contraindicated (most importantly, neuroleptic malignant syndrome and malignant catatonia). Regular illicit use of stimulants including methamphetamine increasingly is seen in the older population. Almost one-third of methamphetamine users in the USA are over the age of 50 [17], and approximately 40 % of regular methamphetamine users will develop psychosis, often complicated by agitation [18]. However, benzodiazepines can precipitate delirium and make preexisting delirium worse both in severity and duration, so benzodiazepine use should be limited [19]. The consulting psychiatrist may be called to the ED to assist in the management of substance-induced psychosis and agitation or

Table 16.3 Comparison of intravenous benzodiazepines for use in severe agitation requiring immediate sedation

	Onset – intravenous	Half-life	Active metabolites	Special considerations	Starting dose in agitated older patient
Lorazepam	15–20 min	14 h	No	Preferred in hepatic dysfunction	0.25 mg IV
Diazepam	5–10 min	Parent drug: 30–60 h Active metabolites: 30–100 h	Yes	Avoid in hepatic dysfunction	1 mg IV
Midazolam	5 min	2.5 h	Yes	Avoid in hepatic dysfunction	0.25 mg IV

may be asked to assist in the management of delirium when the possibility of withdrawal has not been recognized by ED staff.

In extremely agitated patients requiring immediate sedation, a parenteral benzodiazepine will be required; the three most commonly used are diazepam, lorazepam, and midazolam, whose pharmacology is compared in Table 16.3.

Barbiturate use in delirium is limited to maintenance/replacement in barbiturate withdrawal in chronic users. In medically unstable patients due to severe alcohol withdrawal, barbiturates as well as propofol have been shown to reduce the need for intubation [20].

As with benzodiazepines, the use of an antipsychotic for agitation in a delirious geriatric patient may help control behavior in the short term, but may worsen the underlying delirium in the long term [11].

The reader is referred to Chap. 10, Sect. 10.2.1.2 "Management of Delirium" for a detailed discussion of antipsychotic use in delirium. The principle of the lowest possible dose for the shortest possible time should be used. All antipsychotic agents carry an increased risk of mortality in the elderly with extended courses, but the risk of a single or few doses of an antipsychotic in the management of the agitated hyperactive delirium patient is unknown. The use of antipsychotics in a patient with prolongation of the QT interval is associated with a risk of polymorphic ventricular tachycardia (see Chap. 12, Sect. 12.3.6.2 "QTc Prolongation and Ventricular Arrhythmias"), and, ideally, serum potassium and magnesium levels should be normalized prior to administration of an antipsychotic agent. Because of the risk of QTc prolongation, an electrocardiogram prior to administration of the antipsychotic is recommended when not prevented by the patient's agitation, and cardiac monitoring during administration of parenteral antipsychotics (e.g., IV haloperidol) should be started as soon as possible. Both olanzapine and risperidone have an oral disintegrating tablet formulation that may provide a non-parenteral option which may be better accepted by older agitated patients.

Case Vignette 1 (Continued) In the ED, Ms. A was placed in a single room with independent lighting controls and a clock, with calming staff. She had an IV placed and received hydromorphone 0.2 mg IV twice. She required a dose of IV lorazepam

0.25 mg as she was hitting and punching at staff and screaming loudly. She was also given quetiapine 12.5 mg PO. A fascia iliaca compartment block was placed with apparent relief of pain as the patient was able to lie on the fractured hip. She received IV antibiotics for her UTI. She was admitted to the medicine service with an orthopedic consultation and underwent early operative fixation of her hip fracture.

16.2.2 Psychosis in the Geriatric Patient in the ED

The term "psychosis" is defined as the loss of reality testing, often characterized by the presence of (i) delusions, (ii) hallucinations, and/or (iii) disorganized thinking, speech, or behavior. Psychotic symptoms are very common in patients with major NCDs, and these patients often present to EDs for treatment of psychosis, agitation, and disruptive behavior [21]. Ideally, the emergency physician will have assessed psychotic symptoms in the geriatric patient carefully before calling for psychiatric consultation. Accurate clinical assessments (uncovering the etiology of psychotic symptoms) have important implications for patients' clinical outcomes and dispositions from emergency settings.

As a general rule, new-onset psychotic symptoms in geriatric patients should be considered a medical emergency. Primary psychiatric disorders certainly can cause psychotic symptoms in older patients (e.g., schizophrenia, depressive and bipolar disorders with psychotic features), yet these illnesses represent the least common cause of psychosis in older patients presenting to the ED. Neurocognitive disorders (delirium and/or major NCDs – formerly dementia) are the most common cause of psychosis in geriatric patients. For example, more than half of patients with Alzheimer's disease will develop delusions or hallucinations during the first few years of clinical onset [22]. Psychosis related to NCDs is associated with faster cognitive decline and increased risk of agitation and violence in nursing home settings.

16.2.2.1 Neurocognitive Disorder Subtypes Associated with Psychosis

- Alzheimer's disease
- Vascular cognitive impairment
- Traumatic brain injury
- Frontotemporal (Pick's) disease
- Human immunodeficiency virus (HIV) disease
- Lewy body disease
- Parkinson's disease
- Huntington's disease

Psychosis secondary to delirium is very common in older adults, as a high percentage of older patients will develop delirium during medical admissions [21]. Even mild infections (such as UTI) or subtle medication adjustments may cause delirium and psychotic symptoms in the geriatric patients. Psychotic symptoms may often develop related to substance use and/or medication side effects.

Commonly prescribed medications associated with delirium and psychosis include anticholinergic agents, antihistamines, corticosteroids, opiates, tricyclic antidepressants, and dopamine agonists [23]. (See also Chap. 12.)

Psychotic symptoms may occur in a major depressive disorder. Psychotically depressed patients will experience the classic mood, neurovegetative, and cognitive symptoms of a depressive episode, yet they will also have mood-congruent delusions or hallucinations. Delusions of persecution or of having an incurable illness are common in such patients. Hallucinations often have a negative tone and quality and may "command" patients to harm themselves. Depression with psychosis has a much higher risk of suicide than depression without psychotic features, and this should influence recommendations for discharge and follow-up by the psychiatric consultant. These patients require careful safety precautions (increased clinical observation, appropriate use of antipsychotics and antianxiety medications), and hospital admission or admission to a psychiatric unit may be necessary. Schizophrenia may also cause psychotic symptoms in geriatric patients, yet it should be remembered that most cases of primary psychotic illness (schizophrenia, schizoaffective disorder) begin in early life (second and third decade of life in most cases) [24].

Psychosis of acute onset (arising within days) generally should raise suspicion of delirium and the search for a metabolic, infectious, or pharmacological etiology (see Chap. 11). In the absence of a previously diagnosed chronic (long-term) NCD or known psychiatric illness, subacute onset (arising over the course of several weeks) should raise concern about a central nervous system process and warrants hospital admission and cranial imaging by magnetic resonance or computed tomography (preferably with contrast). Lumbar puncture may also be necessary. Subacute psychosis from an encephalitis, although rare, can be seen in diseases like tertiary syphilis, HIV or an infection associated with HIV (e.g., *Cryptococcus*), and neurocysticercosis and a number of viruses (e.g., West Nile virus). Risk factors for these conditions often can be gleaned from informants, if available. Autoimmune conditions like CNS vasculitis, neurosarcoidosis, and limbic encephalitis also have presented as psychosis. The psychiatric manifestations of neurosyphilis and HIV can become chronic.

16.2.3 Substance Abuse in the Geriatric Patient in the ED

On a daily basis in the ED, it is common to see patients of any age present with evidence of substance abuse disorders and withdrawal syndromes. These substances include alcohol, prescription and over-the-counter medications, recreational drugs, or any combination of these. Presentations with alcohol intoxication are usually straightforward. Clinicians in emergency settings may not inquire about or recognize substance use disorder in geriatric patients. In some instances this is because patients have had decades to acquire tolerance and may not appear to be intoxicated or have hidden their substance use from family members. Having a high index of suspicion for withdrawal syndromes is important in all emergency clinical settings.

Addiction to illicit drugs such as marijuana, cocaine, heroin, and methamphetamine does not stop because the patient has passed age 65. In old age the long-term effects of substance abuse are likely to increase, and clinicians should have a low threshold for examination and detection of substance use in their patients. Up to 10 % of trauma patients over the age of 65 had a detectable blood alcohol level in the ED and at least one positive finding on a urine drug screen nearly 50 % of the time [25].

Prescription of opioids for chronic pain has become a topic of considerable controversy due to increased mortality associated with prescription opioid use. In addition to patients using medications as prescribed, some scheduled substances are diverted from their original purpose.

Substance abuse in older patients will continue to be a problem as the demographic bubble of the geriatric "baby boomers" enlarges. Substance use in older patients is not currently a focus of significant research attention. Specific substance abuse patterns in older patients are less clearly described than in younger patients. Clinicians should continue to have a low threshold for direct testing, as well as interviewing of patients and family members to help identify high-risk substance abuse behaviors.

Key Points

- Systemic medical and/or psychiatric emergencies are commonly assessed in the fast-paced setting of a busy ED, with emphasis on triage, stabilization, and rapid turnaround of patients.
- Geriatric patients receiving treatment in the ED setting are at high risk of developing delirium, particularly those with preexisting cognitive impairment, severe pain, severe acute illness, and hip fractures.
- The ED environment is crowded, noisy, and with inadequate orienting stimuli, which further can provoke anxiety, delirium, and agitation in vulnerable geriatric patients, especially those with underlying psychiatric illness, including NCDs.
- As a general rule, new-onset psychotic symptoms in geriatric patients should be considered a medical emergency. In these cases a delirium workup is warranted to search for the underlying cause (metabolic, infectious, pharmacological, or CNS process).
- Geriatric patients with psychiatric illness may be unable to effectively communicate their physical and psychological distress, and their initial needs may go unrecognized or result in increased agitation; the ED staff may not have the time to perform a thorough assessment and may treat the patient's behavior, rather than the underlying cause.
- When a psychoactive medication is required to symptomatically treat the behavior, the goal is to administer a dose sufficient to manage the behavior while avoiding excessive sedation.
- Clinicians in emergency settings may not inquire about or recognize substance use disorders (including prescription and over-the-counter agents) in geriatric patients. Having a high index of suspicion for intoxication and withdrawal syndromes is important in ED settings.

References

1. Carpenter CR, Bromley M, Caterino JM, et al. Optimal older adult emergency care: introducing multidisciplinary geriatric emergency department guidelines from the American College of Emergency Physicians, American Geriatrics Society, Emergency Nurses Association, and Society for Academic Emergency Medicine. Acad Emerg Med. 2014;21(7):806–9.
2. Terrell KM, Hustey FM, Hwang U, et al. Quality indicators for geriatric emergency care. Acad Emerg Med. 2009;16(5):441–9.
3. Han JH, Zimmerman EE, Cutler N, et al. Delirium in older emergency department patients: recognition, risk factors, and psychomotor subtypes. Acad Emerg Med. 2009;16(3): 193–200.
4. Misek RK, DeBarba AE, Brill A. Predictors of psychiatric boarding in the emergency department. West J Emerg Med. 2015;16(1):71–5.
5. Andrew MK, Rockwood K. Psychiatric illness in relation to frailty in community-dwelling elderly people without dementia: a report from the Canadian Study of Health and Aging. Can J Aging. 2007;26(1):33–8.
6. Inouye SK, Westendorp RG, Saczynski JS. Delirium in elderly people. Lancet. 2014;383(9920): 911–22.
7. Young J, Murthy L, Westby M, Akunne A, O'Mahony R, Group GD. Diagnosis, prevention, and management of delirium: summary of NICE guidance. BMJ. 2010;341:c3704.
8. Mouzopoulos G, Vasiliadis G, Lasanianos N, Nikolaras G, Morakis E, Kaminaris M. Fascia iliaca block prophylaxis for hip fracture patients at risk for delirium: a randomized placebo-controlled study. J Orthop Traumatol. 2009;10(3):127–33.
9. Roberts KC, Brox WT, Jevsevar DS, Sevarino K. Management of hip fractures in the elderly. J Am Acad Orthop Surg. 2015;23(2):131–7.
10. Eubank KJ, Covinsky KE. Delirium severity in the hospitalized patient: time to pay attention. Ann Intern Med. 2014;160(8):574–5.
11. Inouye SK, Marcantonio ER, Metzger ED. Doing damage in delirium: the hazards of antipsychotic treatment in elderly persons. Lancet Psychiatry. 2014;1(4):312–5.
12. Rossi J, Swan MC, Isaacs ED. The violent or agitated patient. Emerg Med Clin North Am. 2010;28(1):235–56. x.
13. Coller JK, Christrup LL, Somogyi AA. Role of active metabolites in the use of opioids. Eur J Clin Pharmacol. 2009;65(2):121–39.
14. Power I. An update on analgesics. Br J Anaesth. 2011;107(1):19–24.
15. Kuo YF, Raji MA, Chen NW, Hasan H, Goodwin JS. Trends in opioid prescriptions among part D medicare recipients from 2007 to 2012. Am J Med. 2015;129(2):221.e21–30. doi: 10.1016/j.amjmed.2015.10.002. Epub 2015 Nov 11.
16. Paulozzi LJ, Strickler GK, Kreiner PW, Koris CM. Controlled substance prescribing patterns – prescription behavior surveillance system, eight states, 2013. MMWR Surveill Summ. 2015;64(9):1–14.
17. Chen LY, Strain EC, Alexandre PK, Alexander GC, Mojtabai R, Martins SS. Correlates of nonmedical use of stimulants and methamphetamine use in a national sample. Addict Behav. 2014;39(5):829–36.
18. Glasner-Edwards S, Mooney LJ. Methamphetamine psychosis: epidemiology and management. CNS Drugs. 2014;28(12):1115–26.
19. Pandharipande P, Shintani A, Peterson J, et al. Lorazepam is an independent risk factor for transitioning to delirium in intensive care unit patients. Anesthesiology. 2006;104(1): 21–6.
20. Mirijello A, D'Angelo C, Ferrulli A, et al. Identification and management of alcohol withdrawal syndrome. Drugs. 2015;75(4):353–65.
21. Khouzam HR, Emes R. Late life psychosis: assessment and general treatment strategies. Compr Ther. 2007;33(3):127–43.

22. Piechniczek-Buczek J. Psychiatric emergencies in the elderly population. Emerg Med Clin North Am. 2006;24(2):467–90. viii.
23. Patkar AA, Mago R, Masand PS. Psychotic symptoms in patients with medical disorders. Curr Psychiatry Rep. 2004;6(3):216–24.
24. Targum SD. Treating psychotic symptoms in elderly patients. Prim Care Companion J Clin Psychiatry. 2001;3(4):156–63.
25. Ekeh AP, Parikh PP, Walusimbi M, Woods RJ, Hawk A, McCarthy MC. The prevalence of positive drug and alcohol screens in elderly trauma patients. Subst Abus. 2014;35(1): 51–5.

Acute Inpatient Psychiatric Settings

17

Howard H. Fenn, James M. Ellison,
and Elmira Yessengaliyeva

17.1 Background

The high prevalence of systemic medical comorbidity contributes to complications and/or exacerbations of psychiatric symptomatology in geriatric patients. For example, 95 % of geriatric patients with schizophrenia have concomitant systemic medical illnesses; up to 19 % of bipolar disorder geriatric patients have metabolic, respiratory, cardiovascular, and endocrine abnormalities [1–3]. The variety of health-care delivery models on inpatient psychiatry units adds complexity to the on-call task. Models vary by institution, molded often not by best practices, outcome data, or randomized clinical trials, but by socioeconomic forces, inpatient bed resources, local staff/physician availability, and reimbursement rates specific to the locale, especially in the United States but also in Canada. The effect of Medicare prospective payment, at least in the United States, incentivizes brief hospital admissions, constraining the time needed for adequate assessment and treatment of geriatric patients. Nor will the Centers for Medicare and Medicaid Services (CMS) reimburse hospitals for costs of hospitalization for psychiatric complications of Alzheimer's disease and related disorders.

Some models of inpatient care may blur the borders of clinical responsibility, allowing several clinicians to prescribe medications and other interventions without consensus and without clear lines of communication. An on-call clinician must avoid adding to confusion over treatment by familiarizing herself/himself with the

H.H. Fenn, MD (✉) • E. Yessengaliyeva, MD
Department of Psychiatry and Behavioral Sciences, Stanford University,
Stanford, CA, USA
e-mail: Howard.Fenn@va.gov

J.M. Ellison, MD, MPH
Swank Foundation Endowed Chair in Memory Care and Geriatrics,
Christiana Care Health System, Wilmington, MA 19801, USA

Research Associate, McLean Hospital, Belmont, MA 02478, USA

A. Hategan et al. (eds.), *On-Call Geriatric Psychiatry: Handbook of Principles and Practice*, DOI 10.1007/978-3-319-30346-8_17

unique care model, institutional policies, legal jurisdiction, civil commitment codes, staffing resources, access to consultants, roles of various primary clinicians, and limits/expectations of her/his unique role. This is especially relevant to *locum tenens* clinicians, who practice in unfamiliar settings.

17.2 Common Clinical Problems on Inpatient Psychiatric Unit

The following case vignettes exemplify how the confluence of psychiatric symptomatology, medical conditions, and disruptive behavior may prompt requests for on-call consultation.

17.2.1 Psychotic Disorders

Case Vignette Mr. A, a 77-year-old man with a 50-year history of early-onset chronic paranoid schizophrenia, was admitted to the inpatient psychiatry ward because the board and care (B&C) operator would not take him back until his behavior improved. The patient said "The people in my boarding house don't like me." For 3 months previously, he was disruptive and disorganized, sleeping only 3 h per night, moving about with excessive energy, and screaming about lobotomy and WWIII. He urinated in inappropriate places. The patient was seen and heard apparently responding to internal stimuli. He had a history of self-destructive behavior in response to auditory command hallucinations; at age 52 he cut his neck and, 10 years later, his wrist, in serious suicide attempts.

Medications on admission included divalproex sodium 500 mg BID, perphenazine 16 mg daily, and benztropine 1 mg TID. The patient reported that he was compliant with treatment, but his B&C operator did not agree. There was no recent history of alcohol use, illegal substances, abrupt discontinuation of sedative-hypnotic, antianxiety medications, or others which may have precipitated withdrawal symptoms. Systemic medical problems included benign prostatic hypertrophy with history of obstruction, urinary retention, unilateral inguinal hernia, osteoarthritis of both knees, hyperlipidemia, and atrial fibrillation. The patient complained of needing to urinate frequently; at other times he was unable to urinate. The patient was noted to be drinking fluids excessively.

During his first three inpatient days, the patient was compliant with medications, though agitated, paranoid, and menacing. The perphenazine dose was increased over the course of 3 days to 32 mg daily to control psychosis and threatening demeanor. He received 1 mg of lorazepam once after he tried to hit a staff member, and this resulted in a slight reduction in agitation for 8 h. In the next 24 h the patient complained of stomach discomfort. On the fourth hospital night, he raised his walker high, about to strike another patient who happened to be on anticoagulation therapy.

The on-call physician was called to address the patient's dangerous behavior. The differential diagnosis included (1) schizophrenia, paranoid type, in acute exacerbation or treatment-resistant schizophrenia and lack of full remission of psychotic symptoms; (2) akathisia; (3) new-onset and/or chronic delirium, due to anticholinergic toxicity; (4) urinary retention due to anticholinergic medications, causing discomfort and agitation; and (5) manic or hypomanic episode.

The physical examination revealed dry oral mucosa and tenderness over the lower abdomen. A bladder ultrasound in the emergency department found a urine volume of 326 cc which led to a catheterization of 420 cc of urine; urinalysis and urine culture were sent to rule out a urinary tract infection. Benztropine was discontinued. Perphenazine was held for 24 h to rule out akathisia as well as minimize anticholinergic effects and then restarted at lower dose of 8 mg daily. The patient's agitation diminished, but after 2 days his delusions became more prominent. A crossover taper to risperidone was instituted over the next 2 weeks. Risperidone was chosen as a second-generation antipsychotic (SGA) with a receptor profile at less risk of producing akathisia than perphenazine, parkinsonian adverse effects [4, 5], or anticholinergic adverse effects. A regular dose of acetaminophen was started to minimize pain of osteoarthritis.

This geriatric patient with early-onset schizophrenia (before age 40) presented with hallucinations and delusions consistent in character, content, and intensity with prior psychotic episodes. His psychotic symptoms had clearly disrupted his functional achievement over his lifetime. A patient with *late-onset* schizophrenia (after age 40 years) is more likely to demonstrate organized, fixed, persecutory delusions, auditory hallucinations with a running commentary, lower levels of negative symptoms, more stable occupational and marital history, and higher premorbid functioning than an *early-onset* patient.

The appropriate initial dosing of antipsychotic medication in a geriatric patient age 77 should be at most 50 % of that for a patient under age 60. Geriatric patients with *late-onset* schizophrenia or *very-late-onset* may require doses as low as 10 % of the dose for a younger patient [5, 6]. With first-generation antipsychotic (FGA) medications such as perphenazine, there is a higher risk of extrapyramidal symptoms (EPSs) than SGAs, such as risperidone or quetiapine, due to greater sensitivity of geriatric patients to adverse effects of antipsychotics with high D_1/D_2 blockade. Medications and doses should be chosen to minimize anticholinergic properties, due to increased sensitivity to systemic adverse effects as well as risk of exacerbating cognitive symptoms of major neurocognitive disorders (NCDs) (formerly dementia) and/or precipitating frank delirium [7, 8]. Focused suspicion is required to identify specific anticholinergic adverse effects, such as constipation, dry mouth, and urinary retention, in this case due to rapid dose escalation of perphenazine and excessive use of benztropine. Although positive psychotic symptoms (hallucinations, thought disorder, and paranoid delusions) diminished, agitation and threatening behavior worsened, likely due to distress and anxiety over physical discomfort.

17.2.1.1 On-Call Clinical Recommendations for Psychotic Disorders

- Rule out systemic medical etiologies which might contribute to agitation or exacerbation of psychotic symptoms (whether or not the patient has delirium per se) before considering a diagnosis of a chronic or acute psychotic, depressive, or bipolar disorder. Constipation, urinary retention, exacerbation of chronic pain, akathisia, dystonias, muscle spasms, and confusion from dehydration or nutritional deficiencies are common.

- Consider substance withdrawal and alcohol withdrawal as contributors to agitation, sudden mood changes, or psychotic symptoms in the newly admitted patient. A geriatric patient who was taking sedative-hypnotic or antianxiety medications inappropriately, for example, may have withdrawal symptoms due to abrupt discontinuation or reduction from a higher dose. The history from caregivers, family, or others is crucial. If evidence of alcohol withdrawal delirium, institute the Clinical Institute Withdrawal Assessment of Alcohol Scale, Revised (CIWA-Ar) [9].
- Search for drug-drug interactions and medications with anticholinergic properties [8]; refer to Chap. 12.
- Determine the daily total medication dose received during the prior shift, including pro re nata (PRN) medications, to identify under-medication of psychotic symptoms, resulting in exacerbations, or adverse effects of excessive dosing.
- Minimize adverse effects of antipsychotic medications with age-adjusted doses.
- Scrutinize medication administration records for problems in drug delivery or compliance. Initiate a proactive discussion with nursing staff about any need for a different, more deliverable formulation, which staff may appreciate.
- Assess potential for emerging adverse effects, e.g., prolongation of the QRS interval on the ECG from QRS peak to the ST segment (QTc), hyponatremia (with serum electrolytes), hepatotoxicity (with liver-associated enzymes), and/or laryngeal dystonias, leading to poor swallowing or aspiration.
- QTc of >450 ms in men or >470 ms in women has been associated with sudden cardiac death. Therefore, the following QTc prolongations of antipsychotic medications should be taken into account before choosing an antipsychotic agent: ziprasidone 16–21 ms, quetiapine 6–15 ms, clozapine 10 ms, risperidone 3.5–10 ms, olanzapine 2–6.5 ms, paliperidone and iloperidone 2–4 ms, and aripiprazole −1 to −4 ms [10].
- Discontinue any presumed offending antipsychotic or antidepressant medication as a "drug holiday." If the medication is held for 24 h, this is an efficient and safe intervention to help clarify the etiology of agitation, which cannot otherwise be identified [5, 6]. Institute discontinuation only *after* discussion with staff about their capability to monitor and manage untoward effects, such as withdrawal dyskinesias, suicidality, impulsivity, exacerbation of psychotic symptoms, and/or increase in agitation.

17.2.2 Bipolar Disorder, Depressive Disorders, and Suicidality

Case Vignette Mr. B, an 89-year-old WWII veteran with a history of prostate cancer and radical prostatectomy, chronic right lower extremity lymphedema, and a resection of right leg lymph nodes, was brought to the emergency department by his ex-wife. The patient stated he would shoot himself because he was told last month that he will have to move out of his rental unit due to its pending sale. His ex-wife noted that he owns a shotgun. He had a history of depressive episodes and successful treatment with selective serotonin reuptake inhibitors (SSRIs) during a first psychiatric hospitalization. In his late 20s, the patient had a manic episode but was not hospitalized. Ten years previously, the patient made a suicide attempt by placing a cord around his neck, was found unconscious, and was hospitalized for 7 days; his depression resolved after a course of ECT. The differential diagnosis included (1) adjustment disorder with depressed mood; (2) major depressive disorder, recurrent; (3) persistent depressive disorder; (4) bipolar disorder, most recent episode depressed; and (5) substance-induced depressive disorder.

Among suicide attempts, a higher proportion are lethal in older than in younger patients. Many etiological factors have been proposed to explain this finding, including frailty and systemic medical comorbidity, which increase the risk of death, living alone which prevents timely intervention, and a propensity for the use of lethal means, such as firearms [11]. In addition, systemic medical comorbidity has been found to be a risk factor among geriatric patients who completed suicide: of 42 % who left a suicide note, one-third gave health problems as their reason for suicide [12].

A high prevalence of geriatric inpatients have depressive disorders or depressive episodes of bipolar disorder. For example, admissions for bipolar disorder comprise up to 10 % of geriatric inpatient admissions, and patients with bipolar disorder present more often with depressive rather than manic episodes [13]. In this context, clinicians on call for depressed geriatric inpatients should evaluate for suicidal ideation and encourage monitoring for self-destructive behavior.

17.2.2.1 On-Call Clinical Recommendations for Bipolar Disorder, Depressive Disorders, and Suicidality

- In the United States, health-care insurance plans, health-care delivery systems, Medicare, and preferred provider organizations all impose limitations on inpatient hospitalization days for specific conditions, often truncating time needed for assessment and medication trials. Criteria for inpatient hospital day authorization are likely to become more stringent in the face of the diagnostic specificity of the *International Classification of Diseases, tenth edition* (ICD-10). Constraints on hospitalization days may require mood-stabilizing medications, antidepressants, and combination treatments to be started during on-call shifts.
- Medication initiation and changes are problematic on call in the absence of full informed consent, including explanations and consultation with the (presumed) competent patient or with family/other surrogates of patients with diminished decisional capacity.
- Before a trial of mood stabilizers and/or any modification of antidepressant treatment regimen, search (1) the history for prior manic or hypomanic episodes, (2) evidence of bipolar or depressive disorder in the biological family, and (3) response to past psychotropic medications. A history and strong suspicion of bipolar disorder should prompt laboratory testing (liver-associated enzymes, ammonia, complete blood count (CBC), renal panel, urinalysis, and thyroid-stimulating hormone (TSH)) in preparation for trial of a mood stabilizer.

- Recognize that a trial of a mood stabilizer may allow the diagnosis of bipolar disorder to go unchallenged by subsequent clinicians, continuing current medications without any review of the presumed diagnosis.
- Antiepileptic drugs (AEDs) for mood stabilization [14], or lithium, can be initiated safely on call at low doses, after appropriate laboratory testing [15].
- Lithium carbonate can be started at a dose 75 or 150 mg daily even in the frail elderly—after renal function by laboratory testing is found adequate, with GFR and serum creatinine. Dose adjustments can be followed up by the daytime treatment team.
- Lamotrigine has demonstrated efficacy, in at least 5 randomized clinical trials, for treating bipolar depression. Although its use in geriatric patients has not been thoroughly studied, standard recommendations for its gradual dosing allows it to be started safely during an on-call shift. Geriatric patients should be observed for the onset of life-threatening skin rash such as Stevens-Johnson syndrome, or more common adverse effects such as nausea, dyspepsia, non-serious skin rash, or insomnia. Starting dose: 25 mg/day for two weeks; or 25 mg orally every other day for 2 weeks if the patient is taking valproic acid.
- Divalproex sodium 125 mg daily or BID may be started, if platelets, liver-associated enzymes, and ammonia level are within normal limits and the patient has no history of significant hepatotoxicity or pancreatitis.
- Asymptomatic elevations of serum ammonia require close monitoring of ammonia levels along with cognitive functioning and level of arousal, particularly in patients who are benefiting from treatment with divalproex. If symptomatic hyperammonemia develops, marked by persistent elevation of serum ammonia, onset of hypothermia, unexplained lethargy, vomiting, and/or delirium, consider immediate discontinuation of divalproex.
- Avoid changing antidepressant doses, adding a second antidepressant, or switching to an alternative antidepressant, except for intolerable adverse effects, contraindications, or drug-drug interactions. Exceptions include mirtazapine 7.5 mg or trazodone 25 mg at bedtime for sleep initiation.
- Do not discontinue antidepressants for lack of full response, especially if one does not know the patient's non-depressive baseline. Although markers of inadequate treatment response have been proposed (see below), it is difficult on call to conclude that an adequate treatment trial has been accomplished; this decision is best left to the regular team and/or clinicians who know the patient. A recent study found that lack of response to treatment after 12 weeks of venlafaxine XR up to 300 mg daily correlated with a higher baseline severity of depression and longer duration of depressive episode [16].
- For acute mania in bipolar disorder, or mania with psychotic features, the FDA and Health Canada have approved the following SGAs: olanzapine, risperidone, quetiapine and quetiapine XR (extended release), aripiprazole, ziprasidone, and asenapine.
- In acute bipolar depression, these agents have been approved by the US FDA: olanzapine-fluoxetine combination, quetiapine and quetiapine XR, and lurasidone, whereas risperidone, olanzapine, quetiapine, aripiprazole, and ziprasidone are approved for maintenance phase treatment. Limited data are available about their efficacy in the geriatric population.

- Specific precautions for SGAs in the geriatric population include ziprasidone, quetiapine, and risperidone, QTc prolongation; olanzapine, anticholinergic activity and diabetes mellitus; risperidone, pedal edema and EPS such as parkinsonism; and aripiprazole, akathisia [10].
- If a potentially suicidal patient must be discharged during an on-call shift, document a discharge plan which includes strategies to decrease risk of suicidal behavior, such as monitoring by caregivers and removal of access to lethal means (e.g., opioid medications and firearms).

17.2.3 Neuropsychiatric Symptoms of Neurocognitive Disorders

Case Vignette An 87-year-old divorced man, diagnosed with major neurocognitive disorder (NCD) due to Alzheimer's disease (AD) 5 years earlier, was admitted to the inpatient psychiatry unit for agitation at his nursing home within the prior month. He could perform his basic activities of daily living (ADLs) and some instrumental activities of daily living (IADLs). Medications included donepezil 5 mg daily and memantine 10 mg daily; cognition was stable, without significant decline over the prior 6 months.

On admission, the MoCA score was 15 out of 30, and he was disoriented to time and place. His level of arousal was good and he followed simple directions but forgot information within 5 min. No attentional or concentration deficits were noted, nor were there any laboratory findings suggestive of delirium. During his hospitalization the patient talked about wanting to visit his deceased wife, who passed away 7 years earlier. He said that he heard her voice and believed she was "next door." He tried to find her, was redirected, and often pulled his arm away, making a fist and swinging. He touched patients and asked often about his wife. He awoke nightly, thrashing and/or screaming. One night the patient walked out of his room and returned to lie in his roommate's bed. The roommate pushed the patient, who fell, whereupon the on-call clinician was called.

Disruptive behaviors such as wandering, intrusiveness, and agitation, whether stemming from delirium or other NCDs, place patients at higher risk for injury and/or assault and should be addressed immediately [17]. In collaboration with staff, the on-call clinician must search for contributing cause(s) of any disruptive behavior, aside from the NCD. Evidence should be gathered to rule out undiagnosed systemic medical conditions, pain, discomfort, and/or disrupted sleep. Table 17.1 summarizes the assessment of some contributors to disruptive behavior in NCDs. A non-pharmacological approach (below) is the first line in managing NCD-related neuropsychiatric symptoms (NPSs) [18].

Chronic pain is prevalent in 40–79 % of people aged 85 years or older yet under-reported in patients with NCD [19]. Stepwise treatment with analgesics can reduce the intensity and duration of agitation [20], as rated on the Cohen-Mansfield Agitation Inventory (CMAI) short form [21], and aggressive behaviors as rated on the Neuropsychiatric Inventory (NPI) [22]. For nonverbal NCD patients with NPS, guidelines help in assessing pain [23]. However, wandering as a symptom has *not* been associated with pain and may not respond to analgesic interventions [24].

Table 17.1 Assessment of contributors to disruptive behavior in major neurocognitive disorders

Contributing factors	Workup and information to gather
Medication adverse effects, drug-drug interactions, compliance problems	Scrutinize medication regimen for: Anticholinergic properties Excessive dosing Recent/abrupt medication changes Formulations not easily administered
Interrupted sleep	Nighttime staff notes Parasomnias of LBD History of PLMS, RLS
Medical comorbidity	Vital signs and PE Laboratory studies Medical history Recent surgical history Orthostatic hypotension Bowel, bladder irregularities
Exacerbation of chronic pain and acute pain	PE: signs of recent injury Nonverbal signs of pain Review of analgesic regimen
Cognitive deficits, inability to express needs or complaints, deficiencies in executive functioning	MoCA
Perceptual distortions, e.g., hallucinations, delusions	New onset, quality, frequency of symptoms as noted by staff and family Chronic symptoms and past exacerbations
Adverse staff-patient interactions	Nonjudgmental discussion with staff Observation of bathing, feeding, bathroom activities
Sensory and motor deficits	Audiology reports Vision tests Neurological exam
Milieu and adverse patient-to-patient interactions	Observation of noise level Behavior of other patients on the unit
Nutritional deficiencies and dehydration	Intake and output; fluids and meals

Note: LBD Lewy body dementia, *MoCA* Montreal Cognitive Assessment, *PE* physical examination, *PLMS* periodic limb movement of sleep, *RLS* restless legs syndrome

17.2.3.1 On-Call Clinical Recommendations for Neuropsychiatric Symptoms of Neurocognitive Disorders

- Screen for delirium with scales such as the Confusion Assessment Method (CAM), which can be administered in under 10 min [25].
- Rule out hypoactive, prolonged, or subclinical delirium, even if delirium has previously been ruled out, perhaps prematurely and/or inaccurately. Review the most recent laboratory profile and order STAT laboratory tests as indicated to rule out delirium. Symptoms of inattention and disorganized thinking can precede and/or follow incident episodes of delirium by several weeks. Scrutinize medication regimens for anticholinergic properties to minimize this risk.

- Begin non-pharmacological interventions such as described in the DICE protocol [18]:
  1. *D*escribe: This first step requires a detailed description of problematic behaviors, including antecedents, precipitants, and social context. Rating scales like the Cohen-Mansfield Agitation Inventory (CMAI) help staff identify and describe NPS [21].
  2. *I*nvestigate the NPS to discover underlying causes and exclude treatable conditions.
  3. *C*reate a treatment plan.
  4. *E*valuate the effect of the treatment plan on the problematic behavior. Steps 3 and 4 of the DICE protocol will likely continue after the on-call shift.
- If the DICE protocol is not successful, and disruptive behaviors or NPS constitutes an imminent risk to self or others, consider psychopharmacological approaches.
- Document that full informed consent for medications was obtained from family and/or surrogates (if decisional incapacity is determined). Explain and document any risks to the patient if disruptive behavior is *not* treated pharmacologically [17].

17.2.3.2 Review of Medication Interventions

- Citalopram at 10–40 mg daily dose may decrease agitation, though improvement would not usually be seen within the on-call time frame [26]. An ECG should be obtained to identify any pretreatment QTc prolongation, which may occur above doses of 20 mg daily as per FDA and Health Canada warnings.
- The use of SGAs for NPS of NCD is controversial due to the risk of fatal adverse effects including an increased risk of cerebrovascular accidents (CVAs) [27]. When NPS or related behaviors pose an immediate risk of danger, however, antipsychotics provide the quickest and most effective intervention [28].
- Olanzapine, risperidone, aripiprazole, and quetiapine all have demonstrated evidence of short-term benefit for agitation and aggression, although quetiapine has the least evidence of efficacy [28].
- Immediate-delivery, rapid-disintegrating formulation of olanzapine (2.5–5 mg daily), which can be mixed with food or juice, may reduce agitation within 2 h. But vigilance is needed: Olanzapine has significant anticholinergic properties and should be avoided in diabetes mellitus patients. All patients should be monitored for emergent hyperglycemia [10, 28].
- Risperidone has shown reductions in aggression at 1–2 mg orally daily in AD patients. Although an SGA, it can produce extrapyramidal side effects due to D_2 receptor blockade. Its immediate intramuscular formulation facilitates administration, with improvement in as little as 1–4 h. Aripiprazole has been found effective for agitation and aggression at doses of 2–10 mg, though evidence is sparse [28].
- The FGA haloperidol provides modest efficacy for aggression unresponsive to non-pharmacological approaches [29]. It has also been found beneficial for delirium and can be initiated intramuscularly, though risks of acute dystonia, akathisia, tardive dyskinesia, and sudden cardiac death must be taken into account. For greatest safety, a baseline ECG should be obtained prior to first dose to rule out QTc prolongation (maximum of 450 ms).

- While initiation of AEDs may be considered for bipolar disorder, there is little evidence of their timely efficacy for emergent NCD-associated NPS. AEDs do not usually take effect for days due to the need for titration and monitoring of serum levels, and they require close monitoring to avoid untoward effects. Carbamazepine, for example, has evidence of efficacy for NPS but can produce adverse events (e.g., sedation, hyponatremia due to the syndrome of inappropriate antidiuretic hormone [SIADH], cardiac toxicity, cytochrome P450 enzymatic induction, and likelihood of drug-drug interactions) [14].
- Cholinesterase inhibitors (ChEIs), such as donepezil, galantamine, and rivastigmine, have not demonstrated consistent evidence of benefit for NPS and are less likely to require urgent initiation during on-call shifts. The oral formulation of rivastigmine may produce nausea and vomiting early in treatment and can be discontinued or switched to the rivastigmine patch, with one-third the rate of gastrointestinal adverse effects. Avoid ChEIs in patients with symptomatic bradycardia (pulse less than 60 beats per minute) and/or history of heart block.
- Memantine, an NMDA receptor antagonist, has shown slight but statistically significant improvement of disruptive behavior in AD patients already receiving donepezil [30].
- Dextromethorphan-quinidine 20 mg/10 mg once daily in the morning has shown preliminary evidence of benefit for agitation in NCDs as rated on the NPI [31].
- Benzodiazepines are to be avoided due to risks of anterograde amnesia, gait imbalance, sedation, and falls with resultant fractures.
- Physical impediments to compliance (e.g., impaired swallowing, dehydration, aspiration, inability to open mouth wide, temporal mandibular joint pain, dental problems) can alter delivery of medications and resulting response.

17.2.3.3 On-Call Clinical Recommendations for Neuropsychiatric Symptoms Specific to Subtypes of Neurocognitive Disorders

Differentiating NCD subtypes, though a challenge while on call, may guide more individualized treatment and avoid contraindications.

Delirium

This is the most treatable NCD subtype, identified by the onset within hours to days with deficits in attention, concentration, consciousness, and level of arousal. The more insidious variant of hypoactive, or subsyndromal, delirium should be considered and ruled out [32, 33].

Alzheimer's Disease (AD)

This is marked by a decline of episodic memory for specific events and contexts (such as story recall or list learning), a rapid rate of forgetting, and difficulty recalling or recognizing new information after a delay of 10–20 min. Memories for recent events (such as the meal last eaten) are quickly forgotten. Unlike the normal geriatric population, AD patients may recall the last few words of a supra-span word list immediately after it is read aloud but then make more intrusion and perseverative errors on memory tests. Procedural memory—for overlearned action—is usually intact in early AD [34, 35]. Ultimately, long-term follow-up is needed to discriminate normal aging from symptomatic AD, but some bedside tests can help raise awareness that AD is in the differential diagnosis:

- Word list delayed recall assesses the ability to acquire and retain new information. AD patients forget new information in as little as 5–10 min.
- Trail Making Test Part B assesses executive function, sequencing, problem solving, and mental flexibility.
- The Montreal Cognitive Assessment (MoCA) rates a score of 25 out of 30 or lower as abnormal.

Frontal Variant of AD

This subtype may present with apathy, withdrawal, disinhibition, and subtle personality changes. Observers and family may interpret these symptoms as social disengagement, depression, and disinhibition. The Geriatric Depression Scale (GDS) can screen for depressive illness, help distinguish it from apathy, and thereby minimize staff frustration [33].

Lewy Body NCD or Dementia (LBD)

The second most common degenerative neurocognitive disorder, LBD represents 15–25 % of cases of major NCDs [36].

Early cognitive findings include:

- Impaired performance in copying of overlapping pentagons, clock drawing, spelling WORLD backward, and subtraction of serial sevens. If LBD is suspected, FGAs and SGAs should be avoided, except for quetiapine or clozapine (which have less D2 blockade).
- Deficits in executive functioning and attention, which are tested with Trail Making Test Parts A and B, Wisconsin Card Sorting Test, and category verbal fluency [36].

Clinical hallmarks, even before observable onset of LBD, include:

- Fluctuation in cognition (60–80 % of patients).
- Recurrent, well-formed, detailed visual hallucinations (50–75 % of patients with LBD), which may be abstract or complex, or misperceptions (e.g., an object seems to move). The affected patient may be convinced these are real events and not symptoms of his/her NCD.
- Spontaneous signs of parkinsonism (80–90 % of patients with LBD).
- Episodes of "blanking out," lasting seconds to days, altered cognition, daytime drowsiness, and confusion.
- Parasomnias: 85 % of LBD patients may have rapid eye movement (REM) behavior disorder (RBD) early, years before the onset of other core symptoms. RBD results from a lack of REM suppression of motor behavior. This loss of

atonia during REM sleep can interrupt the patient's sleep with complex motor behavior, acting out dreams, and purposeful-seeming gestures (e.g., throwing a ball) [25, 36]. The patient may awaken confused out of REM sleep, which can also disrupt others. RBD may respond to clonazepam, though it is best to avoid benzodiazepines. Rather consider trazodone 25–50 mg or melatonin 1–5 mg at bedtime for disrupted sleep [36].

- LBD patients with NPS may respond to cholinesterase inhibitors better than AD patients since cholinergic deficit in LBD is greater than in AD [36]. A double-blind, placebo-controlled study of rivastigmine in patients with LBD showed reductions in hallucinations as well as improved cognition [36]. Minimize the predictable risk of falls (up to 1/3 of LBD) with close observation and appropriate environmental safeguards.
- Extrapyramidal syndrome (EPS) in LBD must be avoided; 30–50 % of LBD patients are sensitive to EPS due to FGAs and some SGAs, such as olanzapine. The syndrome may be difficult to identify and lethal; quetiapine and clozapine are the least harmful alternative medications for LBD who demonstrate NPS.

Frontotemporal NCD or Dementia (FTD)

This constitutes 5 % of NCDs, with approximately 50 % of FTD in the *behavioral variant* (bvFTD) category [37], which includes clinical hallmarks such as:

- Progressive change in premorbid personality and behavior.
- Euphoria, disinhibition, apathy, repetitive behaviors, and progressive nonfluent or fluent aphasia. Primary progressive aphasia is generally used to describe nonfluent presentation, whereas semantic dementia is applied to the fluent form.
- Symptoms may precede the correct diagnosis of FTD by several years, onset as early as the second decade, and often in the sixth decade.
- Disinhibition includes inappropriate touching or kissing of strangers, public urination, flatulence without concern, offensive remarks, intruding on others, utilization behavior, playing with objects in the surroundings, or taking personal items without asking.
- Apathy, described as reduced interest and/or motivation for activities and relationships and reduced participation in conversations, may be mistaken for depression, and the patient may be described as cold, unfeeling, or detached. Staff and family interactions with the patient may improve if there is an understanding that the patient's behavior is a result of the disease and that it is labeled correctly as "apathy" rather than it being seen as a personal affront.
- Hyperorality includes unusual eating and drinking, cravings (e.g., for sweet foods), binge eating, and alcohol or smoking excess; patients may eat more than needed or put amounts of food in their mouths that cannot be chewed or swallowed and may try to consume inedible objects (pica).
- Compulsive, perseverative, stereotyped, and/or ritualistic behaviors, such as stereotyped speech, simple repetitive movements, hoarding, cheeking, or cleaning.
- Rigid behavior (e.g., rigid food preferences) and inflexibility to changes in routine.

Major Vascular NCD

This is estimated to comprise 18 % of incident major NCDs [38].

- Compared with AD (on tests of language, construction, and memory registration), such patients are significantly less impaired on tests of recognition memory and more impaired on measures of executive functioning [38].
- Depression should be considered in patients with NCD who appear apathetic or withdrawn, especially in the context of small-vessel cerebrovascular pathology. A trial of antidepressant medication for depressive symptoms may be the only way to determine the presence of depression in this subtype, though symptoms are rarely urgent enough to start treatment during an on-call shift [27].

17.3 Calls Prompting Immediate Attention

17.3.1 Pain, Injuries, and Falls

Complaints of acute pain localized to the limbs or joints should prompt a search for cuts, bruises, and point tenderness indicating an injury and/or a fall. If an injury appears significant, such as a hip fracture, consultation with the on-call hospitalist or internal medicine specialist and/or an emergency department visit with radiological workup should be accomplished. Patients who sustain any trauma to the head, and/or who are on anticoagulation, need a head CT scan or MRI (usually a non-contrast head CT is more immediately available and is easier for the patient to tolerate). Close observation can rule out emergence of a subdural hematoma or subarachnoid hemorrhage, which may present as a new-onset headache of a severity which the patient has not experienced before.

Recommendations The treatment of acute pain should be preceded by an evaluation of its location(s), etiology, frequency, duration, quality, and severity. In the context of cognitive limitations of major NCD or verbal (speech and language) impairments, details may be difficult to determine. Instead, one can observe facial expressions, vocalizations, body movements, changes in socialization, interpersonal interactions, activity patterns or routines, and mental status [23]. Acetaminophen 650 mg every 6 h may be started in the interim unless there is a history or laboratory data which is consistent with liver disease. See Chap. 11 for further assessment and management of complaints of pain.

17.3.2 Disturbances of Sleep and Parasomnias

Disruptive behavior or awakenings at night prompt calls to the clinician on duty; this issue is addressed in Chap. 10. Complaints of disrupted sleep or agitation among the geriatric inpatient population are due, in part, to the high prevalence of systemic medical comorbidity, including chronic pain, physical discomfort, nocturia, and sleep-wakefulness cycle reversal. If underlying medical conditions and environmental-related complaints are ruled out, consider:

- Periodic limb movement disorder (PLMD), due to muscular contractions during sleep, may affect between 30 and 45 % of those over age 60 years, much higher than the 5–6 % of all adults. Clinical hallmarks include excessive daytime drowsiness, insomnia, cold feet, and leg kicking [39, 40].
- Restless legs syndrome (RLS) is marked by an irresistible urge to move the lower extremities; symptoms are worse when the patient is at rest, and movement may relieve the symptoms [39, 40].
- First-line treatment for both RLS and PLMD includes dopaminergic agonists (e.g., pramipexole, ropinirole, or rotigotine transdermal patch). Second-line treatment includes gabapentin and/or benzodiazepines (e.g., clonazepam) [39, 40].
- Avoid initiating treatment with benzodiazepines, especially very long-acting medications, such as flurazepam, which can extend sedation into morning hours, and hypnotics with anticholinergic properties (e.g., diphenhydramine).

17.3.3 Catatonia, Refusal to Eat or Drink, and Dehydration

Catatonia may present on the inpatient psychiatry unit in greater prevalence than in any other setting aside from medical units. The Bush-Francis Catatonia Rating Scale (BFCRS) is in common use as a catatonia diagnostic instrument [41]. If present, catatonia demands prompt attention, as it has a high rate of complications (40 %) and death (20 %) [42].

Clinical hallmarks include a refusal to eat, rigidity, mutism, bizarre postures, excessive motor activity, negativity, staring, echolalia, or a combination thereof. DSM-5 includes diagnoses of either (1) catatonia associated with another mental disorder or (2) catatonic disorder due to another medical condition. Manic episodes with psychotic features, major depressive episodes with melancholic and/or psychotic features, and schizophrenia are common underlying psychiatric conditions. Neuroleptic malignant syndrome (NMS) may present similarly and often can be ruled out in the absence of elevated temperature, elevated creatine phosphokinase (CPK), elevated white blood cell count, and muscular rigidity. If NMS is suspected, medical attention in the emergency department or intensive care unit is needed, and all antipsychotics must be held until NMS symptoms have resolved and CPK is stable in normal range. Milder sensitivity to antipsychotics may be managed by reduction in dose or switch to an alternative antipsychotic agent.

If catatonia and/or poor intake begins or worsens while on call, one must first rule out systemic medical conditions which have precipitated or exacerbated it. Vital signs can identify the malignant form, marked by hyperthermia, hypertension, and/or cardiopulmonary problems, which might require immediate transfer to an ICU unit. Laboratory studies should include serum electrolytes and serial CPK values. Delirium should be ruled out.

When significant dehydration and/or poor nutrition is present, intravenous fluids or parenteral feeding may be needed if the unit policy permits and if no emergency setting is available.

Benzodiazepines, most often lorazepam 1–4 mg IV QID, for the first 24–48 h or until improvement, are the first line of treatment. Antipsychotics should be avoided, due to the risk of precipitating or prolonging catatonia and the risk of NMS. ECT is the definitive treatment for catatonia which does not respond to benzodiazepines.

17.3.4 First Aid After Injuries, Falls, and Altercations

The on-call physician may be called to evaluate a geriatric inpatient who sustained a traumatic injury due to a fall, assault, or similar incident. Please refer to Chap. 11 and 14.

Geriatric patients who have sustained a fall, injury, or physical altercation deserve a full physical and neurological examination. Scrutinize for lacerations, bruises, bleeding from any orifices, tenderness, pain, swelling, new-onset loss of mobility, new-onset loss of range of motion around joints, and pain. Any changes in mental status, especially level of arousal, orientation, attention, and concentration, should be noted. In the case of head injuries, headaches or head pain should be watched, especially in anticoagulated patients. For patients on warfarin, a STAT non-contrast head CT and INR will alert to any high risk of bleeding.

If there has been a fall, the vital signs, especially blood pressure sitting and standing, may rule out orthostatic hypotension and dehydration due to antihypertensive medications, diuretics, alpha-1 adrenergic blockers, alpha-2 adrenergic agonists, and beta-adrenergic blockers. For geriatric psychiatry inpatients, referral to an internal medicine consultation is indicated for excessive sedation, rigidity, confusion and visual changes, suspected fractures, uncontrolled bleeding, need for suturing, persistent low systolic blood pressure, or suspected internal bleeding.

17.3.5 Seizures and Seizure-Like Phenomena

Following report of a seizure-like event, examine for signs of nonconvulsive seizures, e.g., twitching in face or extremities, deviation of eyes, intermittent impaired levels of arousal, and automatisms. After the onset of a seizure, and before the return to baseline mental status, there is a postictal period, lasting from minutes to hours. During this interval the patient is at risk for postictal paresis (Todd's paralysis), falls, confusion, obtundation, and amnesia and should be confined to bed and monitored with direct 1:1 observation. A physical examination should include examination for injuries and lacerations of the tongue.

Events that may look like seizures, but are not, include syncope, non-epileptic seizures, toxic-metabolic encephalopathy, dyskinesias, parasomnias (see previous section on sleep), tremors, myoclonus after a hypoxic event, and rigors. Laboratory examinations include serum electrolytes, calcium, magnesium, complete blood count with differential, urinalysis, urine sample for drugs of abuse, and AED if the patient is receiving AEDs. Noncompliance or intermittent compliance with AEDs is a common cause for increase in seizure frequency [43]. Consider alcohol withdrawal if the patient has been admitted to the psychiatric unit within the prior 72 h. CIWA protocol should be initiated. Following a new-onset seizure, a head CT and/or MRI is indicated to evaluate etiology of the event or any resulting trauma to the head. Treatment for continued seizure activity, and if intravenous (IV) lines are permitted on the unit, consists of lorazepam 2 mg IV over 1 min, repeated after 1 min for maximum dose of 0.1 mg/kg. If seizure activity continues beyond 5 min, the patient may be considered in status epilepticus and transferred to an emergency setting [43].

Key Points

A. *Prior to the on-call shift*
- Learn the care delivery model, unit culture, availability of consultants, access to emergency medical treatment, legal jurisdiction, institutional policies on restraints, resources for sitters and close observation, and policies on documentation of capacity to give informed consent/substituted judgment. This information may also help guide a decision about whether to accept a *locum tenens* assignment in this setting.
- Obtain sign-out from physicians for any anticipated problems, especially new admissions and potential discharges.
- Clarify complicated treatment plans with the signing-out clinicians.
- Attend nurse-to-nurse reports at the end of shifts, which will anticipate on-call requests.

B. *During the on-call shift*
- Meet with nursing staff at the beginning of each shift to identify concerns and to develop a working alliance (see Chap. 9).
- Use geriatric doses, e.g., antipsychotic doses should be less than half of young adult doses for schizophrenia (see Chap. 3).
- Change treatment plans/medication regimens *only* as needed to address adverse effects, contraindications, allergic responses, drug-drug interactions, behavioral management, excess or inappropriate dosing, or strong family objection to specific treatments.
- Meet with families if requested. Proactively offer to answer questions from families, who are often present after-hours; document the discussion.
- Rule out prolonged, subclinical, or subsyndromal, hypoactive delirium, even if previously ruled out. Unexplained or insidious changes in behavior, cognition, attention, or level of arousal, within the past 24–48 h, are suspicious for delirium.
- Document, evaluate, and take precautions to prevent self-harm and risk of harm to others.

- Scrutinize medication lists for (1) medications with anticholinergic properties, (2) drug-drug interactions, (3) recent medication discontinuations, or (4) abrupt dose changes. Identify medications with anticholinergic properties which can prolong delirium.
- Choose medication formulations designed to improve compliance or minimize unique limitations, such as difficulty chewing, swallowing, or tolerating unpleasant tastes. Consider rapid-disintegrating, liquid, or intramuscular formulations. Consider mixing medications in food, on tongue—always with informed consent.

C. *Collaboration with nursing staff*

- Monitor adverse events and encourage prevention protocols, e.g., seizure and fall precautions, aspiration protocols, and prevention of constipation and urinary retention.
- Assess for alcohol withdrawal symptoms with the CIWA protocol.
- Monitor and record medication compliance as well as obstacles to medication delivery; substitute for formulations which better facilitate compliance.
- Encourage accurate, timely, detailed descriptions and the context of behavioral/psychiatric symptoms as well as any precipitating interpersonal interactions.
- Anticipate risk for falls and other injurious behaviors; develop precautions. Assess vital signs several times daily, attend to orthostatic hypotension, and consider discontinuation of medications responsible.

References

1. Fenn HH, Bauer MS, Altshuler L, Evans DR, Williford WO, Kilbourne AM, et al. Medical comorbidity and health-related quality of life in bipolar disorder across the adult age span. J Affect Disord. 2005;86(1):47–60.
2. Pirraglia PA, Biswas K, Kilbourne AM, Fenn H, Bauer MS. A prospective study of the impact of comorbid medical disease on bipolar disorder outcomes. J Affect Disord. 2009;115(3): 355–9.
3. Lala SV, Sajatovic M. Medical and psychiatric comorbidities among elderly individuals with bipolar disorder: a literature review. J Geriatr Psychiatry Neurol. 2012;25(1):20–5.
4. Suzuki T, Uchida H. Successful withdrawal from antipsychotic treatment in elderly male inpatients with schizophrenia—description of four cases and review of the literature. Psychiatry Res. 2014;220(1–2):152–7.
5. Suzuki T, Remington G, Uchida H, Raji TK, Graff-Guerrero A, Mamo DC. Management of schizophrenia in late life with antipsychotic medications: a qualitative review. Drugs Aging. 2011;28(12):961–80.
6. Howard R, Rabins PV, Seeman MV, et al. Late-onset schizophrenia and very-late-onset schizophrenia-like psychosis: an international consensus. Am J Psychiatry. 2000;157(2):172–8.
7. Chew ML, Mulsant BH, Pollock BG, Lehman ME, Greenspan A, Mahmoud RA, et al. Anticholinergic activity of 107 medications commonly used by older adults. J Am Geriatr Soc. 2008;56:1333–41.

8. Gray SL, Anderson ML, Dublin S, Hanlon JT, Hubbard R, Walker R, et al. Cumulative use of strong anticholinergics and incident dementia: a prospective cohort study. JAMA Intern Med. 2015;175(3):401–7. doi:10.1001/jamainternmed.2014.7663.
9. Wan SH, Kyomen HH, Catic AG, et al. Identification and management of alcohol abuse and withdrawal in elders. Clin Geriatr. 2012;20(4):28–34.
10. Jacobson SA. Clinical manual of geriatric psychopharmacology. 2nd ed. Washington, DC/ London: American Psychiatric Publishing; 2014.
11. Yeates C, Thompson C. Suicidal behavior in elders. Psychiatr Clin North Am. 2008;31(2): 333–56.
12. Cheung G, Merry S, Sundram F. Late-life suicide: insight on motives and contributors derived from suicide notes. J Affect Disord. 2015;185:17–23.
13. Depp CA, Jeste DV. Bipolar disorder in older adults: a critical review. Bipolar Disord. 2004;6(5):343–67.
14. Fenn HH, Sommer BR, Ketter TA, Alldredge B. Safety and tolerability of mood-stabilising anticonvulsants in the elderly. Expert Opin Drug Saf. 2006;5(3):401–16.
15. D'Souza R, Raiji TK, Mulsant BH, Pollack BG. Use of lithium in the treatment of bipolar disorder in late-life. Curr Psychiatry Rep. 2011;13:488–92.
16. Smagula SF, Butters MA, Anderson SJ, Lenze EJ, Dew MA, Mulsant BH, et al. Antidepressant response trajectories and associated clinical prognostic factors among older adults. JAMA Psychiatry. 2015. doi:10.1001/jamapsychiatry.2015.1324.
17. Shinoda-Tagawa T, Leonard R, Pontikas J, et al. Resident-to-resident violent incidents in nursing homes. JAMA. 2004;291(5):591–615.
18. Kales HC, Gitlin LN, Lyketsos CG. Management of neuropsychiatric symptoms of dementia in clinical settings: recommendations from a Multidisciplinary Expert Panel for the Detroit Expert Panel on the assessment and management of the neuropsychiatric symptoms of dementia. J Am Geriatr Soc. 2014;62:762–9.
19. Helme RD, Gibson SJ. The epidemiology of pain in elderly people. Clin Geriatr Med. 2001;17:417–31.
20. Husebo BS, Ballard C, Sandvik R, Nilsen OB, Aarsland D. Efficacy of treating pain to reduce behavioural disturbances in residents of nursing homes with dementia: cluster randomised clinical trial. BMJ. 2011;343:d4065. doi:10.1136/bmj.d4065.PMID:21765198.
21. Cohen-Mansfield J, Marx MS, Rosenthal AS. A description of agitation in a nursing home. J Gerontol. 1989;44(3):M77–84.
22. Cummings J, Mega M, Gray K, Rosenberg-Thompson S, Carusi DA, Gornbein J. The neuropsychiatric inventory: the neuropsychiatric inventory: comprehensive assessment of psychopathology in dementia. Neurology. 1994;44:2308–14.
23. Hadjistavropoulos T, Herr K, Prkachin KM, Craig KD, Gibson SJ, Lukas A, et al. Pain assessment in elderly adults with dementia. Lancet Neurol. 2014;13:1216–27.
24. Ahn H, Horgas A. The relationship between pain and disruptive behaviors in nursing home residents with dementia. BMC Geriatr. 2013;13:14.
25. Inouye S, van Dyck C, Alessi C, Balkin S, Siegal A, Horwitz R. The confusion assessment method. Ann Intern Med. 1990;113(12):941–8.
26. Porsteinsson AP, Drye LT, Pollock GG, Devanand DP, Franqakis C, Ismail Z, et al. Effect of citalopram on agitation in Alzheimer disease: the CitAD Randomized Clinical Trial. JAMA. 2014;311(7):682–91.
27. Press D, Alexander M. Management of neuropsychiatric symptoms of dementia. UpToDate. www.uptodate.com. Accessed 29 Jul 2015.
28. Ballard C, Corbett A. Agitation and aggression in people with Alzheimer's disease. Curr Opin Psychiatry. 2013;26:252–9.
29. Alexopoulous GS, Weiden PJ, Preskorn SH, et al. A roadmap to key pharmacologic principles in using antipsychotics in the treatment of older patients. J Clin Psychiatry. 2009;70(1): 131–8.
30. Cummings JL, Schneider E, Tariot PN, Graham SM. Behavioral effects of memantine in Alzheimer disease patients receiving donepezil treatment. Neurology. 2006;67:57–63.

31. Cummings JL, Lykestsos CG, Peskind ER, Porsteinsson AP, Mintzer JE, Scharre DW, et al. Effect of Dextromethorphan-Quinidine on agitation in patients with Alzheimer disease dementia. A randomized clinical trial. JAMA. 2015;314(12):1242–54.
32. Cole MG, McCusker J, Voyer P, Monette J, Champoux N, Ciampi A, et al. Symptoms of delirium occurring before and after episodes of delirium in older long-term care residents. J Am Geriatr Soc. 2012;60:2302–7.
33. Meagher D, Adamis D, Trzepacz P, Leonard M. Features of subsyndromal and persistent delirium. Br J Psychiatry. 2012;200(1):37–44.
34. Albert MS, Dekosky ST, Dickson D, Dubois B, Felman HH, Fox NC, et al. The diagnosis of mild cognitive impairment due to Alzheimer's disease: recommendations from the National Institute on Aging-Alzheimer's Association workgroups on diagnostic guidelines for Alzheimer's disease. Alzheimers Dement. 2011;7:270–9.
35. Grabowski TJ Jr. Clinical features and diagnosis of Alzheimer Disease. UpToDate. www.uptodate.com. Accessed 29 Jul 2015.
36. Farlow MR UpToDate Clinical features and diagnosis of dementia with Lewy bodies. UpToDate. www.uptodate.com. Accessed 29 Jul 2015.
37. Lee SE, Miller BL. Frontotemporal dementia: clinical features and diagnosis. UpToDate. www.uptodate.com. Accessed 29 Jul 2015.
38. Wright CB. Etiology, clinical manifestations, and diagnosis of vascular dementia. UpToDate. www.uptodate.com. Accessed 29 Jul 2015.
39. Rose KM, Beck C, Tsai PF, Liem PH, Davila DG, Klemban M, et al. Sleep disturbances and nocturnal agitation behaviors in older adults with dementia. Sleep. 2011;34(6):779–86.
40. Trenkwalder C, Winkelmann J, Inoue Y, Paulus W. Restless legs syndrome-current therapies and management of augmentation. Nat Rev Neurol. 2015. doi:10.1038/nrneurol.2015.122. [Epub ahead of print].
41. Wong E, Ungvari GS, Leung SK, Tang WK. Rating catatonia in patients with chronic schizophrenia: Rasch analysis of the Bush-Francis Catatonia Rating Scale. Rating scale. Int J Methods Psychiatr Res. 2007;16(3):161–70.
42. Jaimes-Albornoz W, Serra-Mestres J. Prevalence and clinical correlations of catatonia in older adults referred to a liaison psychiatry service in a general hospital. Gen Hos Psychiatry. 2013;35(5):512–6.
43. Roberson ED, Hope OA, Martin RC, Schmidt D. Geriatric epilepsy: research and clinical directions for the future. Epilepsy Behav. 2011;22:103–11.

18 Acute Inpatient Medical Settings

James A. Bourgeois, Deborah C. Francis, and Ana Hategan

18.1 Background

"Acute inpatient medical settings" refer to the general acute care hospital. We will not discuss geriatric patients admitted to psychiatric inpatient units (often called "geropsychiatry units"), which may or may not be physically located within a general hospital. In performing consultations with hospitalized patients, it is helpful for the consultant to be aware of the medical/surgical illness(es) that generated the emergency department (ED) presentation and hospital admission, as adaptation to/coping with illness is often an important element of the patient's experience.

18.2 General Approach to Examination of the Hospitalized Geriatric Patient

Modification of examination procedures is needed in the general hospital setting. Before entering the room, first observe the physical environment (both of the room itself and devices attached to the patient). Look for medical tubes, lines, surgical drains, and other devices that pose not only the risk of infection and other complications but are also safety hazards to the patient with poor cognition and/or

J.A. Bourgeois, OD, MD (✉)
Department of Psychiatry/Langley Porter Psychiatric Institute,
University of California San Francisco, San Francisco, CA, USA
e-mail: james.bourgeois@ucsf.edu

D.C. Francis, RN, MSN, GCNS-BC
Geriatric Clinical Nurse Specialist Co-Chair Bioethics Committee,
Kaiser Permanente South Sacramento Medical Center, Sacramento, USA

A. Hategan, MD
Department of Psychiatry and Behavioural Neurosciences, Division of Geriatric Psychiatry,
Michael G. DeGroote School of Medicine, Faculty of Health Sciences, McMaster University,
Hamilton, ON, Canada

A. Hategan et al. (eds.), *On-Call Geriatric Psychiatry: Handbook of Principles and Practice*, DOI 10.1007/978-3-319-30346-8_18

- Medication lists
- Medication profiling
- Clinical laboratory
- Neuroimaging
- ECG/EEG
- Nursing and interdisciplinary notes

Fig. 18.1 Medical data sources for hospital consultations

behavioral dyscontrol, as the risk of secondary physical injury from medical equipment and other physical items is significant. Pills can be hoarded for an overdose, while intravenous (IV) tubing can be wrapped around the neck and sharps used in a suicide attempt. In the case of ICU patients, self-extubation can be life-threatening, while restraints, including bedside rails, have been attributed to falls with injury and death in hospitalized geriatric patients [1, 2].

Sensory deficits are common in older patients, contribute to delirium risk, and can interfere with patient assessment. Can the patient see and hear you, or does he/she need eyeglasses, hearing aids, and/or dentures to communicate? Some hospital units offer hearing amplification devices and writing or communication boards to facilitate patient communication. For the hearing impaired, it is helpful to eliminate background noise, speak slowly, and enunciate in a low tone at a level where the patient can see your lips.

Ascertain the level of light and sound in the hospital room; see if the window blinds are adjusted to differentiate day and night. Can modifications in the sensory environment be made to compensate for the fact that older adults need more light, contrast, and sensory aids to see? Are noise levels and nursing care interruptions controlled to allow uninterrupted sleep, as medically indicated? A clock and "orientation board" in plain view of the patient with information, such as date, place, physician and nurse names, and family phone numbers/messages, updated every shift is important.

Look for the presence at the bedside of family/significant others or nursing staff, including a sitter assigned to constantly observe the patient, to inquire about agitated behaviors, confusion, and level of arousal. Obtaining baseline functional and cognitive status from those familiar with the older patient is critical. Review nursing and ancillary discipline notes for cognitive, functional, or behavioral issues and to determine the ability of the patient to cooperate with the treatment plan. The psychiatric consultant is advised to acquire clinical data about hospitalized patients from various sources. Examples of these data sources are included in Fig. 18.1.

In addition to the usual elements of the mental status examination, every hospitalized older patient who generates a psychiatric consultation needs to have an assessment of cognitive function, which must include a delirium assessment. The goal is to establish the presence or absence of cognitive impairment, whether it is due to delirium and/or underlying major neurocognitive disorder (NCD) (formerly dementia). Know whether nursing staff assesses for delirium, using standardized screening tools such as the Confusion Assessment Method for the Intensive Care Unit (CAM-ICU), Confusion Assessment Method (CAM), and Neecham Confusion Scale and/or Delirium Observation Screening Scale. If not, ask nurses and family members/visitors about acute onset of mental status and behavioral changes with a fluctuating course, inattention, and either disorganized thinking or altered levels of arousal (consistent with hyper- and hypoactive delirium and abnormal Richmond Agitation-Sedation Scale (RASS) score). Disrupted sleep-wake cycle, perceptual disturbances (hallucination or illusions), delusions, emotional lability, and inappropriate behavior are common in delirium. Consider using simple tests to assess orientation and attention. The latter could include naming the days of the week (allow no errors), or months of the year backward (allow one error), serial 7 s (allow one error on five subtractions), or reciting digit spans backward [3, 4].

Formal standardized cognitive assessments such as the Montreal Cognitive Assessment (MoCA), Mini-Cog, and Short Portable Mental Status Questionnaire are best used to identify a major or mild NCD [3]. The MoCA does not require specialized training to administer and interpret, but results can be affected by the patient's systemic medical symptoms or treatments and ability to cooperate and the presence of delirium. The Mini-Cog (a clock draw and three-item recall) is a good screening tool for cognitive impairment that is brief and easy to administer.

When called to urgently evaluate a hospitalized geriatric patient, it is best to ascertain the acute change in cognition and/or behavior that generated the consultation; current and chronic medical illness(es) and/or surgical procedures, including complications; and any known history of psychiatric illness/medications, cognitive deficits, and substance use. Medications must be reviewed for possible contribution to altered mental status, paying particular attention to medications that have actions on the CNS such as opioids, benzodiazepines, and anticholinergics. The Beers Criteria for medications to avoid in the older adult can be helpful to identify culprits (see Chap. 12, "The Chief Adverse Effects of Medications").

It is necessary to learn if there have been recent or imminently planned major invasive procedures, a terminal diagnosis, or caregiver disruption that may impact on the patient's psychiatric status. For example, excess concern about invasive procedures and caregiver burnout can be manifested in mood and anxiety disturbances; if acutely temporally linked to illness/medical circumstances, many of these episodes will appropriately be diagnosed as adjustment disorders. Often patients must confront a long length of stay due to serious illness and prolonged recovery and/or acceptance of chronic disability, dependence, and institutionalization, which can lead to demoralization.

Geriatric patients with premorbid chronic neuropsychiatric conditions can be particularly difficult to manage in the acute care hospital given the medical, surgical, and nursing restrictions that patients with neurocognitive, psychotic, bipolar, or major depressive disorders must maintain and the potential behavioral dyscontrol that pose staff safety hazards and make discharge problematic.

It is highly recommended that the psychiatric consultant communicate with nursing staff (in any hospital setting) to ensure they are aware of and able to implement the important nursing behavioral interventions that are critical to delirium prevention and management, as well as the management of the patients with major NCDs with behavioral dyscontrol.

Geriatric patients with major NCDs are particularly vulnerable to the adverse effects of psychotropic medications, and all evidence indicates that, except in situations of imminent risk, implementing a non-pharmacologic approach utilizing behavioral and environmental interventions, while identifying and eliminating the etiologies, is indicated prior to administration of medication except to manage acute agitation. Non-pharmacologic delirium prevention measures adopted from the work of Inouye are being disseminated via Hospital Elder Life Program (HELP) and Nurses Improving Care for Healthsystem Elders (NICHE) programs and are being adopted by major health-care systems as they recognize the importance of evidence-based geriatric care in delirium prevention [5]. Inouye et al. and the HELP programs have demonstrated significant reduction in delirium by using structured bedside interventions [3, 5] (see Table 18.1).

18.3 Understanding the Settings

18.3.1 Intensive Care Unit

The intensive care unit (ICU) provides the highest, most complex level of patient care in the general hospital. ICUs are characterized by critically ill patients with multisystem failure, technological sophistication, robust nursing/patient ratios, and interdisciplinary clinical rounding. Often, there are physicians devoted solely to the management of ICU patients (intensivists), while other physicians may also be involved in their care. The environment poses unique challenges due to the 24 h/7 days per week operations including noise and light levels and interruptions related to patient care activity, which is not conducive to restful sleep and directly contributes to delirium.

Rates of delirium in the critically ill geriatric patient range from 45 to 87 %, and delirium is the primary cause of the psychiatric consultation in the ICU [6, 7]. As such, the psychiatric consultant being called by the ICU should consider delirium as the first psychiatric illness to rule out. It is problematic to assume that "ICU psychosis" (a nonspecific term in common use to describe delirium) is "normal" or that the ICU itself causes delirium, as patient and illness variables are much more to blame and the etiology is multifactorial (more often than not). A common example is when the psychiatric consultant is called to "assess depression," when the patient actually is in the hypoactive form of delirium. Older ICU patients are at the greatest risk of chronic cognitive deficits from prolonged delirium, so it is imperative to aggressively and frequently review and treat the potential causes of delirium throughout the hospitalization [8]. The risk of developing permanent cognitive decline after an episode of delirium is high, including acceleration of decline with underlying NCD [9].

When called to evaluate an ICU patient, it is highly desirable for the consultant to attend the interdisciplinary team rounds, which have become routine practice [10]. When speaking to the nursing staff, ascertain how long the patient has been in the ICU and what led to the ICU admission. Since the ICU is where patients requiring ventilator support are managed, the psychiatric consultant may be called on to assess patients who are not only difficult to communicate with but who are difficult to extubate because of anxiety manifest at the time of attempted extubation. This

Table 18.1 Identification and non-pharmacologic management of delirium

Identification of risk for delirium

Implement delirium prevention measures for patients:

- Admitted with altered level of consciousness/delirium or
- with known risk factors for delirium:
  - Age ≥70
  - History of cognitive impairment, delirium
  - Functional impairment
  - Vision impairment
  - History of alcohol abuse
  - Comorbidity burden (e.g., stroke, depression)

Identification of delirium:

- Use formal instrument, such as the Confusion Assessment Method (CAM), CAM-ICU, months of the year backward, to identify delirium [5]
- *Acute* onset (abrupt, within minutes, hours, shifts, days up to 2 weeks) of *any change* in cognition (inattention, memory loss, disorientation, hallucinations, delusions)
  - Altered and fluctuating LOC: hyperactive or hypoactive; remember lethargy, falling asleep, staring off into space, and decreased motor activity is not normal in older adults with dementia (major NCDs)
  - Disorganized thinking, disorientation
  - Inattention: assess by asking to say days of the week backward or spell world backward and by observing for problems in focusing, staring off into space, or losing track of questions

Component	Nursing intervention: identify etiology and provide supportive care
Maintain safety	Maintain airway, prevent aspiration, skin breakdown, falls
Physiologic stability: • Infection • Hypoxia • Dehydration • Electrolyte imbalance • Medications • Pain • Urinary retention • Impaction • Immobility • Sleep deprivation • Sensory impairment	• Reduce psychoactive medications and polypharmacy: avoid benzodiazepines, anticholinergic, and other deliriogenic medications; monitor for side effects, consult pharmacy as needed • Monitor labs to prevent electrolyte abnormalities and infection • Maintain hydration/nutrition: offer fluids with each encounter, if not on IV fluids • Optimize oxygenation with early mobilization, incentive spirometer, and O2 as indicated • Optimize sleep and sensory input, and progressively mobilize per below • Proactively assess/treat pain with ATC non-opiates and opiates for breakthrough pain • Monitor for impaction or retention: ensure scheduled/prompted voiding and bowel regime • Notify physician of any acute change in behavior or mental status
Sleep promotion	Normalize sleep-wake cycle: the goal is to ensure 4–6 h uninterrupted sleep at night • Identify and maintain patient's sleep pattern/routine as much as possible (e.g., identify history sleep disturbance/aides and notify physician) • Optimize sleep-wake cycle with OOB daytime activity/limited napping and quiet at night • Open blinds during day, close at night, adjust lighting to low level at night • Promote bedtime ritual with warm milk/herbal tea, massage, relaxation music • Cluster care and avoid unnecessary awakening; maintain quiet at night • Avoid caffeine, excessive IV/PO fluids after 6 pm

(continued)

Table 18.1 (continued)

Activity	• Progressively mobilize to maximal potential and encourage self-care in ADLs, as appropriate
	  • Ensure/assist patient out of bed for all meals unless contraindicated
	  • Discourage napping during day
	  • Ambulate every shift with goal to regain prior level of function as possible
	• Review for removal of unnecessary lines (catheter, telemetry, IV lines, SCDs, restraint, etc.) every shift; avoid/minimize restraints
	• Engage in age-appropriate, meaningful activities; enlist involvement of family/SO to identify patient-specific routines/interests and incorporate into care plan as possible
	• Use familiar, calm music, relaxation techniques

Communication enhancement	• Assess for communication deficits and provide assistive devices as needed
	• Compassionate communication:
	  – Approach in a calm, nonthreatening manner. Call person by name, introduce self with each encounter
	  – Set the stage for positive interaction; *smile*
	  – Use active listening, one task/command/step at a time; repeat information using exact words, allow patient time to respond
	  – Search for the meaning/emotion in patient's message and respond to patient feelings
	  – Respond to paranoid or delusional thoughts/expressions by providing comfort to the emotions (i.e., "You sound angry/scared/sad. I'm here to help, to keep you safe"); avoid arguing and rationalizing and do not take it personally
	• Redirect agitated patient with validation and distraction (e.g., reminiscence, walk, sweets)

Reality orientation	• Reorient patient frequently within normal conversation; do not quiz patient • Provide simple explanation of nursing care and all activities with each encounter • Foster familiarity: encourage family/friends at bedside, familiar items from home, consistent caregivers and routine as possible; minimize relocations, especially at night • Clock and updated care board with date/orienting information; be sure patient can see it
Sensory stimulation regulation	• Optimize sensory stimulation: ensure patient can see and hear with hearing aide/amplifier, glasses, communication board • Ensure quiet room with good lighting to differentiate day from night (blinds open in day, closed at night) • Turn off TV if patient is not engaged; use familiar music or relaxation tapes • Limit visitors as needed; minimize noise, interruptions, and distractions • Cluster care to limit unnecessary awakening, especially later in day when patient is fatigued

Note: ATC around the clock, *OOB* out of bed, *SCD* sequential compression device, *SO* significant other can be particularly problematic in geriatric patients with cognitive deficits and behavioral disturbances. Recommending non-pharmacological behavioral interventions and incorporating geriatric principles of psychopharmacology is important to optimize patient and staff safety. In addition to routine delirium assessment and management, patients in this circumstance may benefit from careful dosing of non-benzodiazepine sedating medications (e.g., dexmedetomidine) due to the cognitive problems associated with benzodiazepines in geriatric patients. Dexmedetomidine can be particularly helpful with violent, agitated patients. Other non-benzodiazepines can be given immediately prior to planned breathing trials to decrease anxiety and to facilitate extubation.

Case Vignette Mr. A was a 65-year-old Greek immigrant male with hypertension, hyperlipidemia, mild type 2 diabetes mellitus, and insomnia for which he took over-the-counter sedatives. He noted subtle cognitive performance problems (e.g., struggling to recall the names of people and being slightly distractible and less organized than before), but he did not seek out care and had no problems commuting to and from work. He lived at home with his 67-year-old wife. He was intermittently reporting feeling "anxious, depressed," but attributed this to "stress" from managing his chronic illnesses, increasing workplace demands, and challenges with his large family. He presented to a nearby community hospital when he experienced angina for the first time. He had mild ST segment elevations and positive troponins and was admitted, medically stabilized, and taken for cardiac catheterization the next morning. He was found to have a major occlusion of the left anterior descending artery, and a coronary artery bypass grafting was recommended.

The procedure went well, with the normal amount of pump time and a good recovery of cardiac output when revascularized. However, when awakened in the ICU, he experienced profound delirium. He was physically hyperactive, thrashing in the bed and trying to pull out his tubes and lines. The intensivist prescribed 2 mg of lorazepam; thereafter, the patient remained confused and became somnolent, unable to eat or follow directions, and intermittently violent. The consultation psychiatrist determined that the patient was positive on the CAM-ICU and noted an altered sleep-wake cycle, altered level of consciousness (LOC), RASS +2, and a MoCA score of 14/30. He was diagnosed with postoperative delirium. Non-pharmacologic delirium interventions were ordered. He was treated with regular doses of acetaminophen for pain, melatonin 3 mg at night, IV haloperidol 2 mg at night, and 1 mg PRN for agitation not responding to non-pharmacologic delirium management measures. Standard delirium pharmacologic precautions (including avoidance of benzodiazepines, anticholinergics, and minimization of opioids) were initiated.

Within 2 days, his motor behavior had normalized as had his sleep-wake cycle and LOC. His MoCA had improved to 22/30. He was then able to describe his recent illness experience in more detail. He was able to understand that the delirium episode was unlike anything he had experienced before and that the acute episode was improving. However, he was also able to appreciate that he had been feeling anxiously depressed as his cardiac illness had progressed and that his memory and concentration were relatively poor in the previous 2 years. He was advised to be seen in follow-up after discharge for further evaluation of his baseline psychiatric status.

18.3.2 Surgical Unit

When called to evaluate a patient on a surgical unit, in addition to the usual clinical information needed to accomplish a psychiatric consult, the consultant needs to know if the patient is pre- or post-op, what the procedure(s) proposed and/or completed are/have been, and whether there have been surgical complications. Geriatric delirium is particularly common in postoperative patients, affecting up to 50 % of older hip fracture patients [11]. This is partially attributable to the stressors of a surgical illness, the surgical procedure(s), anesthesia, opioid pain medications, inadequate pain control, sleep disturbances, alterations in medication administration and feedings due to *nil per os* status, dehydration, as well as other factors.

Due to the "culture" of surgical wards, surgeons/surgery residents are often in the operating room and thus less immediately available to speak to consultants when they arrive. Some surgical units employ nurse practitioners who comanage patients and are more readily available to communicate the clinical impressions of the surgical team. These nurse practitioners closely coordinate with other members of the surgical and nursing teams and are often able to facilitate implementation of any recommendations arising from the psychiatric consultation.

Case Vignette Mr. C was a 70-year-old retired, divorced white male with two adult children, with a history of hepatitis C virus (HCV) infection complicated by cirrhosis and subsequent orthotopic liver transplant (OLT). He had a history of depression, mild NCD (baseline MoCA of 21/30), opioid dependence, interferon treatment for HCV associated with depression, and 12 months of sobriety and recovery. One year after being listed for transplant, he was admitted to a medical center for the OLT. Initially, he did well postoperatively and was transferred to the surgical ward after an initial stay in the ICU. He was receiving regular IV opioids for postoperative pain, as well as lorazepam for anxiety, and diphenhydramine for sleep. On postoperative day 4, he developed delirium with disorientation, cognitive impairment, visual hallucinations, altered sleep-wake cycle, fluctuating LOC, and motor agitation. He was seeing images of dead relatives in his room criticizing him for his prior drug abuse and saying he was "not worthy" of receiving an OLT. On examination, he had a RASS of +2, was picking at his wound dressings, and was unable to describe his recent surgery and the need for postoperative immunosuppression. His CAM was positive for delirium and his MoCA score was 10/30. He was diagnosed with delirium. Non-pharmacologic delirium interventions were initiated. He was managed with cautious dosing of olanzapine SL 2.5 mg at bedtime and q6h PRN plus standard pharmacologic delirium precautions, including reduction in opioid dosing and holding anticholinergics and benzodiazepines. Over a period of 2 days, his agitation improved, his sleep-wake cycle normalized, and he was no longer hallucinating. His CAM was now negative for delirium and his MoCA improved to 18/30. He was now able to verbalize understanding of his operation and need for compliance with immunosuppression. His opioids were weaned and discontinued. After 5 days in stable condition, his olanzapine was also weaned and discontinued.

18.3.3 Medical Unit

Geriatric patients on medical units pose specific challenges as they tend to be admitted with a broad range of medical diagnoses, levels of acuity, and complex social situations. In addition, these older medical patients tend to be more challenging due to multiple medical comorbidities, polypharmacy, and cognitive and sensory deficits. Medical patients tend to have longer lengths of stay and are more prone than ICU or surgical admissions to have primarily "social" admissions and resultant discharge problems (e.g., chronic homelessness or abandonment limiting safe discharge options). While the risk of NCDs is high in all hospitalized geriatric patients, older medical patients also have high rates of depressive and anxiety disorders, which can often complicate the management of the index systemic medical illness that generated the hospitalization.

Some medical patients require prolonged courses of therapy under medical supervision (e.g., IV antibiotics for persistent infections, chemotherapy infusions, hemodialysis), which leads to excessive time away from the familiar home environment. Challenges coping with such regimens can be associated with depressive and anxiety disorders. Management of patients with underlying psychotic or other neuropsychiatric disorders who must comply with medical restrictions can be particularly challenging, and the psychiatric consultant is often requested when a "code" for violent, agitated, or threatening behavior is called and psychotropic medication and behavioral interventions are warranted to help deescalate the patient.

As with many acutely ill patients, medical patients may face challenges to finance long-term care that can be particularly problematic and contributes to prolonged hospital stay, delayed discharge, and the poorer outcomes associated with adjusting to chronic disease, disability, dependence, and institutionalization. In many settings, a significant problem is the lack of beds in the community especially if a patient has behavioral problems or concomitant psychiatric and/or medical or nursing care needs. The psychiatric consultant is not only a critical member of the health-care team to manage the patient's behavior but can be a vital team member to contribute to the treatment plan and any multidisciplinary patient rounds designed to facilitate discharge to a more appropriate level of care.

Case Vignette Ms. B was a 75-year-old white female, retired real estate agent, married with two adult children who had an episode of major depression around age 50 from which she recovered with a course of a selective serotonin reuptake inhibitor (SSRI). Several years later, she developed multiple motor and sensory symptoms. Workup, including a lumbar puncture and MRI of the head, led to a diagnosis of multiple sclerosis. Two years later, she began to have acute flares of her multiple sclerosis symptoms with subacute worsening of her motor symptoms, more profound weakness and incoordination, and problems with urinary retention. She had several presentations to the ED leading to brief medical admissions, where she received boluses of prednisone and other immunomodulating therapies. These acute treatments did improve her motor, sensory, and urinary symptoms, but were associated with acute deterioration of her mental status.

At the time of consultation, she was admitted for another exacerbation of her multiple sclerosis leading to treatment with prednisone at doses up to 60 mg per day. Her psychiatric status was now characterized by fluctuating LOC, inattention, irritability, visual hallucinations, altered sleep-wake cycle, RASS +1, and mild cognitive impairment (MoCA of 18 out of 30). An inpatient psychiatric consultation led to a diagnosis of steroid-induced delirium. Non-pharmacologic delirium interventions were initiated. She was treated with olanzapine 2.5 mg SL at bedtime plus 2.5 mg SL q6h PRN for confusion/agitation. Standard delirium pharmacologic precautions were initiated. She experienced normalized sleep-wake cycle and recovery of her psychiatric symptoms over 3 days. Her MoCA improved to 25 out of 30 and she was no longer exhibiting irritability or fluctuations of LOC. Once the acute high doses of prednisone could be tapered and discontinued 1 week later, the olanzapine was itself tapered and discontinued.

18.3.4 Emergency Department

Although the emergency medicine setting is discussed elsewhere in this book, the emergency department (ED) is the most common entry portal to the acute care hospital. If the general hospital is also a trauma center, the likelihood of the psychiatric consultant being called to the ED to evaluate trauma victims with premorbid psychiatric illness and/or psychiatric complications of trauma is significantly higher. When called to do a geriatric psychiatric consultation in the ED, it is important to ensure that an adequate physical examination and laboratory assessment have been completed before the presenting complaints are attributed to being "solely psychiatric." In the USA, for patients brought to the ED in restraints placed elsewhere and/or those placed in behavioral restraints in the ED, there is a Joint Commission mandate to be documented in the medical record by a physician (or specially trained RN) within one hour of initiation of restraints.

The culture and operations of the ED is team-based, fast-paced, and focused on triage, stabilization, and appropriate placement as major priorities. As such, assessments of cognitive function, suicide risk, drug intoxication/withdrawal states, and acute change in mental status (which may include acute onset psychosis as well as cognitive impairment) are common. In geriatric psychiatric patients, it is important to remember that acute onset psychosis is far more commonly due to delirium, major NCD, or both, rather than a new-onset primary psychotic or depressive disorder.

Case Vignette Mr. T was a 75-year-old retired Hispanic male, widowed with three adult children, with a known history of major NCD (Alzheimer's disease type) treated with donepezil 10 mg daily and memantine 10 mg daily. He lived in assisted living facility where he had meals prepared and a private room. His family members lived one hour away and would visit monthly. He was brought in by his son due to concerns that he was "not doing well for the last month, not leaving his room much, sleeping and eating poorly, and more irritable" and in the last 4 days "he is saying nonsensical things, like that he thinks people at his residence are stealing his things and plotting to hurt him and that he thinks there is a vicious dog threatening him." His son reported that the patient had never had this presentation before, although he had mild depression 3 years previously (treated with an SSRI) when initially diagnosed with major NCD and needing to leave his own home and enter assisted living for a higher level of care. However, this episode improved with treatment. Per a note in the electronic medical records, his last MoCA at an outpatient psychiatric appointment was 16 two months previously. He had not seen his physician since. Although he had an appointment booked for the next month, the son was alarmed enough to bring him to the ED.

On exam, the patient was alert, with no altered LOC, and with RASS 0. He was dysphoric and tearful, with psychomotor retardation. He did not make good eye contact. While he denied suicidal ideation per se, he said that he was "often tired of living" and "kind of hopeless." He believed that staff at the assisted living facility were stealing his things and "trying to hack my computer to get my money." He could not be dissuaded of this belief. He also mentioned a threatening dog outside his room "that no one else believes is there." MoCA was 14/30. His workup revealed a diffuse cerebral atrophy and ventriculomegaly with white matter disease on CT. Thyroid-stimulating hormone and B12 were normal, urine drug screen revealed no drugs, blood alcohol content was negative, and urinalysis and CXR were normal. He was diagnosed with major depression with psychotic features and major NCD. For stabilization and management, he was admitted to a geriatric psychiatric unit for antidepressant and antipsychotic treatment and an ECT consultation if needed. While awaiting transfer, he was given risperidone 0.5 mg PO/SL q6h PRN for paranoia/anxiety/bedtime insomnia.

18.4 Special Considerations in the Acute Care Medical Settings

18.4.1 Communication Barriers

Common to acute care settings are the challenges posed by multiple communication barriers not commonly seen in other psychiatric settings. Besides the barriers imposed by the psychiatric illness *itself*, the patient may be intubated, not speak the local language, have neurosensory impairments [e.g., vision and hearing deficits, language deficits, aphasia (receptive, expressive, anomic, conduction, global)], have limited education/literacy (exacerbated by the highly jargon-intensive language of

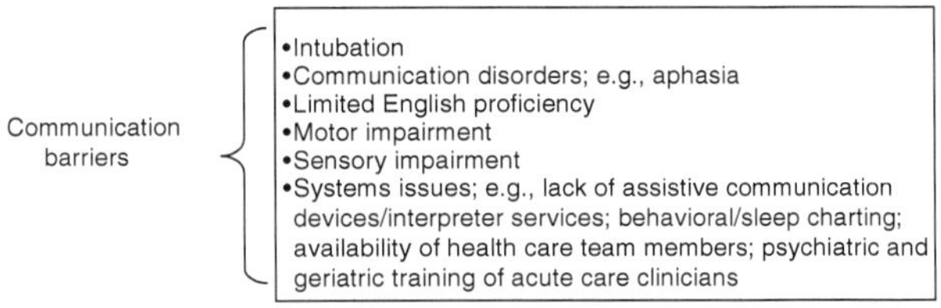

Fig. 18.2 Communication barriers in the acute care medical setting

medical systems), have paralysis (which limits writing), and/or have facial disfigurement (which limits expression and interpretation of affect). Geriatric patients, in particular, commonly have several of these problems simultaneously that the psychiatric consultant needs to address (see Fig. 18.2).

It is critical to work with nursing and rehabilitation staff to identify and utilize appropriate communication techniques and devices. This includes the creative and empathic use of in-person, telephone, or video interpreters, eyeglasses, magnification devices, hearing aids, amplification devices, and communication and writing tools; at times, gesture rather than speech must be used. Consultations will typically require excess time to complete owing to the inefficiency of modified communication methods. Charting should specifically comment on the manifest communication barriers addressed and the means used to address them, and clinical conclusions must take this into account when formulating the case and its disposition.

Other communication barriers that need to be addressed are more systemic in nature. These include the lack of pertinent behavioral charting in acute care settings that makes it especially difficult to get a picture of what the patient's behaviors are throughout the day. More indirectly is the lack of training in psychiatric care by other medical specialists, nursing and ancillary staff that can lead to more behavioral emergencies, staff or patient injuries, and overly aggressive use of pharmacologic (in lieu of behavioral) management or "drugs used as a restraint." Geriatric patients are particularly prone to over-sedation or paradoxical confusion and agitation due to side effects of psychotropic medications (particularly benzodiazepines and antipsychotics) [12, 13]. This is particularly problematic in geriatric patients who are already prone to hospital-acquired disability and other iatrogenic complications related to prolonged hospital stays, which increase the risk of institutionalization [14].

18.4.2 Sitters

Continuous observation by 24-h in-person personal care assistants, or "sitters," or security standby is an important component in managing psychiatrically unstable and/or behaviorally difficult patients in the acute care setting. A physician order may or may not be needed to place a sitter, although hospitals routinely place one when a patient is deemed to be a danger to self or others and/or has a psychiatric commitment order written. Sitters are used to ensure patient safety and are best utilized to actively engage with the patient to reorient, reassure, prevent escalation and constantly observe for acts of self-harm or agitation. Sitters need to be able to quickly call the patient's nurse and/or security for any behavioral disruption and preferably are trained in techniques to prevent behavioral escalation.

Sitters may or may not be involved in physical restraint of the patient, so it is important for the psychiatric consultant to be well informed of the hospital policies on restraint and the roles and responsibility of the sitter and standby security personnel. Particularly important is the ability of the sitter to ensure safety when the suicidal patient is engaged in personal care in the bathroom, as this may be the site of self-harm acts. For all patients at risk of self-harm, as deemed by the psychiatric consultant, the sitter will need to accompany the patient to the bathroom and maintain continuous observation at all times.

18.5 On-Call Psychiatry and Clinical Problems Common in the Acute Inpatient Medical Setting

The on-call psychiatric consultant is called to see a wide variety of clinical syndromes which may be commingled with social issues. Common clinical scenarios include (1) the management of confused/agitated/psychotic behavior associated with delirium (including delirium superimposed on major or mild NCD), (2) major or mild NCD (in the absence of delirium), (3) depression, (4) suicide risk assessment, (5) personality disorders with maladaptive behavior, and (6) assessment of decisional capacity. Specific psychiatric illnesses common in the medical hospital are included in Fig. 18.3.

18.5.1 Delirium

A major geriatric psychiatric problem in acute inpatient medical settings, but particularly in critical care, is delirium. Premorbid cognitive impairment is a major predisposing factor for delirium, e.g., major or mild NCD, history of delirium, or traumatic brain injury. Other predisposing factors include age 70 years and greater, visual deficits, alcohol abuse, and functional impairment. Once hospitalized, factors

Psychiatric illnesses	Delirium (including chronic delirium and terminal delirium) Major or mild neurocognitive disorder (dementia) Depression Delirium superimposed on Dementia/Major or mild neurocognitive disorder ("the double Ds") Dementia, Delirium, and Depression ("the triple Ds") PTSD Non-delirium psychiatric illnesses due to medications Catatonia Serotonin Syndrome Neuroleptic Malignant Syndrome

Fig. 18.3 Specific psychiatric illness in geriatric inpatient medical settings

Table 18.2 Risk factors of delirium [3]

Predisposing factors	Precipitating factors
Cognitive impairment/major or mild neurocognitive disorder	Infection
Functional impairment	Hypoxia
Visual impairment	Medications
History of alcohol abuse	Metabolic abnormalities
Age >70	Sleep deprivation
Morbidity burden (stroke, depression)	Immobility
	Restraints
	Indwelling catheter
	Surgery
	Pain

that will precipitate the development of delirium include multisystem failure (commonly seen in the ICU patient), "psychotoxic" or "deliriogenic" medications, infection, hypoxia, metabolic abnormalities, sleep deprivation, pain, restraints, fecal impaction/urinary retention, brain tumors, and other CNS illnesses.

Because of the high incidence of delirium in hospitalized patients, it is advisable for the on-call psychiatric consultant to speak to the nursing staff about symptoms and behaviors observed, including evidence of acute onset, fluctuating and altered levels of arousal, inattention, disorganized thinking, and/or hallucinations. Inquire about sleep-wake cycles and changes in LOC, cognition, behavior, nutrition, hydration, and elimination patterns that can help to identify the causative factor(s). Identify the index illness(es) that generated the hospital admission and any medical/surgical complications that were proximate to the development of delirium. Whenever possible, talk to family or significant others to identify the presence of potential cognitive or behavioral issues that could be exacerbated by the acute care admission and encourage their involvement throughout the hospitalization, as indicated, to minimize complications [3] (see Table 18.2).

With the detailed hourly patient behavioral observations in the ICU, tracking of circadian rhythm disturbances to substantiate a diagnosis of delirium can be facilitated. Sophisticated applications of electronic medical record systems, although not universally available as of yet, offer significant promise in delirium surveillance and management. Some hospitals have developed delirium screening protocols seeking early case surveillance and diagnosis, as well as prevention by risk factor control. Hospitals that have implemented the HELP programs have shown significant improvement in delirium prevention, patient satisfaction, and shorter hospital stays through the use of clinical rounding and bedside volunteers [15, 16]. NICHE is another national initiative that has improved delirium management in its NICHE hospitals [17]. Psychiatric consultants seeing hospitalized geriatric patients are advised to become familiar with any existing delirium screening, prevention, and management programs at their hospitals. Any data derived from delirium screening protocols (e.g., CAM results, formal cognitive testing) should be integrated into the clinical database when assessing patients for delirium. For further details on the assessment and management of the confused patient with delirium, see Chap. 10.

Any new definitive diagnosis of a comorbid major or mild NCD can only be made after the delirium has resolved. Caution must be taken not to assume that the cognitive or behavioral problems are solely manifestations of an underlying NCD, but may be an episode of delirium superimposed on NCD (or associated with another underlying neuropsychiatric disorder).

When the on-call question is to "evaluate for depression" because the patient has dysphoric affect and psychomotor retardation, recall that hypoactive delirium is more common than the hyperactive form. Since the patient presents with a "depressed" appearance, this often leads to a misdiagnosis of a depressive disorder.

18.5.2 Major or Mild Neurocognitive Disorders

While, ideally, all patients in the acute care hospital will have been admitted to treat acute systemic medical illness or surgical needs, this is not always the case. The acute care hospital also often holds geriatric patients who are not acutely ill, but are nevertheless brought to the ED due to behavioral dyscontrol of major NCD or other underlying psychiatric conditions. Although more appropriately managed on an inpatient psychiatry and/or NCD unit, not all communities have access to these resources, so the ED is often the sole option due to its 24-h availability. Once it is ascertained that the patient with a preexisting NCD is not secondarily delirious, full assessment for possibly reversible causes of NCDs (e.g., hypothyroidism, B12 deficiency, neurosyphilis, human immunodeficiency virus encephalopathy, herpes virus encephalitis) should be accomplished. Many cases of major NCD managed in the community, if and when recognized, will not necessarily have had formal cognitive testing, full laboratory assessment, or neuroimaging accomplished. It is desirable to use the presentation to the ED as a convenient opportunity to accomplish the basic clinical assessment. This is where gathering data from family members regarding cognition and behaviors is critical and developing a non-pharmacological treatment plan is essential.

The role of the on-call psychiatric consultant is to recommend non-pharmacological behavioral interventions and pharmacological treatment when the former is ineffective to optimize function and prevent harm to patient, staff, or others. If hospital admission is required, ongoing consultation may be needed (see Chap. 17 regarding management of neuropsychiatric symptoms due to NCDs).

18.5.3 Depression

Depression is a risk factor for NCDs. Atypical presentation of depression in the older adult is common with more problems associated with memory (commonly known as "pseudodementia" disorder), irritability, illness anxiety disorder (formerly hypochondriasis), "failure to thrive," refusal of medications/food/hydration, "giving up," and sleep and appetite problems. Older adults with depression who progress to psychosis and catatonia are at great risk for medical instability due to poor oral intake of nutrition and fluids, which not uncommonly leads to transfer to the general hospital from an inpatient psychiatry unit. Older adults tend to have less access to community support services, and polypharmacy can lead to difficulties in medication management, which can then lead to ED presentation due to inadequately treated depression.

Depression is also more common in certain systemic illnesses that lead to the hospital presentation, e.g., neurologic disease, diabetes mellitus, cancer, and liver disease/HCV infection. Depression can be a risk factor for, as well as a prodrome of, major or mild NCDs, although the relationship between the two disorders is far from conclusive [18]. Management of depression in geriatric patients must actively address systemic illness(es) as well as metabolic and drug interaction factors affecting psychopharmacological options.

When assessing and treating depression in the context of systemic medical illness in geriatric patients, it can be difficult to completely separate certain physical symptoms that could be representative of the depressive episode, the underlying systemic medical illness, or both. Familiar examples of these "overlap" symptoms are sleep disturbance, poor appetite, low energy, and psychomotor slowing. It is often pragmatic to treat such symptoms as if attributed to depression (particularly if associated with symptoms more specific for a depressive disorder, such as sad mood, tearfulness, and hopelessness) with targeted treatment and close follow-up.

Mirtazapine can be particularly helpful as an antidepressant in older medically ill depressed patients due to its rapid effects on sleep and appetite, which may occur before other improvements in the depressive state [19]. Low-dose methylphenidate has been used to treat depressed, medically frail patients due to its rapid onset of effect. In those with significant cardiovascular disease, methylphenidate can be increased to clinical effect by 2.5–5 mg every one to two days up to maximum 30 mg daily, in divided doses, if well tolerated; if ineffective at the maximum dose, it should be tapered and discontinued. Vital signs should be monitored before and during methylphenidate therapy. In patients with acute/subacute illness, methylphenidate can be discontinued once the condition has stabilized [20].

18.5.4 Suicide Assessment

Suicide risk is well known to increase with age and the risk in older men is concerningly high. If the on-call consultation pertains to suicide risk assessment, it is best to ascertain if there is any prior association between the psychiatric illness associated with the suicide risk and the hospital admission itself. For example, especially in geriatric patients with more medical comorbidity and age-related changes that make them more medically vulnerable, toxic overdoses will frequently lead to ICU admission for fluid/electrolyte management and invasive monitoring.

It is common to be asked to evaluate patients with undiagnosed neurocognitive problems in whom the medication overdose is unintentional or because the patient states or infers she/he "would rather be dead." Nursing staff is expected by the Joint Commission to assess for suicide risk, which may include intent and means, but typically defer to the psychiatric consultant for determination of risk and need for safety observation. Full suicide risk assessment and constant observation until psychiatrically cleared is needed for any patient with evidence of self-harming intent or manifest behavior that generates or develops during the current hospitalization. For on-call suicide risk assessment and management, please see Chap. 10.

18.5.5 Personality Disorders

Another common reason for psychiatric consultation on medical units are personality-disordered patients, especially cluster B personalities (antisocial, borderline, histrionic, narcissistic), who do not cope well with either the index illness or the demands and expectations of hospitalized patients for tolerating nursing routines, interfaces with multiple different health-care personnel, and personal/social disruption. Such patients routinely provoke problematic countertransference reactions in health-care professionals. If the call for psychiatric consultation is primarily in such a context, it is best first to speak to the referring physician and nursing staff about their collective experience of the patient's behavior.

Patients with manifest "splitting" behavior of seeing some medical personnel as "all good" and others as "all bad" will provoke different reactions among staff members, depending on how the patient interacts with them, leading to staff splitting and undue unit stress and anxiety. Such behavior is essentially pathognomonic for cluster B personality disorders, notably borderline, but also narcissistic personality disorder.

Frequently, the consult request from medical teams is (paraphrased) "make (the personality-disordered patient) stop this behavior so that we can properly care for him/her." While understandably reflecting the frustration that these patients engender, this request is impossible to fulfill. A patient with baseline poor psychological coping (the essence of personality disorder) is going to do *worse*, not better, when facing the challenges of acute illness. Such coping problems are usually worse when the patient is facing indefinite or permanent impairment, disability, or impending death. The clinical task is to help the care team understand this and help the patient to *modulate*, not fundamentally *change*, their manifest behavior to "get through" the illness episode.

18.5.6 Decisional Capacity Determinations

Although on-call principles of decisional capacity are detailed elsewhere in the book, these determinations are increasingly common in hospitalized geriatric patients. While all physicians are empowered to accomplish decisional capacity

Fig. 18.4 Decisional capacity determinations and clinical scenarios

Clinical scenarios	Invasive Procedures Against Medical Advice Discharge Requests Placement "Self-Determination" Code Status/Advance Directives Disposition of Property/Assignment of a Power of Attorney

determinations for their proposed investigations and treatment, it is common in hospital settings with access to psychiatric consultation services for the psychiatric consultant to assist in completing these assessments, especially if there is evidence of a neuropsychiatric comorbid illness (including delirium or major NCD) that might impact the patient's ability to consent. Additionally, it is sometimes assumed (incorrectly) that a patient with a recent suicide attempt or one on a psychiatric commitment order is a priori unable to consent for medical procedures as a result. Common types of decisional capacity determinations include informed consent for medical/surgical procedures, the ability to accept/refuse placement (in either psychiatric or non-psychiatric institutions), and being discharged against medical advice (AMA).

Less commonly (and only an issue at academic centers) is the capacity to engage in consent for research protocols. It is important to ensure that clinicians understand that the lack of decisional capacity is different from conservatorship/guardianship and that a patient can have capacity for one decision and not another. The context of the decisional capacity question is important to ascertain as a decisional capacity determination is valid for a specific decision at a specific time and cannot necessarily be generalized to other scenarios (see Fig. 18.4).

While decisional capacity determinations on medical units may be less likely focal to a particular invasive procedure (as would be common on surgical units), they may be somewhat more nebulous and less situation specific, such as "can he/she care for him/herself at home," "can he/she refuse a nursing home placement or assistance at home," "does he/she have capacity to sign an advance directive or POLST (Physician's Order for Life-Sustaining Treatment)," or "will the patient be compliant?" For matters of self-determination and self-care, supplementation of the routine decisional capacity assessment (which should always include a formal cognitive assessment) with in vivo assessment of activities of daily living (ADL) mastery (e.g., KELS assessment) should be routinely accomplished. Ask nursing staff or discharge planners where the documentation of baseline and current functional status is in the medical record, as the latter will be needed to consider admission to acute psychiatric units (as will cognitive status).

Because of the nature of surgical units, requests for decisional capacity are quite common, and the reason is more likely related to the ability to provide informed consent for surgical procedures. It is helpful to initially ascertain the surgical team's impression of decisional capacity, as surgical services who find the patient to lack capacity are usually supported by a psychiatric consultant, while only 50 % of patients who are found to "have capacity" by medical or surgical teams are found to have intact decisional capacity by psychiatric consultants [21].

Against medical advice (AMA) discharge requests are common on-call decisional capacity requests in the acute care hospital [22]. AMA requests are often reflective of conflict between patient and physician preferences or other breakdowns in communication and alliance. AMA should be approached like other decisional capacity consultations, with some assessment of psychiatric history, cognitive status (e.g., MoCA), and an empathic understanding of the disruptions in treatment alliance and communication that led to the AMA request.

Obviously, screening for suicidal/homicidal intent and psychosis are important, but AMA requests *solely* for the purposes of self-destructive behavior are rare. Infrequently, paranoid patients may be fearful of specific aspects of care due to paranoid ideation. This is particularly common in the patient with major NCD who "resists care" when feeling threatened, but may be labeled as "aggressive" or "combative" when nursing staff do not understand the underlying condition, which will lead to more problematic discharge.

Sometimes, cluster A personality disorder (paranoid, schizoid, schizotypal) patients cannot socially accommodate to the routines of hospital care and may seek AMA to escape this conflict. Cluster B personality (especially narcissistic, antisocial, and borderline) patients are prone to angry and emotionally chaotic relationships with medical personnel which may culminate in an AMA request. Patients with substance use disorders (many of whom are also personality disordered) may request AMA when their requests for pain and other controlled medications are thwarted, or when they perceive that their withdrawal states are not managed adequately.

Less emphasized in the literature are AMA requests due to "other than psychiatric illness" factors. This includes patients of illegal immigration status who fear discovery of their legal status; patients who are homeless, impoverished, and cannot pay for care; marginally employed patients who cannot miss time at work; and those who care for dependent family members (and pets) with little or no social support. Any of the aforementioned AMA contexts may present with a geriatric hospitalized patient, especially with increasing numbers of seniors who are responsible for caring for dependents and maintaining employment, often in marginal economic circumstances. It is helpful to consult with hospital social services to see if there are geriatric-specific social supports to help mitigate the requests for AMA discharge.

18.5.7 Social Matters/Placement

Similarly, older adults can be admitted to the hospital (or present to the ED) due to homelessness, abandonment, and other social matters where inadequate family or community services exist. This group of patients primarily need placement in more appropriate levels of care, which can be difficult and time-consuming due to widespread shortages in appropriate placement for geriatric patients. Most notable is a shortage of locked or secure units to manage patients with NCDs and/or psychiatric units that can treat aging patients with coexistent physical, cognitive, or nursing care needs that have resulted in many complex problems in appropriately placing

Fig. 18.5 Social matters presenting as "psychiatric illness"

Social matters	Displacement Adjustment to illness/poor prognosis/want to die Demoralization/existential despair Concerns about costs of care Concern over ill/dependent family members/pets/property Caregiver burden/burnout

patients at the appropriate level of care. In addition, geriatric patients with complex systemic medical, psychiatric, and nursing care needs may require longer inpatient treatment, especially when faced with severe terminal illness, institutionalization, and profound social concerns (see Fig. 18.5).

These patients often have long stays in the general hospital awaiting placement and pragmatic, solution-focused interdisciplinary collaboration with social services and discharge planning, and the treatment team is crucial. As many such patients are cognitively impaired, they are likely to have behavioral problems, especially in a novel and highly stimulating environment, which will lead to requests for on-call psychiatric consultation. Hospitals with targeted multidisciplinary rounds on complex patients appreciate the participation of the psychiatric consultant in the regularly scheduled meetings to assist in optimizing behavior and discharge outcomes; integration of such readily available information regarding management plans is crucial to on-call geriatric psychiatric practice.

Key Points

- The acute care hospital environment represents specific challenges for on-call psychiatric consultation with geriatric patients; the patient's experience of comorbid medical and/or psychiatric illness influences the context and content of psychiatric consultation requests.
- Major NCDs and delirium are prevalent in hospitalized geriatric patients, and these illnesses must always be considered first in on-call hospital consultations on geriatric patients.
- Less common is a consultation request for depression and failure to thrive; ruling out hypoactive delirium is important in such cases.
- Many geriatric patients with suicidal ideation and suicide risk will not necessarily meet full diagnostic criteria for a major depressive episode, but clinical vigilance for suicide risk is needed with a willingness to pursue psychiatric hospitalization for high-suicide-risk patients.
- AMA discharge requests are common on-call decisional capacity requests; AMA should be approached like other decisional capacity evaluations.
- The psychiatric consultant has specific skills to be a leader in the acute care hospital to bring evidence-based geropsychiatric best practice to the bedside. This includes a multidisciplinary role in the pharmacologic and nonpharmacologic management of geriatric patients with neurocognitive, behavioral, and other psychiatric problems.

References

1. Miles SH, Irvine P. Deaths caused by physical restraints. Gerontologist. 1992;32(6):762–6.
2. Parker K, Miles SH. Deaths caused be bedrails. J Am Geriatr Soc. 1997;45(7):797–802.
3. Inouye SK, Westendorp RGJ, Saczynski JS. Delirium in elderly people. Lancet. 2014;383(9920): 911–22.
4. O'Reagan NA, Ryan DJ, Boland E, Connolly W, McGlade C, Leonard M, et al. Attention! A good bedside test for delirium? J Neurol Neurosurg Psychiatry. 2014;85:1122–31.
5. Inouye SK, Bogardus ST, Charpentier PA, Leo-Summers L, Acampora D, Holford TR, et al. A multicomponent intervention to prevent delirium in hospitalized older patients. N Engl J Med. 1999;340(9):669–86.
6. Roberts B, Rickard CM, Rajbhandari D, Turner G, Clarke J, Hill D, et al. Multicentre study of delirium in ICU patients using a simple screening tool. Aust Crit Care. 2005;18(1):6, 8–9, 11–14 passim.
7. Ely EW, Margolin R, Francis J, May L, Truman B, Dittus R, et al. Evaluation of delirium in critically ill patients: validation of the Confusion Assessment Method for the Intensive Care Unit (CAM-ICU). Crit Care Med. 2001;29(7):1370–9.
8. Morandi A, Jackson JC, Ely EW. Delirium in the intensive care unit. Int Rev Psychiatry. 2009;21(1):43–58.
9. Fong T, Jones RN, Shi P, Marcantonio ER, Yap L, Rudolph JL, et al. Delirium accelerates cognitive decline in Alzheimer disease. Neurology. 2009;72:1570–5.
10. Curtis P, Sethi F, Ahmed F. Creating a high quality consultant led psychiatric intensive care unit multidisciplinary team ward round. J Psychiatr Inten Care. 2014;10(1):13–22.
11. Francis J. Delirium in older patients. J Am Geriatr Soc. 1992;40(8):829–38.
12. Saïas T, Gallarda T. Paradoxical aggressive reactions to benzodiazepine use: a review. Encéphale. 2008;34(4):330–6. Review. French.
13. Lindsey PL. Psychotropic medication use among older adults: what all nurses need to know. J Gerontol Nurs. 2009;35(9):28–38.
14. Pierluissi E, Francis DC, Covinsky KE. Patient and hospital factors that lead to adverse outcomes in hospitalized elders. In: Malone ML, Capezuti E, Palmer RM, editors. Acute care for elders: a model for interdisciplinary care. New York: Springer Science and Business Media; 2014.
15. Inouye SK, Baker DI, Fugal P, Bradley EH. Dissemination of the Hospital Elder Life Program implementation, adaptation, and successes. J Am Geriatr Soc. 2006;54(10):1492–9.
16. Yue J, Tabloski P, Dowal SL, Puelle MR, Nandan R, Inouye SK. NICE to HELP: operationalizing National Institute for Health and Clinical Excellence guidelines to improve clinical practice. J Am Geriatr Soc. 2014;62(4):754–61.
17. Fulmer T, Mezey M, Bottrell M, Abraham I, Sazant J, Grossman S, et al. Nurses Improving Care for Healthsystem Elders (NICHE): using outcomes and benchmarks for evidenced-based practice. Geriatr Nurs. 2002;23(3):121–7.
18. Bennett S, Thomas AJ. Depression and dementia: cause, consequence or coincidence? Maturitas. 2014;79(2):184–90.
19. Alam A, Voronovich Z, Carley JA. A review of therapeutic uses of mirtazapine in psychiatric and medical conditions. Prim Care Companion CNS Disord. 2013;15(5):PCC.13r01525. doi:10.4088/PCC.13r01525.
20. Hardy SE. Methylphenidate for treatment of depressive symptoms, apathy, and fatigue in medically ill older adults and terminally ill adults. Am J Geriatr Pharmacother. 2009;7(1): 34–59.
21. Kahn DR, Bourgeois JA, Klein SC, Iosif AM. A prospective observational study of decisional capacity determinations in an academic medical center. Int J Psychiatry Med. 2009; 39:405–15.
22. Alfandre DJ. "I'm going home": discharges against medical advice. Mayo Clin Proc. 2009; 84(3):255–60.

Subacute or Intermediate Medical Settings

19

Debra Bakerjian, Rebecca Anglin, and Calvin H. Hirsch

19.1 Background

This chapter describes settings that fall in the overarching category of "intermediate care," which essentially means care between acute hospital inpatient care, traditional long-term care, and ambulatory care. This has been a rapidly expanding but poorly defined category of care with a lack of international consensus as to what it encompasses and which patients are most appropriate for care in these settings [1]. Patients receiving care in subacute settings are deemed too stable for acute inpatient care yet too unstable for home or ambulatory care or traditional long-term care. The term "intermediate care" stems from the British National Health Service, who developed this service to reduce hospitalizations and provide a setting to receive and promote early hospital discharges [2, 3]. The literature describes a variety of settings that seem to fall into this category including subacute or post-acute care settings that may be freestanding or part of a skilled nursing home in the USA or intermediate care facilities in Japan. The Canadian Health Act defines extended health-care services as "nursing home intermediate care," which is similar to the US skilled nursing home. In Europe, there has been an

D. Bakerjian, PhD, APRN, FAAN, FAANP (✉)
NP/PA Clinical, Education and Practice, Betty Irene Moore School of Nursing, University of California, Davis, 4610 X Street, Suite 4202, Sacramento, CA 95817, USA
e-mail: dbakerjian@ucdavis.edu

R. Anglin, MD, PhD
Department of Psychiatry and Behavioural Neurosciences, McMaster University, Hamilton, ON, Canada

Division of Gastroenterology, Department of Medicine, McMaster University, Hamilton, ON, Canada

C.H. Hirsch, MD
Department of Internal Medicine, Division of General Medicine, University of California Davis Medical Center, Sacramento, CA, USA

A. Hategan et al. (eds.), *On-Call Geriatric Psychiatry: Handbook of Principles and Practice*, DOI 10.1007/978-3-319-30346-8_19

increase in the number of respiratory intermediate care units to support long-term ventilator-dependent patients (European Respiratory Society Task Force) that also fall into this category.

Patients in intermediate care settings have a wide variety of medical and psychiatric health needs. Common medical conditions include acute exacerbations of chronic illnesses (e.g., diabetes mellitus, heart failure), an acute event (e.g., stroke, acute myocardial infarction), or some type of trauma (e.g., motor vehicle accidents, burns, gunshot wounds). These patients often have psychiatric illnesses superimposed on their medical problem. Additionally, due to international efforts to deinstitutionalize mental health care, the need for psychiatric community-based care has increased, and therefore the prevalence of patients with acute and chronic psychiatric illnesses in many models of community-based care has increased as well [4]. These cases might include patients with uncontrolled schizophrenia, other psychotic episodes, manic episodes in bipolar disorder, severe/melancholic/psychotic depression, or other psychiatric disorders. Because of the variability in the types of settings and differences internationally, the settings below are described based on the US standards, which seems to have the most different types of settings with the greatest number of regulatory requirements. Where international differences could be found, explanations are provided.

19.2 Understanding the Settings

Long-term care hospitals (LTCH) provide hospital-level care for medically complex, long-stay patients; regulations and standards are the same as acute care hospitals, but lengths of stay are significantly longer (average 25 days or longer). They can be organized within a hospital or freestanding care setting; the patients typically are ventilator dependent or have some type of respiratory failure, have complex wounds, have significant and chronic infections, and/or have experienced severe trauma.

Intermediate care in Great Britain and some other European countries and subacute care in the USA consists of specialized units that provide care to medically fragile patients or those with complex medical needs. In the USA, patients qualify for this level of care if they are transferred immediately after hospitalization or admitted as an alternative to acute care hospitalization, depending on the type of insurance coverage they have and may qualify if they have acute mental health needs as well. In Canada, patients who are not ready for discharge from the hospital but who no longer need acute services may be admitted to complex continuing care or chronic care units. These settings typically provide ongoing access to multidisciplinary care, and the facilities may be within a hospital or freestanding care setting. They may be colocated or separate from rehabilitation units that typically admit patients following orthopedic surgeries or injuries, brain injuries including stroke, or other medical patients who require rehabilitation. The requirements in other countries may be quite different.

In the past several years, US skilled nursing facilities (SNF) have begun to differentiate between post-acute care, subacute care, and long-term care. Patients admitted for subacute care, similarly to post-acute care, have complex medical needs, may be recently discharged from the acute care hospital, and need intensive follow-up care that might include rehabilitation (these facilities have extra staffing requirements). One way in which these two types of care might be differentiated is that post-acute patients are short stay and are expected to be discharged home after intense rehabilitation (e.g., total hip replacement), while subacute patients may be long stay with an expectation of prolonged or even lifetime care (e.g., severe traumatic brain injury, massive stroke, ventilator dependence).

19.3 Approach to Care

Psychiatric and/or behavioral symptoms are common in patients in subacute or intermediate care settings who are often admitted with traumatic brain injuries, major strokes, anoxic events, or severe cardiopulmonary events; many also have moderate to severe pain. Depression, anxiety, and even psychosis are common secondary conditions and, in this way, management is similar to acute care settings (see Chaps. 17 and 18). Behavioral causes can also include adverse drug reactions, delirium/confusion secondary to hypoxia or metabolic imbalances, neurologic disorders, other medical illness, pain, neurocognitive disorders, and environmental and social triggers (see Chap. 18).

In general, the initial goal of care is to treat the primary underlying cause of the behavior, which may include pain, hypoxia, metabolic or electrolyte abnormalities, and adverse drug events versus a major psychiatric illness. The on-call consultant needs to partner with the nursing staff to try to determine underlying cause. Of course, the actual behavior or psychiatric disorder may also need to be treated early on, particularly if the patient is a danger to himself/herself or others. Similar to the acute settings, patients admitted with major psychiatric disorders frequently have significant comorbid conditions such as heart failure, diabetes mellitus, hypertension, and chronic obstructive pulmonary disease.

In subacute settings, the staffing model is likely not to be as comprehensive as it is in acute inpatient settings. While there are typically several registered nurses on duty, licensed vocational nurses and certified nursing assistants are also part of the care team. Most of these facilities will have full-time physical, speech, and occupational therapy and at least a part-time respiratory therapist. Some, particularly the long-term care hospitals, will have physician staff during daytime hours, but on-site psychiatrists or mental health professionals are less common.

19.3.1 Pharmacological Management

This may need to be a first-line approach in emergency situations, particularly if the patient has serious or life-threatening medical conditions that must be managed.

Therefore, on-call psychiatric consultants should first call the regular general clinician (physician, nurse practitioner, or physician assistant) to discuss the use of psychotropic medications, if at all possible. If the regular general clinician is not available, the use of short-acting medications is preferable, and close monitoring and follow-up is necessary.

19.3.2 Non-pharmacological Management

This option may be limited, again due to the seriousness of the immediate or life-threatening conditions. However, non-pharmacologic approaches are often preferable in most minor or routine psychiatric situations and some urgent situations if the patient's medical condition is relatively stable. Examples of this might be using music therapy or purposeful diversion for patients who have anxiety or engagement in focused activities for patients with depressive symptoms.

19.3.3 Emergency Situations

Most true psychiatric emergency situations (e.g., suicide attempts, danger to self or others, severe psychosis) will require the patient to be transferred to the emergency department with a subsequent acute inpatient psychiatric admission.

19.3.4 Urgent Situations

Treatment of urgent psychiatric conditions is dependent upon the resources available in the specific site (see Chaps. 17 and 18). If the facility is a long-term care hospital, they may have the ability to manage some situations, particularly adverse drug events or conditions that can be managed with medications. Psychotherapy is likely not available. In subacute units in nursing homes, resources are scarcer and decisions about whether to send patients to the hospital or emergency psychiatric services will depend on the severity of the problem and the resources of the facility. Diagnostic resources (laboratory or radiology) may also be limited as these services are often provided by outside vendors. In nursing homes, intermediate or subacute facilities, STAT laboratory tests may take 4–6 h to get results. If the patient's diagnosis or management is dependent upon laboratory results, on-call clinicians may have no choice but to send the patient to the emergency department.

Case Vignette Ms. M, a 68-year-old woman previously in good health, was admitted to the hospital with an aggressive necrotizing pneumonia that rapidly progressed to respiratory failure requiring intubation. Her hospitalization was complicated by a bronchopulmonary fistula requiring video-assisted thoracoscopic surgery, a right upper extremity deep venous thrombosis, critical illness myopathy, pneumothorax, and delirium. Her intensivist managed frequent agitation and attempts to pull out her intravenous lines and tracheostomy tube with a continuous infusion of midazolam 3.5 mg per hour. Because she could not be weaned from the ventilator, a tracheostomy was performed, along with placement of a gastrostomy tube for nutrition. After 33 days she was discharged to a freestanding subacute hospital 20 miles away, still ventilator dependent. At the subacute facility, Ms. M was continued on her bronchodilators and hydrocodone 7.5 mg/acetaminophen (paracetamol) 325 mg every 4 h PRN for pain. Her midazolam was stopped and replaced with lorazepam 5 mg IV every 6 h with an additional 2 mg IV every 4–6 h PRN for breakthrough anxiety and agitation.

Over the ensuing 2 weeks, the pulmonologist tried to hold the lorazepam during daily weaning trials, but she would start thrashing about, staring wide-eyed, and would not follow commands. The pulmonologist considered starting dexmedetomidine but was informed that the drug was unavailable on the formulary. The on-call psychiatrist was called to assist in the management of agitation and confusion. After reviewing the case, the psychiatrist recommended in his note to give olanzapine 5 mg IM x 1, then 2.5 mg dissolved in water per PEG tube every 24 h, with an additional 2.5–5 mg every 8 h PRN for severe agitation. Concurrently, the psychiatrist recommended reducing the scheduled per dose amount of lorazepam by 1 mg every other day for 8 days, then giving 1 mg BID for 2 days, then discontinuing. The pulmonologist, concerned about new-onset QT_c prolongation to 482 msec, stopped the olanzapine after the second day but did not recontact the psychiatrist about alternative medications. The bedside nurses continued to follow the PRN order for lorazepam to treat anxiety, so that Ms. M continued to receive an average of 8 mg per day 10 days later. In addition, the nurses responded to the patient's facial grimacing by administering PRN hydrocodone/acetaminophen (paracetamol), for an average daily dose of 22.5 mg of hydrocodone. The family expressed anger and frustration over the inability of the facility to wean Ms. M from the ventilator; the use of antipsychotics, about which they had learned only from the nurse; and the apparent failure to control Ms. M's pain and anxiety. After 30 days at the subacute facility, they arranged for an air ambulance to transport her to a university-affiliated subacute facility in a different state.

Case Analysis Ms. M was experiencing agitated delirium, to which the benzodiazepines, given initially as sedation because of the patient's resistance to mechanical ventilation, were a principal contributor. A physician order for PRN lorazepam conflicted with the psychiatrist's taper protocol. Poor communication among physicians and between the family and physicians is common in subacute facilities, in part because of the sporadic rounding schedule of physicians, whose principal offices may be elsewhere.

This case illustrates several challenges for the on-call psychiatrist in subacute and intermediate care facilities, where a small census of patients with psychiatric illnesses does not justify daily rounds. In this case, ongoing management of the patient's delirium would have benefitted from an active interdisciplinary team approach involving close collaboration between the pulmonologist, the psychiatrist, and the bedside nurses. Instead, lack of follow-up communication between the psychiatrist and pulmonologist resulted in a poor outcome. Management of psychiatric and behavioral disturbances in the long-term care environment also requires good communication with family, whose understanding and acceptance of the treatment plan can help engage them as part of the therapeutic intervention. As this case illustrates, freestanding facilities (and even large hospitals) may not offer preferred, evidence-based pharmacological options (e.g., dexmedetomidine) because of budgetary constraints. The choice of medications also may be determined by the patient's insurance plan.

Key Points

- Subacute and intermediate care settings provide care for patients with extremely complex care needs.
- Approach to care should balance the needs of the patients with the resources of the specific facility.
- Treatment of underlying causes of behavioral or psychiatric problems is essential.
- Diagnostic services (laboratory or radiology) may limit some options in subacute or intermediate care settings.

References

1. Melis RJ, Rikkert MG, Parker SG, van Eijken MI. What is intermediate care? BMJ. 2004;329(7462):360–1.
2. Glasby J, Martin GP, Regen EL. Older people and the relationship between hospital services and intermediate care: results from a national evaluation. J Interprof Care. 2008;22(6): 639–49.
3. Godfrey M, Keen J, Townsend J, Moore J, Ware P, Hardy B, et al. An evaluation of intermediate care for older people. Leeds, UK: Institute of Health Sciences and Public Health Research; 2005.
4. Thomas K, Rickwood DJ, Bussenschutt G. Adult step-up step-down: a sub-acute short-term residential mental health service. Int J Psychosoc Rehabil. 2015;19(1):13–21.

Residential Medical Settings 20

Debra Bakerjian and Glen L. Xiong

20.1 Background

There is a high prevalence of patients with mental health disorders and behavioral symptoms in residential care settings (nursing homes (NHs), board and care facilities (B&C), and assisted living communities (ALCs)) internationally [1]. A majority of studies about the prevalence and available treatment has come from the USA, with many authors citing poor quality and lack of access to mental health services [1, 2]. In a longitudinal study of US NHs, Li [2] found that almost half of US NHs had either only "on-call" services (24 %) or no (22 %) on-site mental health services. Canada and Great Britain have also reported insufficient mental health services in long-term care [1]. Additionally, nursing staffing may be minimal to nonexistent in some settings. Patients in these settings often have multiple other comorbid conditions, which increases complexity of care. In particular, patients with major neurocognitive disorder (NCDs) (formerly termed dementia) with psychotic features and/or behavioral manifestations can be particularly challenging to care for and are the cause of many after-hours calls to physicians.

This chapter describes various residential care settings and highlights differences in the care management of older adults with psychiatric disorders and behavioral disturbances. A general approach to care is described along with both

D. Bakerjian, PhD, APRN, FAAN, FAANP (✉)
NP/PA Clinical, Education and Practice, Betty Irene Moore School of Nursing,
University of California, Davis, 4610 X Street, Suite 4202, Sacramento, CA 95817, USA
e-mail: dbakerjian@ucdavis.edu

G.L. Xiong, MD, CMD
Department of Psychiatry & Behavioral Sciences, University of California,
Davis Medical Center, Sacramento, CA 95818, USA
e-mail: gxiong@ucdavis.edu

A. Hategan et al. (eds.), *On-Call Geriatric Psychiatry: Handbook of Principles and Practice*, DOI 10.1007/978-3-319-30346-8_20

pharmacological and non-pharmacological management strategies. Crosswalks highlight setting differences as well as emergent, urgent, and routine conditions and management strategies.

20.2 Understanding the Settings

Three main types of community-based organizations provide services to older adults, NHs, B&C, and ALCs. Table 20.1 provides key information and highlights the main differences among these settings. As can be seen, NHs are the most "formal" of these settings, in terms of their organized medical and nursing care models being more similar to that of hospitals, while ALCs are designed to be independent living but allow for some assistance with activities of daily living (e.g., bathing, dressing) and medication administration. Residential care facilities (RCFs) are somewhere in the middle and are typically much smaller in size. It is common to receive frequent calls from NHs for after-hours urgent issues, while ALCs and RCFs often send patients to the hospital ED for urgent problems. On-call psychiatric consultants should become familiarized with the different settings and the regulations that govern care, even if they do not often make visits to the sites.

20.3 Approach to Care

20.3.1 General Approach to Disease-Specific Conditions

In the following section, we focus on emergency, urgent, and routine manifestations of common conditions prevalent in older adults in long-term care settings with a focus on management limitations of the settings. Table 20.2 lists specific psychiatric and behavioral conditions that require emergent, urgent, and routine management approach. Due to limitations of ALC and B&C settings, clinicians have rarely been called to provide "on-call" or telephone management of acute medical emergencies. Nevertheless, it is expected that community care will expand in the coming years indicating a growing need for geriatric psychiatric staff to be available to provide medical and behavioral consultations for additional settings. We define *emergency* issues as those that require referral to the emergency department (ED) or same-day visit by the treating clinician; *urgent* issues would need to be address with face-to-face evaluation in the next 2–5 days; then *routine* evaluations may be managed by phone and face-to-face evaluation within 2–4 weeks.

Most emergency issues will require imminent referral to local ED or emergency psychiatric services. When addressing emergencies, a few general principles apply to all settings:

- *Medical stability.* For obvious reasons, if a resident is having a medical emergency, referral to the local ED is indicated. Therefore, vital signs, status, level of consciousness, and current behavior are important to ascertain.

Table 20.1 Crosswalk of residential settings of care

Setting characteristics	Medical and pharmacy	Staffing	Comments
Nursing homes Size: < 50 beds to >1,000 beds; NHs cluster patients in "units" or "wards" comprised of private and semiprivate rooms; many residents live there for prolonged periods; many have either major neurocognitive disorders (formerly dementia) and/or other psychiatric illnesses in addition to chronic diseases: behavioral symptoms (physical aggression) are common. Care is highly regulated	Professional medical services provided by physicians, nurse practitioners, and physician assistants visiting at least monthly; psychiatric services follow a consultative model Most NHs obtain drugs through a regional pharmacy making frequent deliveries; medications ordered after hours may be available through an "emergency medical kit"	Team of licensed and unlicensed nurses provide 24 h care; staffing varies widely; most direct care provided by unlicensed, certified nursing assistants (CNAs); numbers of registered nurses (RN) or licensed vocational nurses (LVN) are limited. In some cases, only one RN or LVN may be available	Some NHs utilize a staff model similar to hospital with formal medical services available in daytime *US NHs also provide short stay, post-acute care after hospitalization. Discussed in Chap. 19* A few NHs have a PIXUS-type machine that provides expanded choice of medications after hours
Board and care Much smaller than NHs, sometimes with only 4–10 beds. Care is informal, primarily to provide assistance with ADLs. Residents are usually stable but may require a lot of care; psychiatric illnesses are common. Care is minimally regulated	Almost all medical services require patients to be brought to office; home health nurses available for nursing care; requires medical director oversight; no on-site psychiatric care; pharmacy usually through community source	Most do not have access to licensed nurses except through home health; CNAs or home health aides provide care	
Assisted living communities Individual apartments, common spaces, and dining rooms where residents get prepared meals. Some have an attached NH; various levels of support services available (ADL assistance, meds). ALCs have minimal regulatory oversight in the USA, although regulations are increasing	Most medical services provided through regular office visits; some have attached "clinic" with medical services provided for limited hours. No on-site psychiatric care	Uncommon for licensed nurse on-site; many ALCs hire licensed nurses to provide oversight for multiple facilities; medication aides can *pass* or assist with medications	Aide "hands" medications to residents who need to be able to take their medications independently in order to qualify for ALCs

Table 20.2 Crosswalk of emergent, urgent, and routine situations by diagnosis and behaviors

Diagnosis	Emergent	Urgent	Routine
Major depression	Suicidal ideation Suicidal attempt	Suicidal ideation without plan Reduced oral intake Refuses to participate in care delivery	Other depressive symptoms Start and titrate antidepressants
GAD/OCD		Panic attacks with vital sign (VS) changes Skin picking resulting in wound infection Insomnia	Panic attacks – stable VS Stable OCD behaviors
Schizophrenia	Suicidal ideation/attempt Acute paranoia posing danger to self/others Disorganized or bizarre behaviors that pose danger to self/others	Paranoia and other delusions Insomnia Disorganized or bizarre behaviors that are new from baseline	Medication side effects Routine dose reduction of antipsychotics Start or titrate existing antipsychotic medications
Bipolar disorder	Suicidal ideation with plan or attempt Irritable or manic behaviors that pose danger to self/other	Pacing, persistent agitation with or without insomnia Moderate to severe depressive symptoms Suicidal ideation without plan	Anxiety, intermittent insomnia Mild to moderate depressive symptoms
Personality disorder	A self-harm behavior that requires emergency medical treatment (e.g., swallowing of razor) New suicidal ideation/attempt	New aggressive behaviors Suicidal ideation without plan	Stable comorbid psychiatric conditions such as major depression or bipolar disorder Stable known behaviors
Delirium	Acute change in level of alertness that has medical etiology and that requires medical work-up and treatment (not available at NH)	Onset of hallucinations or delusions with or without hyperactivity	Decreased cognition without behavior changes Intermittent confusion without change in level of consciousness Mild, intermittent disorientation
Major NCD/ dementia	New behavior that is dangerous to self/ others	Behaviors involving confusion that impact others but are not dangerous or respond to redirection or reorientation	Confusion or behavior that does not pose a danger to self
Huntington's chorea	New behavior that is dangerous to self/ others	Dangerous behaviors that respond to additional staff monitoring	Behaviors are not dangerous to self/ others

Parkinson's disease	New behavior that is dangerous to self/ others	Dangerous behaviors that respond to additional staff monitoring	Symptoms that respond to reduction of Parkinson's medications Behaviors are not dangerous to self/ others
Traumatic brain injury	New behavior that is dangerous to self/ others	Dangerous behavior that responds to additional staff monitoring	Mild confusion or disorientation Mild anxiety
Behavior	**Emergent**	**Urgent**	**Routine**
Agitation	Progressive increase associated with significantly elevated VS or physical aggression	Verbal aggression	Mild to moderate anxiousness and agitation
Physical aggression	Physically aggressive behaviors that pose a danger to resident or others	Physically aggressive behaviors that are not dangerous but that are not responsive to redirection	Physical aggression that responds to redirection
Repetitive behaviors	Rarely a problem	Behaviors disrupt ADLs and fail to respond to redirection	Behaviors disrupt ADLs but temporarily respond to redirection
Sundowning	Usually chronic and do not require emergency treatment unless associated with dangerous behaviors	Behaviors disrupt ADLs and may require treatment of insomnia if present	
Sexually inappropriate behavior	Often requires 1:1 monitoring until behaviors improve, rarely require ED referral	May require 1:1 monitoring	Medication may be helpful Behavioral treatment plans need to be implemented
Verbal aggression	May become an emergency if there's risk of assaultive behavior	May require temporary medication administration until anxiety or agitation improves Often interferes in ADL care and quality of life of affected resident and peers	Often will improve if symptoms are associated with primary psychiatric disorder such as depression, anxiety, or other mood disorders Will likely improve using behavior analysis and behavioral treatment plan

- *Assaultive behavior.* Most suicidal behaviors can be managed by increasing staff monitoring, and most behavioral problems can be managed through short-term interventions followed by behavioral analysis and corresponding behavioral treatment. However, assaultive and other behaviors where a resident poses danger toward staff and others may require referral to local ED or even law enforcement.
- *Safety monitoring.* If one-to-one monitoring is required to prevent injury to the resident and/or others, sites have varying ability to respond to acute behavioral disturbances. If one-to-one staff is not readily available, increased observation by family may be considered until additional staff arrives.
- *Medical causes of behavior or psychiatric symptoms.* If delirium or other psychiatric symptoms could be due to an acute *systemic medical* disorder, then a work-up may include urinalysis, blood work, and perhaps even chest X-ray to rule out infection. At times, laboratory work is not feasible because some residents will not permit laboratory tests or take prescribed medications; the resident may need to transfer to the hospital ED. On-call clinicians should follow antibiotic stewardship principles when managing infections [3].
- *Referral to emergency services.* It is important to note that while ED referrals may serve as a reprieve for NH staff, the benefits of these referrals may be minimal for nonemergency conditions and may in fact increase the behavioral and health risk to the residents. Therefore, it is important to have a clear treatment goal in mind when sending patients out for emergency medical treatment.

For urgent psychiatric conditions, it is assumed that the NH has the capacity to manage most acute psychiatric symptoms and behaviors that are not life threatening and that the resident will likely need an immediate telephonic consultation and may need to be evaluated within a week. B&C and ALCs may not have that capability and residents will likely need to be sent for emergency services. For new acute symptoms, a basic medical work-up is recommended, although laboratory studies are not always medically necessary.

Routine management of major psychiatric symptoms is outlined in Table 20.1. The general approach is to use a biopsychosocial approach with considering the initiation of new medications or titration of an existing medication, followed by psychosocial treatments. On-call clinicians should use a cautious approach and begin with conservative measures.

20.3.2 Pharmacological Management

Arriving at a primary diagnosis to help guide initial medication selection is just as important as maintaining a reasonable broad differential diagnosis. Reduction of polypharmacy may be an important first step prior to starting new medications to target psychiatric symptoms, especially for patients that are recently transferred from hospital settings (see Chap. 3 for specifics on pharmacotherapy principles). Due to both morbidity and mortality risks of antipsychotics along with the general public's concern about the use of psychotropic medications as "chemical restraints," in the USA, there are active initiatives led by the Centers for Medicare and Medicaid Services (CMS) to reduce the use of antipsychotic medications in NHs [4, 5]. As a result, informed consent and documentation of benefits versus risks of "psychotropic" medications are heavily regulated, more so in NHs than in acute hospitals. A specific, large group of patients where long-term antipsychotic use is *unlikely* to be beneficial are patients who were hospitalized and acutely treated with antipsychotics for delirium, which then has resolved. Many of these patients have been improved from delirium on low doses of antipsychotics that can be reduced or discontinued without major adverse events soon after discharge from the hospital. On the other hand, patients with other comorbid or undiagnosed psychiatric disorder in addition to major NCDs require careful medication and symptom monitoring and often referral to neuropsychiatric evaluations and management.

20.3.3 Non-pharmacological (Psychosocial) Management

Detailed psychosocial treatment is beyond the scope of this chapter, although these approaches are commonly used in residential settings. Music therapy, quiet rooms, massage, biofeedback, aromatherapy, and light therapy have been found to be helpful treatments in some instances [6]. Antecedent or behavioral triggers may include an "unmet need" or another resident getting lost and wandering into the room of the "problematic" resident causing fear and the urge to defend his/her living space. Some consequences or responses from staff members may lead to increased occurrence of the behavior, and therefore such responses should be reduced and eliminated. Obvious responses that tend to work to reduce behaviors should be shared among staff and family members such as calm voice, positive emotional affect, and warmth/empathy.

Social activities are often the highlight of most residential settings. Residential facilities should be discouraged in using psychotropic medications unless necessary and encouraged to use non-pharmacological approaches when possible. Remember, staff members may need positive support as non-pharmacological approaches are more staff intensive. Routine exercise, outings, and group games can play an important role in the overall management of behavioral problems while leading to resident well-being. While there are ample evidence-based approaches for the non-pharmacological treatment of behavioral symptoms, unfortunately, the translation and wide implementation of those treatments have not reached long-term care settings [7, 8].

Case Vignette 1 The NH nurse contacted the on-call clinician. Mr. J was an 84-year-old male NH resident with Parkinson's disease, hypertension, constipation, dysphagia, weight loss, osteoarthritis, and depression. He had worsening major depression with suicidal ideation and anxiety and received lorazepam 1 mg orally 2 h previously for insomnia, but it was ineffective as he became extremely agitated, reporting seeing "dead people" in his room. Mr. J was calling out that he needed "something" so he could kill himself. He had no history of NCD. There were no acute reasons to suspect delirium. The nurse requested medication to calm him or an order to send him to the hospital. The on-call clinician's concern was that patients with suicidal ideation are an emergent problem and may need to be hospitalized; however, older patients often get worse when hospitalized.

Mr. J's routine medications were carbidopa/levodopa CR 25–250 mg twice daily, entacapone 200 mg recently increased from three to five times daily, lisinopril 10 mg daily, and paroxetine 40 mg daily. Vital signs were BP 138/80 mmHg, HR 92 BPM, RR 20/min, and T 98.7 °F (37 °C). The on-call clinician made a diagnosis of antiparkinsonian medication-induced psychosis. The nurse reaffirmed Mr. J had no means to harm himself and that his room location allowed for direct observation. The clinician's order was to hold entacapone and give quetiapine 25 mg at bedtime and every 8 h as needed. However, quetiapine was not in the emergency kit, but his family agreed to purchase medication at the 24-h pharmacy. The nurse assigned a certified nursing assistant (CNA) to sit with Mr. J until his family brought quetiapine from the off-site pharmacy. The nurse was directed to call the on-call clinician back in 2–3 h if Mr. J was not improved or sooner if he worsened.

In a follow-up visit at the NH in 2 days, the clinician examined Mr. J's gait and determined that entacapone 200 mg three times daily may be sufficient to manage his Parkinson's disease; he was no longer suicidal or psychotic, was less anxious, and was sleeping better without daytime sedation from quetiapine. He had continued this medication regimen with plan to reduce the quetiapine dose in the following 3–4 months.

Case Vignette 2 The NH staff called you, the on-call clinician, about Mr. B, a 75-year-old male resident, who was admitted 2 weeks previously with a history of anoxic brain injury, type 2 diabetes mellitus, hypertension, failure to thrive, and two stage 2 decubitus pressure ulcers. He apparently groped a female resident's breast in the dining room. The NH was reporting the incident to the local regulatory authority. You saw this patient 1 week prior and noted some cognitive impairment and possible major NCD. However, there was minimal past medical and psychiatric history available as this patient was discharged from the hospital after he was found on the floor at home. No family members were available to give collateral information. The NH staff reported that the patient denied the incident, although he told another staff that he did not do anything wrong and that he would do this again. At the recommendation of the staff, you decided to place the patient on one-to-one staff monitoring due to concern about another incident. You ordered a urinalysis, complete blood count, and comprehensive metabolic panel as a work-up for possible acute medical issues that were contributing to the patient's behavior. Staff reassured you that the patient did not look ill, although he did have a bladder catheter when he was in the hospital.

On exam 2 days later, Mr. B displayed rapid speech and was tangential and grandiose. His vital signs and physical exam were unchanged. Basic laboratory studies were unremarkable. He admitted the incident that he touched a female peer but he would not state whether he had done anything wrong. He stated that he owned the hospital and that you worked for him. He asked that you help him get out of bed and that his limousine was waiting for him outside. The patient, however, declined to answer any cognitive questions despite multiple attempts. He refused to tell you his birthday or age, citing that you were very rude.

Medical records on admission to NH indicated that his quetiapine 200 mg in the morning and 400 mg at bedtime were discontinued shortly after admission due to concern about oversedation. Mr. B seemed to have "awakened" as per nursing staff's reports and had been much more active several days after his medication change. He had been resistive to care and increasingly more argumentative with staff and peers. Although you were unable to obtain prior treatment records, you suspected that Mr. B may have had a history of bipolar disorder with psychotic features. You started him on valproate 500 mg twice daily and quetiapine 100 mg in the morning and 200 mg at bedtime, with an additional 25–50 mg every 8 h as needed.

In follow-up visit, Mr. B's manic symptoms improved 7 days after initiating treatment and regarded you as the "doctor." Staff were also more comfortable with taking the patient off one-to-one monitoring; he had also become more agreeable and less resistive to care. Another week later, he reported continued early morning sleepiness but stated that he was doing okay otherwise. You ordered a serum valproate level for monitoring and future reference and lowered his quetiapine to only 200 mg nightly to reduce morning sedation, with no extra doses of PRN quetiapine. The patient was able to recall his own birthday and some basic orientation questions. However, he was unable to answer questions about his prior history except that he recalled taking lithium and haloperidol in the past.

Key Points

- US NHs are highly regulated with new regulations that focus on psychoactive drugs; antipsychotic medications are strongly discouraged in patients with major NCDs.
- Staffing and pharmaceutical resources are often minimal in residential care settings requiring the on-call clinician to be creative with solutions to urgent or emergent issues.
- Calling on family members to help in some situations can be extremely useful.
- Hospitalization of older adult residents should be considered only when local measures are unsuccessful or when there is clear acute reasons.
- While psychotropic medications are generally discouraged, some long-term care residents may have history of chronic psychiatric illness such as bipolar disorder, recurrent major depression, and schizophrenia. These residents will need careful monitoring of symptoms and use of pharmacological and behavioral treatments.
- Antipsychotics (usually at low doses) that were prescribed in hospital settings for the treatment of delirium can often be discontinued in long-term care settings.

References

1. Snowdon J. Mental health service delivery in long-term care homes. Int Psychogeriatr. 2010;22(7):1063–71.
2. Li Y. Provision of mental health services in US nursing homes, 1995–2004. Psychiatr Serv. 2010;61(4):349–55.
3. Center for Disease Control. 2013. http://www.cdc.gov/getsmart/healthcare/learn-from-others/factsheets/nursing-homes.html. Accessed 18 Sept 2015.
4. Center for Medicare and Medicaid Services. https://www.cms.gov/Newsroom/MediaReleaseDatabase/Press-releases/2014-Press-releases-items/2014-09-19.html. Accessed 18 Sept 2015.
5. Kales HC, Valenstein M, Kim HM, McCarthy JF, Ganoczy D, Cunningham F, et al. Mortality risk in patients with dementia treated with antipsychotics versus other psychiatric medications. Am J Psychiatry. 2007;164(10):1568–76.
6. O'Neil M, Freeman M, Christensen V, Telerant A, Addleman A, Kansagara D. Non-pharmacological interventions for behavioral symptoms of dementia: A systematic review of the evidence. VA-ESP Project. 2011;5:e225.
7. Ayalon L, Gum AM, Feliciano L, Areán PA. Effectiveness of nonpharmacological interventions for the management of neuropsychiatric symptoms in patients with dementia: a systematic review. Arch Intern Med. 2006;166(20):2182–8.
8. Gitlin LN, Marx K, Stanley IH, Hodgson N. Translating evidence-based dementia caregiving interventions into practice: state-of-the-science and next steps. Gerontologist. 2015;55(2): 210–26.

21 Community and Outpatient Settings

Tricia Woo and Julia Baxter

21.1 Background

There is considerable variation in terms of the composition, context, and direction of outpatient or geriatric psychiatry community programs. The models of care can include (a) solo geriatric psychiatrist in an individual practice or working singly in a clinic-based outpatient setting, (b) geriatric psychiatrist embedded in a community-based health service (e.g., community health center, family health team, primary care physician's office, shelter) that works collaboratively with the other staff/practitioners available in that setting, (c) geriatric psychiatrist providing consultation service to a community via videoconferencing, or (d) geriatric psychiatrist that is part of a mobile outreach multidisciplinary team doing home visits to patients in their natural settings (e.g., individual residential home, retirement home, long-term care home). The models of care can also reflect variations in services and supports available to the patient or family. Specialized assessment, diagnosis, treatment, and/or management planning is provided but may or may not be inclusive of interventions such as case management, specific therapies (e.g., cognitive behavioral, interpersonal, problem-solving, behavioral activation), supportive counseling, health teaching, caregiver support, and education. Other variations of practice could include whether the psychiatrist provides recommendations or consultative service to a primary care physician or whether the psychiatrist functions in a primary care role in which they order or prescribe medications, and investigations related to the psychiatric presentation [1].

T. Woo, MD (✉)
Division of Geriatric Internal Medicine, McMaster University, Hamilton, ON, Canada
e-mail: twoo@hhsc.ca

J. Baxter, BSc. HK, MHS
Department of Psychiatry and Behavioural Neurosciences, McMaster University, Hamilton, ON, Canada
e-mail: jbaxter@stjoes.ca

A. Hategan et al. (eds.), *On-Call Geriatric Psychiatry: Handbook of Principles and Practice*, DOI 10.1007/978-3-319-30346-8_21

It is recognized that a large number of marginalized older adults are unlikely to use traditional clinic-based mental health services for a variety of reasons including physical frailty, psychiatric symptoms, transportation difficulties, isolation, and stigma. While a continuum of community geriatric psychiatry service options is promoted to meet the diverse needs of the older adult population, outreach services have been promoted as a means of improving access to service for those who cannot or will not seek traditional ambulatory services. Outreach programs with psychiatry consultation are designed with psychiatrists providing direct patient home visits and/or indirect consultation via outreach clinicians who interact with the patient face-to-face [2].

21.2 Crisis Prevention

Case Vignette Mrs. A was a 90-year-old woman living in the community with her son. She was a frail woman with a long history of major neurocognitive disorder (NCD) secondary to Alzheimer's disease. She also had poorly controlled diabetes mellitus, osteoporosis, and hypertension. Her son also had a history of bipolar disorder which had required two hospitalizations in the previous 3 years. Mrs. A had been attending her outpatient clinic on a regular basis, and as her cognition had declined, she began to have symptoms of paranoia that her neighbors wanted to break into her house. The primary care physician was involved but having difficulty in maintaining consistent control of Mrs. A's blood pressure and blood glucose levels.

Case Analysis The role of community psychiatry is to prevent a crisis in the above case. Given the changes in Mrs. A's cognition, presenting paranoia, uncontrolled blood pressure and blood glucose levels, and the potential increasing strain on the son's caregiving role and responsibilities, an urgently scheduled comprehensive assessment and documentation inclusive of assessing for physical or mental health risks of potential crisis is paramount. Inclusive of this process would be to communicate crisis risks to the patient and family, encourage contingency planning (e.g., "in the case of a crisis, we will/could") and development of an individual community crisis plan to increase awareness of what problem situations look like, what possible triggers may exist, what family, friends, and/or clinicians supports can be called upon, and importantly when to call or access crisis or emergency services.

It is critical to work in close partnership with the individual patient, family, and others. Anchoring intervention plans to the patient and family's goals and perceived needs is critical as insufficient relationship or patient engagement will only cause possible harm and delays.

While communicating with other clinicians via notes and faxes is often common, in order to prevent a crisis, a proactive one-to-one phone call with a primary care physician is reasonable. Given the complexity of Mrs. A, her caregiving situation, and the potential for a crisis, a phone call can assist in establishing a shared understanding of psychiatric assessment, rationale for treatment and intervention, and immediate planning and prioritization of actions inclusive of risk reduction. Outlining when and how to access supports related to the patient's acute and chronic medical illness is critical. Patient, family, and others also need to be informed of the psychiatric crisis services inclusive of when and how to access the services of mobile mental health teams (e.g., telephone, home visit) and when to access hospital-based psychiatric emergency services. While the patient and family have not accepted outside service help, the recent changes and risks to the current living situation create the opportunity to represent community support services (e.g., adult day programs, in-home assistance, respite stay, caregiver relief options) as viable risk reduction strategies possibly aligning with the patient and family's overall goals of wanting to stay at home. Specific on-call or crisis intervention is limited primarily due to the limited availability of the geriatric consultant. In a team setting, on-call intervention can be handled by other members of the clinical outpatient or outreach team during regular business hours. After-hours crisis intervention needs to be clearly communicated to patients, families, and others. In general, the psychiatrist and/or team will often provide secondary support to a primary crisis system and need to establish the local relationships to do so. There can be arranged peer-to-peer phone calls with the primary care physician or possibly an ad hoc call if the patient is presenting in the primary care physician's office in an urgent situation. There can be chronic crises in which an urgent home or office visit is planned and scheduled for the purpose of crisis assessment and planning; visit could result in possibility of involuntary detention under the psychiatric commitment statute specific to the local jurisdiction if that patient is at imminent risk and cannot be further assessed and treated in the current community context and requires a hospital setting. Outpatient settings and outreach programs need to establish a process in this instance and be prepared for what to do if the patient requires an involuntary (or "civil") commitment to hospital.

The role of the geriatric psychiatrist in the community setting is one of anticipating crises and emergent issues based on the knowledge and patient/family experiences and communicating this with others, increasing the collective understanding of the illness, the impact, and the resulting biopsychosocial needs and often advocating with and for the patient and family [3].

21.3 Role of Community Psychiatry in Crisis Management

Case Vignette (Continued) Mrs. A continued to have worsening paranoia about her neighbors and had started to move her dresser to barricade herself into her bedroom each evening. On one occasion, moving the heavy dresser resulted in an acute back injury. Her son brought her to the emergency department and she received acetaminophen for her pain. The emergency physician did not feel that hospitalization was warranted, and Mrs. A was discharged home with her son. The stress of the situation had caused her son to have a decompensation of his bipolar disorder, and he had started to shout at his mother. Mrs. A missed her outpatient appointment as she was unwilling to get out of bed and travel to the clinic with her son.

Case Analysis (Continued) The role of community psychiatry in the management of a crisis consists of assessment, planning, intervention, and follow-up. Mrs. A and her son were in a crisis state. Having the ability to respond urgently and with flexibility is essential. While Mrs. A was typically seen in an ambulatory clinic setting, accommodating a home visit in this instance is critical. Where the psychiatrist cannot urgently go out on a visit, other team members could be used to conduct the visit, directly assessing the situation and working remotely with the psychiatrist to appropriately plan.

Once a patient is identified as being at risk of a crisis in the community, the psychiatrist, often working alongside the team/other community agencies, uses a number of approaches to de-escalate the crises and potentially avoid hospitalization. A key question for the psychiatrist to consider is whether the patient can be safely assessed, treated, and managed in the current community context. In the case vignette, the community psychiatrist plays a key role in flagging and treating modifiable acute or chronic medical illness in the patient working in partnership with the primary care physician or community-based nurse practitioners; reassessing the presenting psychiatric illness and adjusting the management plan; advocating for an increase in community support services to provide direct patient care and monitoring, caregiver relief, and increased supervision given the increased risk for caregiver violence; or initiating the application for a more supervised setting for the patient (e.g., retirement home, skilled nursing facility). Working with others can also facilitate access and review of documentation allowing one to cross-check information, fill in historical disease or treatment history gaps, and may also indicate how past crises were handled and resolved. While a crisis can often cause clinicians to act quickly, the geriatric psychiatrist promotes a sense of responsiveness without compromising a systematic approach acknowledging the biopsychosocial complexity of the geriatric patient.

Key Points

- While crisis is universal and can affect all people, culture can influence how individuals express crisis reactions and how they ask for and accept help. Clinicians need to be multicultural competent.
- It is critical that responders/clinicians possess familiarity with the community setting. The ability to direct people to local shelters, senior respite services, and other safe places and to locate appropriate help and intervention is crucial in this work.
- It is also noted that vulnerability is often exacerbated in that community care is not always well coordinated among an array of agencies and clinicians. The community psychiatrist can advocate for improved coordination and collaboration of services and supports surrounding the patient and family by requesting processes such as urgent case conference, complex case review, establishment of a community lead, development of a community safety plan, and/or the implementation of crisis protocols.

- Although we cannot predict crisis, we can anticipate how people may react to them. The aim is to focus on the "here and now" with a goal to establish immediate coping skills, provide support, and hopefully restore to previous or improved functioning. The assessment of the family and/or caregiver is critical given the patient's reliance on the relationship.
- Crisis prevention, intervention, and management supported by the community geriatric psychiatrist can provide opportunities for older adults, their families, and others to learn new coping skills while identifying, mobilizing, and enhancing the skills they already possess.

References

1. Stolee P, Le Clair JK, Kessler L. Geriatric psychiatry consultation in the community. Can J Psychiatry. 1994;39(8 Suppl 1):S27–33.
2. Van Citters AV, Bartels SJ. A systematic review of the effectiveness of community-based mental health outreach services for older adults. Psychiatr Serv. 2004;55(11):1237–49.
3. Kennedy GJ, Lowinger R. Psychogeriatric emergencies. Clin Geriatr Med. 1993;9(3):641–53.

Correctional Settings 22

Emily MacKillop and Gary Chaimowitz

22.1 Background

The scope of the problem and classification of older adults in correctional settings are herein explored. Incarcerated psychiatrically ill older inmates are even more vulnerable and disenfranchised than younger inmates with psychiatric illness. It is well understood that incarcerated older adults have typically been exposed to a harsher set of life circumstances relative to non-incarcerated and non-psychiatrically ill older adults. This would include increased exposure to communicable diseases, drug and alcohol abuse, higher rates of psychiatric illness, higher rates of traumatic brain injury, reduced access to medical care, stress associated with incarceration, and homelessness. As a consequence, it has been suggested that they are prone to a process of "accelerated aging." As such, "geriatric," or older adults, is commonly defined as ages greater than 50 years within forensic settings and in the context of this chapter [1, 2]. The combination of age, psychiatric illness, and incarceration poses a complex burden which can challenge effective treatment and drain financial and staffing resources. For example, incarcerated older adults have higher rates of psychiatric and physical illness relative to community-dwelling older adults and their younger incarcerated counterparts. They are often socially isolated within the prison setting as well as from friends and family [2]. In addition, individuals with psychiatric illness are particularly vulnerable to victimization inside prison, and they may not be willing to provide information on their attackers for fear of further victimization from being labeled a "snitch" [3–5]. They may be dealing with

E. MacKillop, PhD, ABPP (✉)
Department of Psychiatry and Behavioural Neurosciences, McMaster University, Hamilton, ON, Canada
e-mail: emackill@stjosham.on.ca

G. Chaimowitz, MD
Department of Psychiatry and Behavioural Neurosciences, Division of Forensic Psychiatry, McMaster University, Hamilton, ON, Canada

A. Hategan et al. (eds.), *On-Call Geriatric Psychiatry: Handbook of Principles and Practice*, DOI 10.1007/978-3-319-30346-8_22

end-of-life concerns and fears of dying alone in an undignified manner [6, 7]. Fear, a deep-seated distrust of the correctional system, social isolation, physical and cognitive limitations, and high rates of deleterious life events, in addition to psychiatric illness, are all factors contributing to their vulnerability and their need for timely access to mental healthcare and intervention. However, little attention has been given to investigating the utility of crisis intervention services for the incarcerated older adults with psychiatric illness.

In addition to the complex unmet needs of older psychiatrically ill inmates, there is an undisputed rise in the aging prison population. A report published by the American Civil Liberties Union (ACLU) asserted that the population of prisoners aged 55 and older in the USA has already climbed 1,300 % since the 1980s and is expected to increase by 4,400 % by the year 2030 [8]. For example, from 1984 to 2002, the number of state and federal prisoners serving life sentences in the USA more than quadrupled [1, 8]. This international trend is documented in the USA, Canada, and throughout Europe; however, the problem is most prevalent in the USA [5, 9–12]. As such, this age group is the fastest-growing prison subgroup [2, 13]. The escalating incarceration rate of older adults is thought to be influenced by longer sentences, stricter criteria for release, and "tough on crime" initiatives in addition to a longer life span and aging of the general population.

Despite the rise in the aging prison population and the drain on correctional system resources, managing older offenders' acute psychiatric symptoms is a generally untapped area of investigation and intervention [8]. While there is an obligation to provide reasonable access to healthcare in conformity with professionally accepted standards of practice [14–16], the delivery and timely access to mental healthcare services has fallen short due to the growth of the prison population, insufficient infrastructure (e.g., lack of immediate psychiatric care units), and difficulties recruiting and retaining qualified psychiatrists and other mental healthcare professionals to manage geriatric inmates with psychiatric illness [17, 18].

22.2 Medical and Psychiatric Needs in the Older Incarcerated Adults

22.2.1 Medical Needs

As noted, the prevalence of older offenders is steadily on the rise, and this population has more physical and psychiatric care needs than their younger counterparts. According to the ACLU report, more than 16 billion USD is spent annually in the USA to incarcerate offenders over the age of 50. A meta-analysis of existing studies revealed that it costs about twice as much to incarcerate prisoners aged 50 years and older as opposed to an average aged prisoner ($68,000 vs. $34,000, respectively (USD)) [8]. This rise in cost is largely due to more chronic health problems in older inmates linked with accelerated aging. In the USA, an estimated 45 % of older offenders over the age of 50 and 82 % over the age of 65 have chronic health problems, with similar rates reported in Canada [18]. The prevalence rate of physical problems in the UK has been estimated to be around 2.6 per older inmate [19]. While many of the actual medical and physical needs of the incarcerated older inmates are similar to younger inmates, they can be more difficult to manage given their age, number of concerns, and a lengthier history of suboptimal healthcare [20]. The chronic health conditions are often related to lifestyle choices, such as smoking, obesity, alcohol and drug abuse, sexually transmitted diseases, and insufficient preventative healthcare [21, 22]. Cardiovascular and endocrine (e.g., diabetes mellitus) problems, arthritis, cancer, and sensory deficits are the most common in the geriatric forensic population [23–25].

22.2.2 Psychiatric Needs

The rate of psychiatric illness in incarcerated older adults is higher than the community-dwelling older adult population [11, 20, 26]. Older inmates are also burdened by an increased risk for multiple health concerns in addition to contending with the risk for the development of major neurocognitive disorders (NCDs) (formerly dementia), which are rarely assessed [19, 23, 27, 28]. They are more likely to be diagnosed with major NCD or depressive disorder, such as a major depressive episode with psychotic features, than schizophrenia or personality disorder relative to younger offenders [11]. In addition, psychiatrically ill and older inmates are at a higher risk for self-harm, suicide, and victimization relative to other inmates [29]. Suicide rates within prisons are three times higher than the general population and are higher in the incarcerated older adults. Suicide rates have been shown to be particularly high in psychiatrically ill female offenders serving life sentences [30, 31].

Depressive disorders, substance dependence (primarily alcohol), and personality and psychotic disorders are among the most common occurring diagnoses reported in older offenders, and the comorbidity of major NCDs with psychiatric illness is striking. Large-scale demographic studies have estimated that approximately 50 % of incarcerated older adults meet the criteria for psychiatric illness, and 12–50 % meet the criteria for major NCDs [19, 20, 32]. One small study examined older male offenders involved in violent crime and found that the majority had a history of psychiatric hospitalization, primary psychotic, bipolar, or depressive disorder, cognitive impairment, traumatic brain injury, neurologic disorder, and/or alcohol abuse [23]. In a report examining older offenders in southern states in the USA, major NCDs (22 %) and paranoia due to psychotic disorders (61 %) were the two most prevalent conditions at the time of their arrest. Additionally, nearly a third were using alcohol or drugs at the time of their arrest [32]. The coexistence of a substance use disorder and psychiatric illness presents diagnostic and intervention challenges, as substance use disorders can mimic or mask underlying psychiatric conditions, including major NCDs, and poses an increased risk for developing neurodegenerative disorders in later life.

22.3 The Role of the On-Call Psychiatric Consultant in Correctional Settings

Given that the majority of older inmates have several co-occurring chronic physical and psychiatric problems, immediate intervention by readily available geriatric psychiatry services could mitigate the costs associated with preventable emergency department visits and lengthy hospitalizations. This model has been cost-effective in community-dwelling populations with access to acute mental health services [33]. Acute management could also help to reduce the costs of off-site treatment, which accounts for the majority of all healthcare costs spent on aging prisoners [34]. However, despite the explosive rise in the number of incarcerated older adults and the prevalence of major NCDs and other psychiatric illness within this group, the availability of services for older psychiatrically ill offenders remains low [35].

Acute assessment and diagnosis could assist in identifying vulnerable individuals and making intervention and treatment recommendations. Additionally, the system would benefit from a range of other services provided in the context of the acute assessment, such as providing an opinion on consent and involuntary treatment issues, identifying and making recommendations for segregated housing for vulnerable and at-risk individuals, avoiding lengthy isolation (e.g., solitary confinement), medication reconciliation and review, threat assessment to self and others, assessment of the impact of chronic conditions, overseeing the utilization of restraints when appropriate in acute situations, recognizing the need for palliative or alternative care, intervening in instances of grave disability, and referring to supportive programs. Psychiatric consultants with expertise in geriatric psychiatry may also assist in making recommendations to parole boards for medical parole/compassionate release for low-risk individuals and in making recommendations about the appropriate level of supervision and behavioral management to minimize acute risks [2, 36]. In summary, the psychiatric consultant with expertise in geriatric psychiatry responding to a crisis situation could assist in operational, treatment and intervention, and resource allocation decisions regarding the needs of the patient as well as assist in communicating the psychiatric care needs with frontline correctional staff.

Once the hurdle of appropriate and timely referral to a psychiatric consultant for acute services is overcome, a second barrier presents. Intervention and assessment can be challenging given that there is very little in the way of empirical research in this area or training in the standards of care for treatment with the forensic population in psychiatry residency programs [37]. One way to assist in intervention would be to develop and implement clinical standards and screening protocols for psychiatric illness geared toward the incarcerated older adult, which would necessarily include the assessment of current symptoms, substance abuse, mental (including cognitive) status, and potentially untreated (or undertreated) physical problems as contributing factors. Rapid screening tools (e.g., Correctional Mental Health Screen [38], Brief Jail Mental Health Screen [39], and Referral Decision Scale [39]) have been developed to identify psychiatric symptoms and threat assessment within the correctional settings; however, more research is needed to apply them to the area of geriatric forensics. Such tools may be helpful within the context of an assessment by a qualified clinician. In addition, using standardized brief cognitive screening tools (e.g., Montreal Cognitive Assessment (MoCA, www.mocatest.org) [40] and Mini-Mental State Examination (MMSE) [41]) as part of clinical assessment assists in quantifying cognitive function and helps to screen for the presence of suspected neurocognitive impairment, as is done outside correctional settings.

As noted, the older incarcerated psychiatrically ill have different needs than community-dwelling older adults and their younger incarcerated counterparts. Special consideration of additional factors should be made during assessment, including, but not limited to, a history of developmental delay, intellectual disability, traumatic brain injury, severe psychotic/bipolar/depressive illness, substance abuse, cardiovascular disease and/or stroke, obesity, and diabetes mellitus (particularly undertreated). Not only are these prevalent within the incarcerated population, but they can be risk factors for development of mild and major NCDs in later life, especially when combined with the consequences of adverse psychosocial factors (e.g., education and socioeconomic factors).

In summary, psychiatry consult services with expertise in geriatric psychiatry would support, at least, the psychiatric care needs, particularly for those older inmates in a crisis situation, through accurate diagnosis, management of acute symptoms, and by making appropriate follow-up recommendations. Research geared toward exploring the implications for better and faster intervention by increasing access to on-call psychiatry services in corrections (e.g., cost-effectiveness, improving long-term outcomes, enhancing quality of life) is warranted.

Case Vignette Mr. A was a 60-year-old male inmate serving a life sentence who had been incarcerated in the same facility since his mid-twenties. He was well known to correctional staff and generally enjoyed a good relationship with them and other inmates. He did not have a history of behavioral problems and was entrusted with janitorial tasks throughout the facility. He was noted to have been withdrawn for the past several weeks but there had been no acute behavioral concerns. He was also known to be taking several medications for medical conditions that were unknown to the guards on duty. During a routine count, he refused to participate and became agitated. He became aggressive with the correctional staff when asked to comply, which was out of character for him. Given the rapid escalation of his behavior and feeble attempt to hit one of the guards, they immediately restrained him and placed him in solitary confinement. Officers noted that the man was incoherent and was not responding well to the restraints, while his aggressive behavior had continued to escalate to the degree of significant harm to self and others. Thus, the psychiatric consultant was called to assess this crisis situation and provide management as necessary.

Case Analysis There are several questions a clinician must answer when assessing and providing an urgent management plan for Mr. A.

A. *Is Mr. A's current behavior consistent or inconsistent with previous behaviors and known preexisting psychiatric illness?* This could be answered by reviewing the medical file to determine psychiatric and medical history. In addition, in this scenario the inmate had been housed in the same facility for many years, and the correctional staff may be a source of information as they might have noticed a change in behavior or circumstance. Gathering other information, for example, any recent changes in routines, medications, disciplinary sanctions, recent visits by family, and/or recently diagnosed conditions, will also help in determining the etiology of the behavioral change.

B. *What procedures might be utilized to assess his psychiatric and/or physical needs?* A multicomponent approach would likely be necessary. First, as previously stated, assessment of physical status in addition to careful review of his medical records to determine whether a physical contribution is warranted. Next, using rapid screening tools such as Correctional Mental Health Screen [38], Brief Jail Mental Health Screen [39], and Referral Decision Scale [39] may be helpful within the context of a psychiatric assessment, whereas brief cognitive screening tools (e.g., MoCA, MMSE) could evaluate acute mental status changes and screen for the presence of suspected neurocognitive disorders (including delirium).
C. *What are Mr. A's primary diagnostic differentials?* Several could be considered, including major depressive episode, psychotic disorder, major NCD and/or delirium secondary to acute infection, or cerebrovascular event. In addition, substance abuse and/or overdose should be investigated (e.g., ingestion of illegally acquired contraband, overdose by hoarding prescription medications). Also, consider the contribution of sensory deficits to the clinical presentation (e.g., hearing loss in the midst of a psychotic episode or acute physical concern).
D. *What might be some considerations when assessing this geriatric inmate relative to a community-dwelling individual with similar symptoms?* In older inmates, there are increased rates of chronic health problems due to accelerated aging, psychiatric illness, suicide rates, social isolation within the prison setting from friends and family, vulnerability to victimization inside prison, and hesitancy to disclose symptoms to correctional personnel due to distrust. Other factors such as lower intellect, history of traumatic brain injury, or sensory deficits should also be considered when assessing geriatric inmates.
E. *What recommendations might be made?* These would depend on the outcome of the assessment and might include a hierarchical approach, starting with the most acute needs. For example, if a medical contribution is determined, such as delirium secondary to acute infection, then antibiotic intervention and monitoring may be most appropriate initially with a follow-up neurocognitive assessment depending on his response to treatment. Transfer of an inmate with suspected delirium to the prison infirmary/hospital is an urgent need for psychiatric and general medical workup and monitoring. A prison infirmary/hospital is advised to follow a comprehensive program of delirium surveillance, screening, and non-pharmacological management as is described in Chap. 18. On the other hand, if an NCD was suspected, based on ruling out a physical or other psychiatric contribution and the results of the assessment, then the inmate may benefit from the initiation of medication for behavioral and/or cognitive symptoms (see Chap. 17). If behavioral symptoms continue or escalate, the

psychiatric consultant could recommend appropriate interventions to manage them in the context of an NCD rather than as willful noncompliance (e.g., placement in segregated housing for vulnerable individuals, referring to supportive programming). Once delirium has been ruled out, if the clinical examination is most consistent with a recurrent psychotic disorder, the patient can be transferred to the prison inpatient psychiatric unit for definitive care (provided the prison has such a unit). Monitoring while his symptoms are treated and stabilized may be the most appropriate initially with follow-up as necessary depending on the outcome. Apprising the correctional staff of the outcome and intervention strategies so they are better informed to manage future events would also be advisable, when possible.

Key Points

- There will continue to be an inevitable rise in older psychiatrically ill inmates.
- These older inmates will have complex needs, with overlapping physical and psychiatric illnesses.
- Victimization of older inmates and abuse from other inmates are likely.
- Correctional settings will pose unexpected barriers to timely and appropriate medical care.
- Consideration for medical/psychiatric units for older inmates in correctional settings should occur.
- Planning for the delivery of geriatric services to the correctional system will require more active involvement of the subspecialty of geriatric psychiatry.

References

1. Human Rights Watch. Old behind bars: the aging prison population in the United States. 2012. https://www.hrw.org/report/2012/01/27/old-behind-bars/aging-prison-population-united-states. Accessed 27 Nov 2015.
2. Aday RH, Krabill JJ. Older and geriatric offenders: critical issues for the 21st century. In: Gideon L, editor. Special needs offenders in correctional institutions. Thousand Oaks (CA): Sage Inc; 2013: 203–32.
3. Blitz CL, Wolff N, Shi J. Physical victimization in prison: the role of mental illness. Int J Law Psychiatry. 2008;31(5):385–93.
4. Teplin LA, McClelland GM, Abram KM, Weiner DA. Crime victimization in adults with severe mental illness: comparison with the National Crime Victimization Survey. Arch Gen Psychiatry. 2005;62(8):911–21.
5. Gal M. The physical and mental health of older offenders. Ment Health (Lond). 2003; 38:12–7.
6. Deaton D, Aday RH, Wahidin A. The effect of health and penal harm on aging female prisoners' views of dying in prison. Omega (Westport). 2009–2010;60(1):51–70.
7. Aday RH. Aging prisoners' concerns toward dying in prison. Omega (Westport). 2005–2006;52(3):199–216.

8. At America's expense: the mass incarceration of the elderly. 2012. https://www.aclu.org/files/assets/elderlyprisonreport_20120613_1.pdf. Accessed 27 Nov 2015.
9. Harrison PM, Beck AJ. Prisoners in 2003. Bur Justice Stat Bull. 2004. http://www.bjs.gov/content/pub/pdf/p03.pdf. Accessed 28 Nov 2015.
10. James DJ. Profile of jail inmates, 2002. Bur Justice Stat Spec Rep. Revised 10/12/2004. http://www.bjs.gov/content/pub/pdf/pji02.pdf. Accessed 28 Nov 2015.
11. Fazel S, Grann M. Older criminals: a descriptive study of psychiatrically examined offenders in Sweden. Int J Geriatr Psychiatry. 2002;17(J10):907–13.
12. Uzoaba JHE. Managing older offenders: where do we stand? Ottawa. 1998. http://www.csc-scc.gc.ca/research/092/r70_e.pdf. Accessed 28 Nov 2015.
13. Sabol WJ, Minton TD, Harrison PM. Prison and jail inmates at midyear 2006. Bur Justice Stat Bull. Revised 03/12/2008. http://www.bjs.gov/content/pub/pdf/pjim06.pdf. Accessed 28 Nov 2015.
14. Corrections and Conditional Release Act (S.C. 1992, c. 20). 1992. fhttp://laws-lois.justice.gc.ca/eng/acts/C-44.6/. Accessed 27 Nov 2015.
15. Estelle v. Gamble, 429 US. (97) (1976).
16. Ruiz v. Estelle, 503 F. Supp 1295 (1980).
17. Anno BJ, Graham C, Lawrence JE, Shansky R, Bisbee J, Blackmore J. Correctional health care: addressing the needs of elderly, chronically ill, and terminally ill inmates. Washington DC: National Institute of Corrections; 2004.
18. Sterns AA, Lax G, Sed S, Keohane P, Sterns RS. Growing wave of older prisoners: a national survey of older prisoner's health, mental health, and programming. Correct Today. 2008;70(4): 70–6.
19. Kingston P, Le Mesurier N, Yorston G, Wardle S, Heath L. Psychiatric morbidity in older prisoners: unrecognized and undertreated. Int Psychogeriatr. 2011;23:1354–60.
20. Fazel S, Hope T, O'Donnell I, Jacoby R. Hidden psychiatric morbidity in elderly prisoners. Br J Psychiatry. 2001;179:535–9.
21. Marquart JW, Merianos DE, Doucet G. The health-related concerns of older prisoners: implications for policy. Ageing Soc. 2000;20:79–96.
22. Shimkus J. Corrections copes with care for the aged. Correct Care. 2004;18(1):16.
23. Rayel MG. Elderly sexual offenders admitted to a maximum-security forensic hospital. J Forensic Sci. 2000;45(6):1190–2.
24. Loeb SJ, Abudagga A. Health-related research on older inmates: an integrative review. Res Nurs Health. 2006;29(6):556–65.
25. Maruschuk LM. Medical problems of prisoners. Washington, DC: US Dept. of Justice, Bureau of Justice Statistics; 2008. http://www.bjs.gov/index.cfm?ty=pbdetail&iid=1097. Accessed 28 Nov 2015.
26. Diamond PM, Wang EW, Holzer CE, Thomas C, Cruser DA. The prevalence of mental illness in prison. Adm Policy Ment Health. 2001;29(1):21–40.
27. Regan JJ, Alderson A, Regan WM. Psychiatric disorders in aging prisoners. Clin Gerontol. 2003;26(1–2):117–24.
28. Yorston GA, Taylor PJ. Commentary: older offenders – no place to go? J Am Acad Psychiatry Law. 2006;34(3):333–7.
29. Kuhlmann R, Ruddell R. Elderly jail inmates: problems, prevalence and public health. Calif J Health Promot. 2005;3(2):49–60.
30. Fazel S, Grann M, Kling B, Hawton K. Prison suicide in 12 countries: an ecological study of 861 suicides during 2003–2007. Soc Psychiatry Psychiatr Epidemiol. 2011;46(3):191–5.
31. Dye MH, Aday RH. "I Just Wanted to Die": preprison and current suicide ideation among women serving life sentences. Crim Justice Behav. 2013;40(8):832–49.
32. Lewis CF, Fields C, Rainey E. A study of geriatric forensic evaluees: who are the violent elderly? J Am Acad Psychiatry Law. 2006;34:324–32.
33. Guo S, Biegel DE, Johnsen JA, Dyches H. Assessing the impact of community-based mobile crisis services on preventing hospitalization. Psychiatr Serv. 2001;52(2):223–8.
34. Price CA. Aging inmate population study. North Carolina Dept. of Correction Submitted by. 2006. https://www.ncdps.gov/div/adultcorrection/AgingStudyReport.pdf. Accessed 28 Nov 2015.

35. Tomar R, Treasaden IH, Shah AK. Is there a case for a specialist forensic psychiatry service for the elderly? Int J Geriatr Psychiatry. 2005;20(1):51–6.
36. Lamberti JS, Weisman R, Faden DI. Forensic assertive community treatment: preventing incarceration of adults with severe mental illness. Psychiatr Serv. 2004;55(11):1285–93.
37. Fisher CE. General psychiatric residents and corrections: moving forensic education beyond the classroom. Acad Psychiatry. 2014;38(6):680–4.
38. Ford JD, Trestman RL, Wiesbrock VH, Zhang W. Validation of a brief screening instrument for identifying psychiatric disorders among newly incarcerated adults. Psychiatr Serv. 2009;60(6):842–6.
39. Steadman HJ, Scott JE, Osher F, Agnese TK, Robbins PC. Validation of the brief jail mental health screen. Psychiatr Serv. 2005;56(7):816–22.
40. Nasreddine ZS, Phillips NA, Bédirian V, Charbonneau S, Whitehead V, Collin I, et al. The Montreal Cognitive Assessment, MoCA: a brief screening tool for mild cognitive impairment. J Am Geriatr Soc. 2005;53(4):695–9.
41. Folstein MF, Folstein SE, McHugh PR. "Mini-mental state". A practical method for grading the cognitive state of patients for the clinician. J Psychiatr Res. 1975;12(3):189–98.

23 Disaster Psychiatry

Caroline Giroux

23.1 Background

Like the firefighters, the police, and the military, healthcare professionals can also be first responders after a disaster. Such trauma occurs both on the collective and the individual level [1]. A disaster mental healthcare response requires the collaborative efforts of the public mental health system, general medical care system, and emergency response systems. Among other vulnerable groups, the older adults are at greater risk of developing psychiatric sequelae of traumatic experiences [2], but the risk may differ based on cultural background [1]. Although some degree of stress inoculation from life experiences can be protective in old age, having a physical injury increases the risk of acute stress disorder (ASD) and post-traumatic stress disorder (PTSD) [3]. Other risk factors for negative outcomes in the older adults include cognitive impairment, physical or mental disability, poor health, sensory impairment, and lack of social supports [1]. The clinicians involved in disaster response should gear their management toward ongoing safety while assessing losses or changes on the following levels: physical, cognitive, behavioral, social (support network), and spiritual (personal beliefs).

Case Vignette 1 Your usually quiet emergency department (ED) of a remote community in Minnesota was called one Saturday late evening by the police sheriff who requested that your team participate in a rescue operation. A tour bus for the seniors had been hijacked by an armed man, who escaped on foot after being subdued by a senior and locked outside. The driver was unfortunately killed, and there were some

C. Giroux, MD
Department of Psychiatry and Behavioral Sciences, APSS Stockton Clinic, Davis Health System, University of California, Sacramento, CA, USA
e-mail: cgiroux@ucdavis.edu

A. Hategan et al. (eds.), *On-Call Geriatric Psychiatry: Handbook of Principles and Practice*, DOI 10.1007/978-3-319-30346-8_23

people who were severely injured but it was not possible to specify how many. The bus was located in a forest but due to a major snow storm, the roads were not plowed and emergency responders would have to go on site via helicopter.

23.2 An Organized Response

Even though the population in general is aware of the variety of calamities that are possible, including children who get trained with fire drills and lockdowns in US elementary schools with a regular frequency, various situations will occur but for which most people may not be prepared.

A catastrophe will force mobilization of resources, and medical professionals should be ready to become "disaster leaders." Assigning tasks to resource persons based on their level of expertise (e.g., physician, social worker, psychologist), triaging, and communicating within all levels of the emergency responders are likely to take place while at the same time caring for the injured.

In cases of overwhelming disasters, planning involves doing a quick estimate of the number of casualties and the available resources. As needed, other groups should be solicited (such as the military, medical, or nursing students as volunteers).

Catastrophic Situation Application Based on the number of phone calls from anxious relatives the sheriff received, there were at least 20 people on the bus. You contacted your physician colleagues and urged them to come to the ER for coverage, while you diligently gathered your "disaster team." A resident physician in primary care who was trained in disaster response procedures by the Red Cross (as you were) agreed to join you and a couple of nurses. While grabbing your first aid kit and some medications (e.g., analgesics, anxiolytics), you asked the nurse manager to work with the social worker on call to gather flashlights and as many blankets as possible, as well as hot beverages and food. On the way there, you asked the police who will be in charge of caring for the driver's body. A preparatory communication should teach about the stresses of first responders who are engaged in body recovery [4].

Case Vignette 1 (Continued) When you arrived on site, a man with a shotgun wound on the upper arm approached you for help. You asked your team to distribute blankets and food to others while triaging each one of them. While your physician colleague carefully removed the bullet from the wounded person, the man next to him reported feeling very nervous and shaky. He was watching the police removing the driver's body. You directed him to go to the rear of the bus to avoid re-traumatization and conducted a health questionnaire (including the CAGE because of his tremor and tachycardia noted by a nurse), but before he could answer, he fell to the ground and started seizing. A few seniors next to him became panicked. You tried to reassure them while you asked a nurse to bring the medication supplies.

23.3 On-Site Management

While enhancing the level of safety:

(a) Do advanced trauma life support (ATLS), including IV lorazepam for seizure, or primary survey [3] and prevention of hypothermia.
(b) Triage: this may come first in large-scale disasters [2]; determine who would not survive the helicopter trip and needs interventions now.
(c) Provide for basic needs (e.g., temperature regulation, hydration, nutrition, rest, pain control [2]).
(d) Administer psychological first aid (PFA) to reduce immediate distress and improve adaptive functioning [2, 5]. Nonintrusive, this practical, individualized assistance will focus on immediate needs such as safety (through evacuation or protection from re-traumatization) and comfort and establishing connections with support networks and resources [5, 6]; the program of post-traumatic stress management (PPTSM) is essentially a community-based prolongation of PFA, using cognitive-behavioral principles taking place within 24 h, such as identification of resources, nonverbal and verbal processing of the trauma narrative, psychoeducation regarding the neurophysiology of traumatic stress, planning, problem solving, and self-care [6]. Critical incident stress debriefing (CISD) is *not* recommended. Not only CISD's theorized prevention of long-term negative psychiatric outcomes has not be supported by studies, there are some robust data that report a higher incidence of negative psychiatric outcomes in those who received CISD compared to the group who did not receive intervention [6]. Some studies suggest that the process might be harmful [2].
(e) Assess and screen to prevent the development of ASD and later PTSD [2]: pay special attention to others who are in the vicinity to prevent secondary trauma upon hearing others' terrifying experiences. There is evidence that brief, early cognitive-behavioral therapy (CBT) interventions can help curb the development of PTSD in injured trauma survivors [7].
(f) Provide education regarding:
    (i) Post-trauma responses: hypervigilance and difficulty sleeping are prominent early on and show rapid recovery for most [8].
    (ii) Reactions as *expectable and understandable* (as opposed to signs of personal failure or weakness).
    (iii) Circumstances under which they should consider seeking further clinical intervention (e.g., persistent/worsening symptoms of depression, altered perceptions, decreased memory and concentration, substance misuse).
    (iv) How and where to access additional help.
    (v) Increase use of social supports and other healthy coping skills; locating loved ones is the first and paramount concern after a disaster [8].
    (vi) Forms of coping to avoid, e.g., problematic alcohol or other drug use and excessive isolation.
    (vii) Ways to help family members cope.

(viii) Accurate and timely information: this can correct cognitive distortions (such as overgeneralization of threat levels); for instance, there should be an ongoing communication with law enforcement to obtain updates on the status of the gunman who fled.

(g) Provide trauma-informed care (see Chap. 14) during all the steps:
   (i) Provide physical assistance (e.g., lifting, transferring) with care sensitivity.
   (ii) Conduct the clinical interview to allow for the progressive elaboration of symptoms in a manner sensitive to the emotional needs of the patient at the time of assessment.
   (iii) Discuss the treatment plan; care management procedures that elicit and address patients' most pressing post-trauma concerns have the potential to initially engage traumatized patients in a shared decision-making process [7].

23.4 The Team Approach: Individual Roles

Emergency care clinicians will discriminate between physical and anxiety symptoms. Mental health clinicians must respond to a range of emotional and behavioral demands (e.g., anger, fear), manage acute anxiety, and use evidence-based interventions (e.g., brief CBT) to decrease the risk of subjects developing ASD/PTSD, understand the special stresses of *quarantine* in epidemics or bioterrorism, and do empathetic disclosure of upsetting news in the case of serious injury or death.

23.5 Pharmacotherapy

Preliminary studies of beta-blockers administered acutely after trauma exposure have demonstrated reductions in physiological correlates of ASD/PTSD and trends in the reduction of ASD/PTSD symptoms but have not yet demonstrated efficacy in preventing the development of symptoms numerous and severe enough to meet criteria for ASD/PTSD [2]. Due to the lack of evidence with pharmacological agents in the acute phase post-trauma, experts recommend use of pharmacology for symptomatic relief only (e.g., prolonged insomnia, suicidality, psychosis, intense anxiety, mania). Medications to avoid in acute phase post-trauma with geriatric patients are [9]:

- Tricyclic antidepressants (e.g., amitriptyline) due to anticholinergic activity
- Atypical and typical antipsychotics (except for maintenance treatment for schizophrenia-spectrum disorders and bipolar disorders) due to anticholinergic, neurologic, cardiovascular, and other adverse effects
- Benzodiazepines due to risk of falls and cognitive impairment

Safer options (see Chap. 3) are:

- Sertraline, citalopram, escitalopram, and mirtazapine for anxiety and/or depression (if history of chronicity)
- Trazodone and mirtazapine (if insomnia)

Case Vignette 2 In a suburb of Quebec City, during early spring, you were the physician on call at a nursing home. The director called you in the middle of the night because of a fire incident. Most residents were evacuated to a nearby school gymnasium, and those who had major respiratory issues were sent to the ED. The director explained that some residents might need support and that four residents were still missing. All of the residents' relatives have been contacted.

Catastrophic Situation Application Since most basic needs were quickly cared for (food from a local pizzeria, clothing and cots by a second-hand store will be delivered to the school), you arrived on site as a physician and also as a leader for the nursing home night shift staff. You triaged the 37 residents and asked for their vitals to be obtained and with the help of the staff, you identified medical conditions (e.g., diabetes mellitus, hypertension) and other special requirements (e.g., anti-coagulotherapy, IV antibiotics). While you did the assessments, taking detailed notes on flashcards with each resident's name and date of birth, it helped narrow down the most pressing issues that could not wait until the morning. You contacted a 24-h pharmacy and a nearby hospital to get medications as needed. Since after the disaster, survivors lose their sense of "place" [10], PFA should be done as needed to help establish a connection between the person and the socio-physical environment. At another level, the leader should communicate with local government administrators (e.g., mayor, public health minister) to know to which ED direct the patients necessitating acute care and to know how to provide shelter after the fire.

Case Vignette 2 (Continued) While you listed the medications you needed to the pharmacist on duty, a journalist with camera people approached you and asked about the specific injuries the residents had suffered so far. They also heard a rumor that this tragedy might have been from an act of arson.

23.6 The News Media

In every extreme situation, the presence of the news media is highly likely and can be experienced as intrusive and insensitive. Regardless of the circumstances, a professional attitude (e.g., declining interview because of your medical duties) and confidentiality should be maintained. Ideally, identify a clinician who had media training or appoint a public affairs person.

Catastrophic Situation Application The personal health information should be kept on you until new records are assembled or left in a secure area (e.g., locked office at school). Nobody from the team should be allowed to share personal information about the residents without their consent. To avoid misinformation, the director or someone else should be designated as the spokesperson and share the most accurate (even if limited) information with the residents prior to involving the news media.

Risk communication is a useful part of the collaboration with news media. It describes effective communication before, during, or after a crisis. When the information conveyed and advice shared are accurate, they may mitigate adverse effects and enable those who have been exposed to take protective actions [4]. For instance, clinicians should provide information about the human factors associated with the event, their time course, about potential grief reactions, and ways to obtain help. Also, it is important to emphasize the fact that most survivors are resilient. Clinicians should decline media interviews when it is not clear what will happen with the information or when the information may not be helpful to the public or may even cause harm [4].

23.7 Disaster Psychotherapy Principles and Optimal Communication

In addition to the listening and presence of skills emphasized in Chap. 4, there are guidelines [4] to communicate with disaster survivors. Among them, Stoddard [4] emphasized the following: since people are risk averse, when upset they tend to focus on the negatives; therefore, (a) words such as *no*, *never*, and *nothing* should be avoided; (b) be caring and empathetic (e.g., people want to know that the doctor cares before they care what the doctor knows); (c) be honest and open while avoiding mixed or inconsistent verbal/nonverbal messages.

Table 23.1 summarizes the recommendations for *clinician self-care* during post-disaster interventions [11]. Figure 23.1 illustrates the on-site safety-enhancement interventions in immediate post-disaster management.

Table 23.1 Clinician self-care at the disaster site

Physical well-being	Psychosocial strategies
Pace yourself Take frequent rest breaks away from the area Watch out for each other Maintain as normal a schedule as possible (e.g., a normal sleep-wake cycle) Drink plenty of fluids (water and juices) and eat a variety of foods	Accept what you cannot change Use mindfulness techniques (e.g., deep breathing) as needed Allow yourself to feel badly Stay in contact with loved ones at home as much as possible

Adapted from Ref. [11]

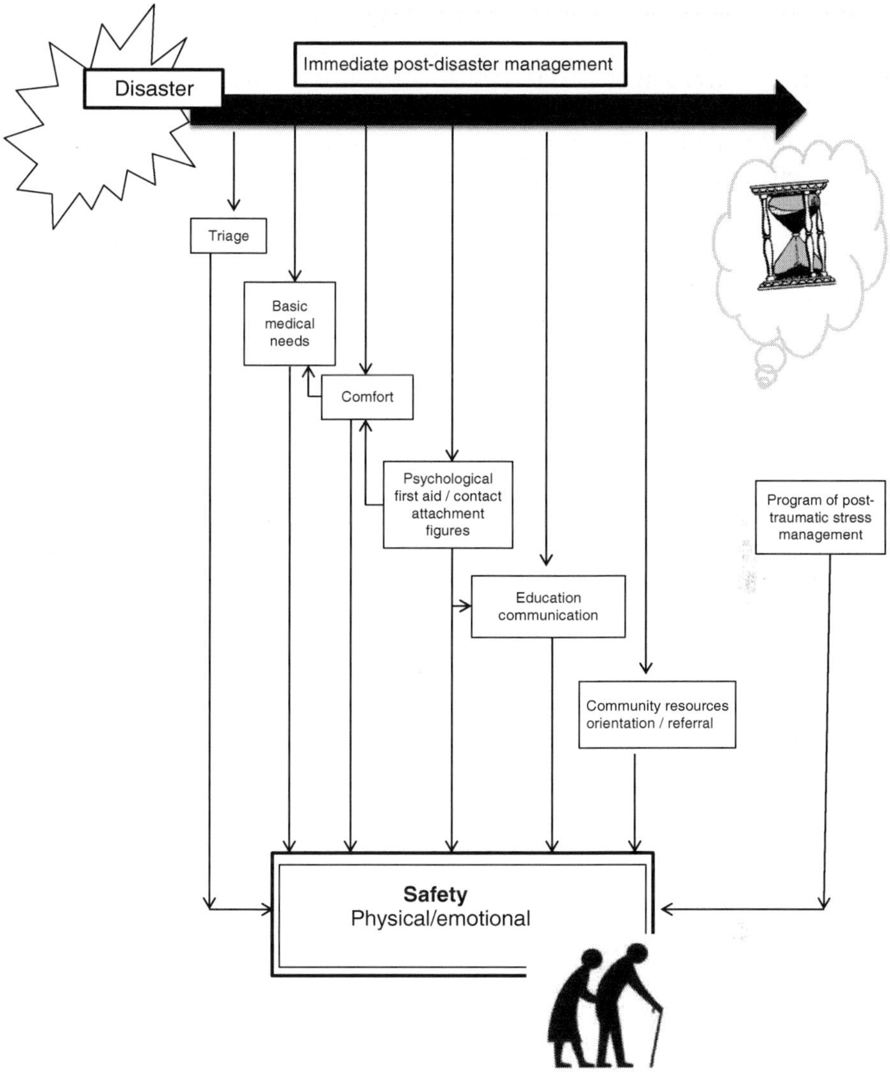

Fig. 23.1 On-site safety-enhancement interventions in immediate post-disaster management

Key Points

- Although most clinicians are not formally prepared for leadership under extreme circumstances, they might be designated as mass crisis leaders to multitask during disaster response.
- Management of catastrophic situations in groups of persons, including older adults, relies mostly on basic principles such as safety and comfort and providing them mental health resources for clinical intervention in case they have stress-related manifestations within days or weeks after the trauma.
- Management skills and systemic considerations such as mobilizing resources (e.g., army, public safety personnel, local clinicians, medical students) are as important as the clinical duties.
- Triaging, identifying crises or decompensation, administering psychological first aid, delegating, and directing to proper services within the local or neighboring communities are examples of tasks specific to disaster response.
- CISD is not recommended; instead, education combined with support or PPTSM is more appropriate.
- All clinicians deployed on a disaster scene should pay attention to their own needs and do appropriate self-care.

References

1. Dowling FG, Jones K. Special populations. In: Stoddard FJ, Pandya A, Katz CL, editors. Disaster psychiatry – readiness, evaluation, and treatment. Washington, DC: American Psychiatric Publishing Inc; 2011. p. 89–110.
2. Benedek DM. ASD and PTSD in the disaster environment. In: Ursano RJ, Fullerton CS, Wiesaeth L, Raphael B, editors. Textbook of disaster psychiatry. London: Cambridge University Press; 2007. p. 140–63.
3. Rundell JR. Management of medical and surgical disaster casualties. In: Ursano RJ, Fullerton CS, Wiesaeth L, Raphael B, editors. Textbook of disaster psychiatry. London: Cambridge University Press; 2007. p. 164–89.
4. Stoddard FJ. Communicating risk before, during, and after a disaster. In: Stoddard FJ, Pandya A, Katz CL, editors. Disaster psychiatry – readiness, evaluation, and treatment. Washington, DC: American Psychiatric Publishing Inc; 2011. p. 19–33.
5. Jones J, Ardern H, Briere J, Scott C. Treating the effects of acute trauma. In: Briere JN, Scott C, editors. Principles of trauma therapy: a guide to symptoms, evaluation, and treatment. 2nd ed. Thousand Oaks, CA: Sage; 2014.
6. Watson P. Early intervention for trauma-related problems following mass trauma. In: Ursano RJ, Fullerton CS, Wiesaeth L, Raphael B, editors. Textbook of disaster psychiatry. London: Cambridge University Press; 2007. p. 121–39.
7. Zatzick D. Interventions for acutely injured trauma survivor. In: Ursano RJ, Fullerton CS, Wiesaeth L, Raphael B, editors. Textbook of disaster psychiatry. London: Cambridge University Press; 2007. p. 190–205.
8. Ursano RJ, Fullerton CS, Weisaeth L, Raphael B. Public health and disaster mental health planning. In: Ursano RJ, Fullerton CS, Wiesaeth L, Raphael B, editors. Textbook of disaster psychiatry. London: Cambridge University Press; 2007. p. 311–25.

9. American Geriatrics Society 2015 Beers Criteria Update Expert Panel. American Geriatrics Society 2015 Updated Beers Criteria for potentially inappropriate medication use in older adults. J Am Geriatr Soc. 2015;63(11):2227–46.
10. Pillay SS. Psychotherapies. In: Stoddard FJ, Pandya A, Katz CL, editors. Disaster psychiatry – readiness, evaluation, and treatment. Washington, DC: American Psychiatric Publishing Inc; 2011. p. 227–39.
11. Merlino JP. Rescuing ourselves. In: Stoddard FJ, Pandya A, Katz CL, editors. Disaster psychiatry – readiness, evaluation, and treatment. Washington, DC: American Psychiatric Publishing Inc; 2011. p. 35–48.

Part IV

Innovations, Teaching, and Future Directions in the On-Call Geriatric Psychiatry Practice

On-Call Telepsychiatry Services: Interventions, Outcomes, and Innovations

24

Donald M. Hilty and Terry Rabinowitz

24.1 Background

Patient-centered care emphasizes quality, accessible, and timely care in a variety of settings. The proportion of older adults is growing faster than any other age group due to longer life expectancy and declining fertility rates [1]. Over 75 % of people with depression, major neurocognitive disorders (NCDs) (formerly dementia), and other psychiatric conditions are cared for at home [2]. Similarly, there is a significant burden of care in rural communities [3].

One of the best options for leveraging psychiatric expertise is telepsychiatry (TP) [4]. Participants, both patients and providers, as well as loved ones, are highly satisfied with assessment, consultation, and a range of treatments in many populations (e.g., adult, child, older adult), settings, and cultures [4, 5]. TP outcomes are comparable to in-person care, and it has been used with a variety of models of care (i.e., collaborative care) [4, 6]. TP competencies for trainees and clinicians are now available (Table 24.1) [7]. Data on care for older adults are emerging, including many for patients in nursing homes and other medical settings [8]. Acceptance of TP is generally quite high, and it was better for older adults than younger adults in one study treating depression in rural populations [9].

D.M. Hilty, MD (✉)
Department of Psychiatry & Addiction Medicine, Kaweah Delta Medical Center and Keck School of Medicine at USC, 400 West Mineral King Avenue, Visalia, CA 93291, USA
e-mail: donh3032612@gmail.com

T. Rabinowitz, MD, DDS
Division of Consultation Psychiatry and Psychosomatic Medicine, Psychiatry and Family Medicine, Telemedicine, University of Vermont College of Medicine, University of Vermont Medical Center, Burlington, VT, USA
e-mail: terry.rabinowitz@uvmhealth.org

A. Hategan et al. (eds.), *On-Call Geriatric Psychiatry: Handbook of Principles and Practice*, DOI 10.1007/978-3-319-30346-8_24

Table 24.1 Abbreviated telepsychiatric (TP) competencies for patient care (adapted from reference [7])

Area/topic	Novice/advanced beginner (e.g., advanced medical student/early resident)	Competent/proficient (e.g., advanced resident/graduating resident/faculty/attending/interdisciplinary team member)	Expert (e.g., advanced faculty/attending/interdisciplinary team member)
Patient care			
History taking	Standard history	Informed consent for telehealth Contextualized history (e.g., aware of geographic and cultural specificity)	Address informed consent problems In-depth, well-paced, and concise interview
Engagement and interpersonal skills	Therapeutic alliance with trust and rapport	Identify and manage problem(s) Adjust interview to technology	Resolve problems and adjust assessment contextually
Assessment and physical examination	Stratify risk and protective factors based on epidemiology Learn tools (e.g., MMSE)	Assess danger risk and adjust follow-up plan vs. in-person Ensure full MSE or alternative Administer tools with adjustments	Synthesize information Adjust tools contextually (e.g., substitute score item) Teach on distance MSE vs. in-person
Management and treatment planning	Treatment plan based on who will do Follow-up with others (e.g., PCP)	Contextualize to patient and PCP Awareness of care continuum Medication recommendations (i.e., side effects) with PCP instructions to initiate, titrate, and augment Follow-up with PCP by TP or phone	Tailors recommendations to resources, culture and patient preference Engages patient and referring doctor Select "best" mode: e-mail, telephone, or other (and if it changes the process) Refines medication recommendations
Documentation	Draft TP note hard copy or rudimentary EHR draft	Initial/revised draft with consultation model; complex EHR (e.g., Epic)	Balance findings/detail with plan; uses variety of documentation options
Privacy and confidentiality	Learn in-person basic regulations	Be aware of regulations; TP, cell phone, and other technology (e.g., HIPAA)	Practice within all standards; be aware of technology option limitations; make recommendations to optimize these parameters
Communication			
Communication	Clear communication with patient and professionals	Amplify communication based on TP	Trouble-shoot communication difficulties; optimal telepresence; ability to teach/enhance others' telepresence

Cultural, diversity, and social determinants	Consider diversity of oneself and patients	Adjust to patient culture and preference Check language fluency to confirm	Follow cultural formulation frameworks Adjust interview, assessment and care
Language/interpreter ability	Use the interpreter	Manage time and pick best option (e.g., professionals > staff and family)	Verbal and nonverbal dimensions
Systems-base practice			
Outreach to community	Participate and engage	Identify relevant resources and needs within community	Visit, establish and maintain relationships Integrate in-person and TP care events
Interprofessional education issues	Participates in and experiences different roles	Work with IPE team and begin to teach within IPE framework	IPE provider and teacher Support interdisciplinary team care Expert level knowledge of the extant telemedicine database
Care models	Grasp care provider vs. consultant role	Employ traditional referral (i.e., management) and consultation TP Begin to learn collaborative care	Has facility with models of consultation, integrated, stepped and hybrid care; practices with one that fits context
Rural health	Learn about rural access, epidemiology, $, and other	Learn rural health basics	Practice and role model
Special populations	Learn differences (e.g., veterans, child/adolescent/parent/family, geriatric)	Recognize differences and adapt assessment and management approaches accordingly	Practice and role model
Licensure regulations for TP and model used	Learn in-person regulations and that states differ	Be aware that in-person and TP regulations may/may not differ	Practice within TP regulations state-to-state or within system (e.g., VA)
Professionalism			
Attitude	Learn/be open to technology	Openness to technology, IPE, and consultation process	Lead in groups/teams
Integrity and ethical behavior	Demonstrate behavior with respect for others	Role model	Role model and give feedback

(continued)

Table 24.1 (continued)

Area/topic	Novice/advanced beginner (e.g., advanced medical student/early resident)	Competent/proficient (e.g., advanced resident/graduating resident/faculty/attending/interdisciplinary team member)	Expert (e.g., advanced faculty/attending/interdisciplinary team member)
Scope	Become aware of scope issues	Practice within scope(s)	Provide feedback on scope and boundary issues; trouble-shoots problems
Practice-based learning			
Administration	Learn basics of in-person care	Be aware of important differences between in-person and telemedicine care	Practice with adjustments to telemedicine care
Safety and QI	Systematic assessment; learn how to participate in QI	Identify risks; apply QI information to cases and system	Adjust treatment plan; analyze QI options, selects and evaluates
Teaching and learning	Participates and contributes	Organize and further educate	Provide context and steps for learning
Knowledge			
	Relevance, history	Relevance, history, and evidence base	History, evidence-based and clinical guidelines
Technology			
Adapt to technology	Project self 15 % more by TP; realize nonverbal issues	Plan for differences, identify barriers, and put patient at ease	Additional ways to engage and express empathy
Remote site design	Observe	Identify problems and solutions Add toys or furniture for child TP	Pre-planning: iterative improvement Modification based on care options
Technology operation	Microphone, camera, and other	Operate hardware, software, and accessories; basic troubleshooting	Optimize components based on context and manage all trouble-shooting

Footnotes: *HER* electronic health record, *HIPAA* health information privacy and accountability act, *IPE* interprofessional education, *MMSE* mini-mental status examination, *MSE* mental status examination, *PCP* primary care provider, *QI* quality improvement, *VA* veterans affairs

TP is most often compared to in-person care, but it is one end of a spectrum of e-Mental Health (MH) care that has emerged – the other end of the spectrum involves patients, families, and caregivers accessing health information on the Internet. This spectrum has a range of options from health education to peer/group chats, tips for self-assessment, health promotion strategies, social media, psychiatry/psychology apps, and informal online clinician consultation [10]. E-MH options may provide resources, connections, and meaningful activities for people facing particular obstacles to care such as geographic distance from services, special needs (e.g., autism-spectrum, sensory), and immobility (e.g., housebound due to physical disabilities or MH problems such as panic disorder or phobias) [10].

This chapter will help the clinician care for older adult patients through technology by describing:

1. How TP leverages a wide range of treatments at a distance to clinics, nursing homes, and patient homes, with outcomes as good as in-person care
2. How geriatric TP is similar to and different from that for other population ages
3. Telemedicine innovations, in general, that may be inroads for TP services for patients, clinicians, and caregivers

24.2 An Update on Telepsychiatry's Evidence Base and Its Application to Patient-Centered Care

TP improves access to care, enables a wide range of treatments at a distance, and provides outcomes as good as in-person care [4]. Comparison and non-inferiority studies show TP is as good as in-person care in terms of diagnosis and treatment [4]. Guidelines and systematic reviews for psychotherapy by TP exist [11, 12]. Telepsychiatry has been studied in culturally diverse populations including Hispanics/Latinos, Asians, Native American, Eastern Europeans, and other populations (e.g., those using sign language) [4, 5]. Special settings and populations including involuntary inpatient, and incarcerated persons – and those in emergency rooms – are not yet well studied. Child and adolescent TP is advancing, too, by providing a telepsychiatrist to co-lead MH care with remote primary care physicians (PCPs) (i.e., collaborative care) for patients with attention-deficit hyperactivity disorder (ADHD) [13] and guidelines that summarize key clinical, administrative, and technical issues for this population [14].

Data on older adult patients are emerging, but more studies are needed related to access to service, challenges related to day-to-day functioning, and attitudes of PCPs [8]. There are many descriptive, non-randomized nursing home TP studies with positive outcomes, usually for depression or major NCDs, and these show that consultant time is efficiently used (see Table 24.2) [15]. Other assessment, cognitive intervention, and outcome studies – many done in medical settings – have direct in-person comparison groups with outcomes being similar (see Table 24.2) [8]. In order for a TP program to be embraced, outreach to local PCPs, nurses, and other community healthcare workers is needed; a long-standing relationship between

Table 24.2 Summary of telepsychiatric clinical/outcome studies for older adult patients (References for those mentioned in chapter manuscript only)

Study	N	Location	Technology	Description	Comments
Nursing home					
Jones (1999) [16]	2	USA	ISDN 128 KBS	Case reports	Able to provide care sooner and staff felt supported
Lee et al. (2000) [17]	140	South Korea	T1	Prospective over 2 years: CDR, SBT, BDS	TP = in-person; nurses satisfied; caregiver distress reduced; improved patient behavior
Tang et al. (2001) [18]	45	Hong Kong	ISDN 512 KBS	Prospective over 1 year	Satisfaction high with learning curve; some savings in costs
Johnston et al. (2001) [19]	40	USA	ISDN 128 KBS	Descriptive study: MMSE	Satisfaction high; efficient use of psychiatrist's time
Lyketsos et al. (2001) [20]	–	USA	Standard telephone	Descriptive study	Reduced hospitalization rate compared to past
Rabinowitz et al. (2004) [21]	24	USA	ISDN 384 KBS	Pilot study: DCM	Satisfaction high; communication between providers and staff good
Yeung et al. (2009) [22]	9	USA	ISDN 384 KBS	Descriptive study: CGI-I	Satisfaction high; significant improvement in 6/9
Rabinowitz et al. [15]	106	USA	ISDN384 KBS	Descriptive study	Cost and time savings exceeded the start-up costs
Other					
Montani et al. (1997) [23]	15, medical inpatient	USA	Coaxial cable	TP vs. in-person: MMSE, clock drawing	Nearly equal, with 0.95 correlation; all preferred in-person, though
Menon et al. (2001) [24]	24, medical inpatient	USA	Standard telephone	In-person (twice) vs. in-person/video: HDRS, GDS-15	TP as reliable as in-person
Grob et al. (2001) [25]	27, veterans home	USA	ISDN 384 KBS	In-person (twice) vs. in-person/video: BPRS, MMSE, GDS	TP as reliable as in-person

Saligari et al. (2002) [26]	20, primary care	USA	ISDN 384 KBS	TP vs. in-person: MMSE, GDS	Equal, with MMSE 0.9 and GDS 0.78 correlation
Shore et al. (2004) [27]	16, veterans home	USA	T1	TP vs. in-person: DSM-IV, clock drawing	TP equal to in-person
Loh et al. (2005) [28]	20, community population	USA	ISDN 384 KBS	TP vs. in-person: MMSE, GDS	Nearly equal with 0.8 correlation for dementia
Collum et al. (2006) [29]	33, primary care	USA	–	TP vs. in-person: MMSE, clock drawing, digit span	High correlations (>0.60) for all, though only 0.48 for clock drawing
Turvey et al. (2007) [30]	118, home	USA	Home monitoring system	Screening for depression with PHQ-2	96.6 % completed the screen; helped with triage and treatment
Sheeran et al. [37]	19, home	USA	ISDN 384 KBS	Descriptive: DCM, English & Spanish	For severe depression, all patients improved to mild depression

Footnotes: *BDS* blessed dementia scale, *BPRS* brief psychiatric rating scale, *CDR* clinical dementia rating, *CGI-I* clinical global impressions-improvement scale, *DCM* depression care management module, *GDS-15* geriatric depression scale-15, *HDRS* Hamilton depression rating scale, *KBS* kilobits per second, *MMSE* mini-mental state examination, *PHQ-2* patient health questionnaire-2, *SBT* short blessed test

PCPs and a local geriatric MH outreach team is helpful [31]. A Canadian national survey of TP programs found that the number of geriatric consultations was low relative to adult and child/adolescent consultations [32].

24.3 Telepsychiatric Assessment Compared to In-Person Care

A good geriatric mental health history not only includes the patient's point of view but also collateral information from all other stakeholders and medical professionals – largely dependent on where the patient generally resides and is cared for (e.g., home, family and caregiver, nursing home, staff, and others). Cognition, pain severity, physical/other limitations, and environmental factors that may affect assessment are important to understand. Screening of older adult patients via self-report questionnaires or clinician-rated instruments is virtually the same as for in-person assessments (e.g., Patient Health Questionnaire – 9 items, Geriatric Depression Scale – 30 items).

There are some important additional items to keep in mind when using TP, including:

- Informed consent: verbal or written, depending on the jurisdiction.
- Pre-visit event summary: an accounting of general events and the patient's attitude, comments, complaints, sources of information, and clinician observations (e.g., olfactory/vision/hearing limitations, gait/balance problems) need to be communicated before the patient enters the room.
- The clinical examination, in general: this may require staff assistance (often a nurse facilitator) to complete, particularly if a patient is delirious, combative, or agitated, has a low level of formal education, or suffers from aphasia, poor hearing, or vision impairment.
- Cognitive examination: may require item substitution if clock drawing or sentence writing cannot be uploaded to see or held visually in the camera; again, staff are better in assisting here so as to not answer questions for the patient.
- Physical examination: camera control at the far end enables easy wide angle, close-up, and focused viewing to detect tremors, micrographia, and other abnormalities, but staff may need to be trained to check for extrapyramidal side effects (EPS) like cogwheel rigidity.
- We encourage family member to attend in general and when there is significant cognitive impairment, as this enhances patient acceptance. Families are very welcoming of TP interventions and are grateful for the extra time and effort put forth to facilitate a TP encounter [15].
- We recommend that most or all TP encounters for nursing home residents or older adults in similar environments include the primary nurse for their care and, when possible, a member of the social work staff to give input on family of origin, family dynamics, and past family and social history [15].

24.4 Culture, Diversity, and Language Issues

There are advantages in using TP related to management of culture, diversity, and language issues [33]. First, by doing something different than in-person care, there is increased pre-visit scrutiny of care delivery due to the Hawthorne effect. Second, in order to make TP as good as an in-person encounter, some mindful matching of patients and clinicians is beneficial, or if in the case of an emergency, one should at least be aware of:

- Language issues mainly related to limited English proficiency, such that an interpreter may be needed. As with in-person care, congruent language fluency increases trust, confidence, and other dimensions of the alliance with the clinician [34], particularly in refugee or asylum-seeking populations.
  - The presence of a third person (i.e., an interpreter) in a confidential relationship affects patient satisfaction and influences both transference and countertransference [33].
  - Formally trained interpreters are less prone to distortion/omission than family members and less prone to conceptual misunderstandings that might affect nurses or others involved in patient care [35]. Such interpreters, however, may not be available in all locations.
- Culture, ethnicity, and other matching of diverse qualities are easier with TP, in that one may access or leverage clinicians and other team members at a distance [36].
- Lesbian, gay, bisexual, and transsexual (LGBT) older adults may have suffered from marginalization and stigmatization and have fear of disclosing their sexuality to their PCP for fear of judgment and discrimination. Some patients have also suffered significant losses in their social networks due to AIDS; on the other hand, LGBT older adults in urban areas are networked better for healthcare, political, social, and other causes. Of note, in one study of adult gay men and lesbians, although 70 % disclosed their sexual orientation to their PCP, only 29 % were asked their sexual orientation by their care clinician [33].

24.5 Telepsychiatry Questions Related to Older Adults: Where Is the Patient, What Is the Model, Who Are the Clinicians, and Who Provides the Actual Care?

Ideally, mental health (MH) service delivery in primary care has a continuum of clinicians: the care coordinator-medical assistant-social worker-nurse-PCP-MH clinician-telepsychiatrist [6]. Patients learn to use care managers (to monitor follow-up plans, for interventions based on risk stratification, and for patient tracking). Optimally, in MH service delivery, the psychiatrist better attends to more complicated cases, provides clinical oversight, and reviews cases in team formats. Overall, this ensures that a range of effective, non-pharmacologic, health psychology-based treatments is employed.

The key elements are:

- The patient and others
  - The patient's setting is key, including inpatient vs. nursing facility vs. emergency room vs. outpatient vs. home; as is relevant, MH vs. general medical setting location informs the plan.
  - It is important to be aware of legal standing (e.g., surrogate decision-makers, power of attorneys, conservatorships).
  - Who else is helping from the patient's end? Spouse/partner, child/children, other family/siblings, nurse, social worker, therapist, or others may be involved.
- The model of care
  - Low-intensity options: these are telephone doctor-to-doctor "curbside" consultations, typically; rarely these are performed by e-mail or text messaging.
  - Psychiatric care (free-standing, as if a patient came to a clinic). This will involve follow-up plans, prescriptions, and contingencies for emergencies for which one is directly responsible.
  - Consultation care model: consultation to a PCP or other clinician, who provides the care. This will involve follow-up plans, prescription instructions (with specifics, back-up options), and contingencies for emergencies for which the PCP/clinic is directly responsible. It is very helpful to be familiar with local MH standards, services, and expectations.
  - Collaborative care model: joint provision of care by specialist and PCP. This involves a mixture of the two models above, often with care coordinators and other interdisciplinary clinicians helping.
- Legal/consultation-liaison issues for evaluation: legal hold, capacity evaluation, or other surrogate decision-making questions

Case Vignette Using Low-Intensity Interventions on the Way to High-Intensity Ones. Models of TP care may be combined with models of care to forge intensity of care interventions, based on technology complexity, specialist time, and service delivery model care [6]. The outline below organizes in-person and TP interventions into low-, moderate-, or high-intensity options.

History of Present Illness. A PCP called from the medical emergency room about onset of psychosis in a 71-year-old Caucasian male, who had a history of major depression and dyslipidemia. There was an 8–12-week wait/delay to see a psychiatrist in-person who worked 60 miles away, as there were no local psychiatrists in the city of 25,000 residences; a videoconference could be set up during weekday daytime hours, but only limited access was available. Medication included venlafaxine extended release 75 mg in the morning and temazepam 15 mg at bedtime.

Reason for Consultation. The patient's auditory and visual hallucinations concerned the PCP, and he was considering a psychiatric admission. As an alternative, the patient could be taken by ambulance to a facility nearby that had a synchronous TP unit if the psychiatrist wanted to evaluate him.

Day 1: Telephone consultation. The contact comprised a 10-min PCP and telepsychiatrist discussion. The PCP was unaware of any recent acute medical problems. When asked by the telepsychiatrist, the PCP was initially unsure of the potential for bipolar disorder, not having thought or inquired about it; he did not recall the patient having had a history of severe insomnia and mood swings. The PCP reported that the patient's wife had not complained about memory problems, but cognition had not been checked. The initial plan was to (1) continue the venlafaxine; (2) replace the temazepam with olanzapine (rapidly orally dissolving) 5 mg qhs; (3) hold off on the psychiatric admission (it was unclear if beds were available anyway); (4) order a comprehensive metabolic panel, complete blood count, thyroid stimulating hormone, and a rapid plasma reagin to screen for neurosyphilis; and (5) have a follow-up appointment in the PCP's office the next day.

Day 2: PCP reevaluation in the office. When asked, the patient and wife denied racing thoughts, trouble sitting still, and spending sprees associated with mood elevations between 3 and 14 days in duration. The depression, though, had worsened with more ruminations and hopelessness, but no suicidal ideation. Memory was a little problematic, but there were no waxing and waning mental status changes. Initial laboratory results revealed no clinically significant abnormalities. A 5-min reconsultation by phone to the telepsychiatrist led to the following recommendations: (1) progressively raising the venlafaxine extended release to 150 mg in the morning, (2) continuing the olanzapine, and (3) follow-up TP visit in 4 weeks which could be a brief evaluation in light of "knowing" the patient already.

Day 30: TP consultation. The patient was scheduled for a 30–60-min evaluation. By that time, he was reportedly about "two-thirds" better in terms of his mood, but he was still not back to normal and his enjoyment, drive, and energy remained low; the latter had not been different with the olanzapine. Consultation suggestions included (1) gradually raising the venlafaxine to 225 mg in the morning or adding bupropion sustained release 150 mg in the morning for inducing more energy and better mood and (2) continuing the olanzapine. Time spent is 30-min telepsychiatrist evaluation of patient by video and 5-min discussion with PCP by video.

Case Analysis The telephone consultation may have prevented an unnecessary medical or psychiatric hospitalization; more important, it aided the PCP and increased his self-efficacy in decision-making. It also almost made the full TP evaluation unnecessary, but there was an important shift in the medications carried out. Some PCPs shy away from antipsychotic medications, due to worry about metabolic disturbances or for other reasons. This process, though, helped the PCP feel more comfortable with the plan.

24.6 Telemedicine and Telepsychiatry Options for Older Patients, Clinicians, and Caregivers

24.6.1 TP to Older Adult Populations [33]

- Nursing home TP non-randomized studies have been effective for depression or major NCDs, making evaluation easier and more efficiently using consultant time [15].
- Assessment, cognitive intervention, and outcomes have been similar to in-person. A new development is telemonitoring of depression in the home, which facilitates connectedness [37].

- Neurocognitive assessment via TP using a Spanish-language battery was comparable to in-person (IP) testing for rural Latino patients in a sample of Spanish-speaking older adults in a rural setting [38].
- Adding a geriatric nurse practitioner via videoconferencing to an outpatient diagnostic multidisciplinary facility for patients with NCDs reduces subjective burden of the informal caregiver [39].
- Telehealth problem-solving therapy (tele-PST) for low-income homebound older adults in a 6-month, randomized controlled trial showed that both tele-PST and in-person PST were associated with reduced depression severity and disability, but tele-PST benefits lasted significantly longer than those gained through in-person PST [40].
- In older adults with chronic illness and depression, compared to regular in-home nursing with education, a telehealth nurse intervention (daily telemonitoring of symptoms, body weight, and medication use; eight weekly sessions of problem-solving treatment; and communication with patients' PCPs prescribing antidepressants) significantly reduced depression scores (50 % less at 3- and 6-month follow-up) and improved self-efficacy with care management [41].

24.6.2 Telehealth and Caregivers

In the USA, 79 % of caregivers have access to the Internet and, of those, 88 % search online for health information. Education (89 % of those with a college degree vs. 38 % who have less than a high school education) and income (95 % of adults with household income $75,000+ vs. 57 % with household income less than $30,000) affect use [42].

- Telehealth to "digital illiterate" patients (i.e., no interest in using, or capacity to use, computers and smartphones) found digital pens for daily reporting of their health state – in the form of a virtual health diary – easy to use, and caregivers felt that improved contact led to more "security" at home.
- Older adults may be challenged to use new technologies due to aging-related cognitive changes, lack of experience, and different attitudes toward their use. One-on-one training/instructions and use of a telemonitoring application help older adults and caregivers adapt to new healthcare technologies in the treatment of major NCDs.
- Geriatric (mean age 80 years) outpatients with heart failure, with an average ejection fraction of 46 %, randomly received control or a telemonitoring system (oxygen saturation, heart rate, and blood pressure readings) over 6 months, office hours telephonic support provided by a geriatrician. The program was feasible, and hospitalizations and risk of death were reduced for the intervention group [43].
- Technology-enhanced nurse monitoring for assessment, diagnosis, and triage of older adults living in community-based settings included biometric and nonbiometric sensors to a data management system. Challenges included (1) data interpretation, (2) clinical inferences from nonbiometric data, (3) integrating

data generated by three different telehealth applications into a clinically meaningful cognitive framework, and (4) determining how best to use nursing judgment to make valid inferences from online reporting systems. Nurses developed expertise over the course of the current study [44].

- A review of Internet-based interventions for medical and MH disorders showed that approximately two-thirds of open or randomized controlled trials reduce caregiver stress and improve quality of life [45] and outcomes [46]. Family caregivers located in rural areas found e-health support to be beneficial compared to conventional caregiver support. The interventions range from interactive communities to bulletin board therapy groups. The population of patients cared for varied from mental health (major NCDs, schizophrenia, anorexia) to medical (older adults/aging, heart transplant, traumatic brain injury, hip fracture, cancer, stroke). Services included webcasts, discussion boards, online classes, learning modules, and chat rooms.

Key Points

- Telepsychiatry is as effective as in-person care in terms of outcomes. It enables a wide range of treatments at a distance to clinics, nursing homes, and patient homes.
- TP with older adults is more similar to, than different from, in-person care and TP for other population ages. The clinician needs to consider the patient population, model of care, collateral sources of information, and a range of cultural issues including language.
- There is steady growth of the TP evidence base, and older adult patients are as open to using TP as other populations and report high satisfaction.
- Telemedicine and TP overcome geographical, physical limitations and access to care obstacles.
- Telemedicine innovations, in general, may be inroads for TP services for patients, clinicians, and caregivers. More formal TP research studies and health service effectiveness studies are needed for older adult patients in culturally diverse populations, team-based or interdisciplinary care, and stepped or integrated care interprofessional models.

Acknowledgements American Telemedicine Association Telemental Health Interest Group

References

1. World Health Organization. Health topics: Ageing. (Online). 2012. www.who.int/topics/ageing/en. Accessed 30 Sept 2015.
2. Schulz R, Martire LM. Family caregiving of persons with dementia: prevalence, health effects, and support strategies. Am J Geriatr Psychiatry. 2004;12(3):240–9.
3. Todman JPF, Law J, MacDougall A. Attitudes of GPs towards older adults' psychology services in the Scottish Highlands. Rural Remote Health. 2011;11(1):1496.

4. Hilty DM, Ferrer D, Parish MB, Johnston B, Callahan EJ, Yellowlees PM. The effectiveness of telemental health: a 2013 review. Telemed J E Health. 2013;19(6):444–54.
5. Yellowlees PM, Odor A, Iosif A, Parish MB, Nafiz N, Patrice K, et al. Transcultural psychiatry made simple: asynchronous telepsychiatry as an approach to providing culturally relevant care. Telemed J E Health. 2013;19(4):259–64.
6. Hilty DM, Yellowlees PM, Parish MB, Chan S. Telepsychiatry: effective, evidence-based and at a tipping point in healthcare delivery? Psychiatr Clin North Am. 2015;38(3):559–92.
7. Hilty DM, Crawford A, Teshima J, Chan S, Sunderji N, Yellowlees PM, et al. A framework for telepsychiatric training and e-health: competency-based education, evaluation and implications. Int Rev Psychiatry. 2015;27(6):569–92. doi:10.3109/09540261.2015.1091292.
8. Sheeran T, Dealy J, Rabinowitz T. Geriatric telemental health. In: Myers K, Turvey CL, editors. Telemental health. New York: Elsevier; 2013. p. 171–95.
9. Hilty DM, Marks SL, Wegelin J, Callahan EJ, Nesbitt TS. A randomized controlled trial of disease management modules, including telepsychiatric care, for depression in rural primary care. Psychiatry (Edgmont). 2007;4(2):58–65.
10. Hilty DM, Chan S, Torous J, Matmahur J, Mucic D. New frontiers in healthcare and technology: internet- and web-based mental options emerge to complement in-person and telepsychiatric care options. J Health Med Informat. 2015;6:200. doi:10.4172/2157-7420.1000200.
11. Backhaus A, Agha Z, Maglione ML, Repp A, Ross B, Zuest D, et al. Videoconferencing psychotherapy: a systematic review. Psychol Serv. 2012;9(2):111–31.
12. Nelson EL, Duncan AB, Lillis T. Special considerations for conducting psychotherapy via videoconferencing. In: Myers K, Turvey CL, editors. Telemental health: clinical, technical and administrative foundations for evidenced-based practice. San Francisco: Elsevier; 2013. p. 295–314.
13. Myers KM, Vander Stoep A, Zhou C. Effectiveness of a telehealth service delivery model for treating attention-deficit hyperactivity disorder: results of a community-based randomized controlled trial. J Am Acad Child Adolesc Psychiatry. 2015;54(4):263–74.
14. Hilty DM, Shoemaker EZ, Myers KM, et al. Issues and steps toward a clinical guideline for telemental health for care of children and adolescents. J Child Adol Psychopharm 2016 Feb 12 [Epub ahead of print]. PMID 26871510.
15. Rabinowitz T, Murphy KM, Amour JL, Ricci MA, Caputo MP, Newhouse PA. Benefits of a telepsychiatry consultation service for rural nursing home residents. Telemed J E Health. 2010;16(1):34–40.
16. Jones III BN. Telepsychiatry and geriatric care. Curr Psychiatry Rep. 2001;3:29–36.
17. Lee JH, Kim JH, Jhoo JH, et al. A telemedicine system as a care modality for dementia patients in Korea. Alzheimer Dis Assoc Disord. 2000;14:94–101.
18. Tang WK, Chiu H, Woo J, et al. Telepsychiatry in psychogeriatric service: a pilot study. Int J Geriatr Psychiatry. 2001;16(1):88–93.
19. Johnston D, Jones III BN. Telepsychiatry consultations to a rural nursing facility: a 2-year experience. J Geriatr Psychiatry Neurol. 2001;14:72–5.
20. Lyketsos C, Roques C, Hovanec L, et al. Telemedicine use and reduction of psychiatric admissions from a long-term care facility. J Geriatr Psychiatry Neurol. 2001;14:76–9.
21. Rabinowitz T. Minimum data set facilitates telepsychiatry consultations for nursing home residents. Ninth annual meeting and exposition of the American Telemedicine Association. Tampa, Florida, May 3, 2004.
22. Yeung A, Johnson DP, Trinh NH, et al. Feasibility and effectiveness of telepsychiatry services for Chinese immigrants in a nursing home. Telemed E-Health. 2009;15:336–41.
23. Montani C, Billaud N, Tyrrell J, et al. Psychological impact of a remote psychometric consultation with hospitalized elderly people. J Telemed Telecare. 1997;3:140–5.
24. Menon AS, Kondapavalru P, Krishna P, et al. Evaluation of a portable low cost videophone system in the assessment of depressive symptoms and cognitive function in elderly medically ill veterans. J Nerv Ment Dis. 2001;189:399–401.
25. Grob P, Weintraub D, Sayles D, et al. Psychiatric assessment of a nursing home population using audiovisual telecommunication. J Geriatric Psychiatry Neurol. 2001;14:63–5.

26. Saligari J, Flicker L, Loh PK, et al. The clinical achievements of a geriatric telehealth project in its first year. J Telemed Telecare. 2002;8:53–5.
27. Shore JH, Manson SM. Telepsychiatric care of American Indian veterans with post-traumatic stress disorder: bridging gaps in geography, organizations, and culture. Telemed J E Health. 2004;10 Suppl 2:64–9.
28. Loh PK, Maher S, Goldswain P, et al. Diagnostic accuracy of telehealth community dementia assessments. J Amer Ger Soc. 2005;53:2043–4.
29. Cullum CM, Weiner MF, Gehrmann HR, Hynan LS. Feasibility of telecognitive assessment in dementia. Assessment. 2006;13(4):385–90.
30. Turvey CL, Willyard D, Hickman DH, Klein DM, Kukoyi O. Telehealth screen for depression in a chronic illness care management program. Telemed J E Health. 2007;13(1):51–6.
31. Conn DK, Madan R, Lam J, Patterson T, Skirten S. Program evaluation of a telepsychiatry service for older adults connecting a university-affiliated geriatric center to a rural psychogeriatric outreach service in Northwest Ontario, Canada. Int Psychogeriatr. 2013;25(11):1795–800.
32. Urness D, Hailey D, Delday L, Callanan T, Orlik H. The status of telepsychiatry services in Canada: a national survey. J Telemed Telecare. 2004;10(3):160–4.
33. Hilty DM, Seritan AL, Ureste P, et al. Geriatric patients in medical settings: assessment of common behavioral health problems, impact of culture and diversity issues and telecare innovations. Jacobs J Gerontology (in press).
34. Mutchler JE, Bacigalupe G, Coppin A, Gottlieb A. Language barriers surrounding medication use among older Latinos. J Cross Cult Gerontol. 2007;22(1):101–14.
35. Elderkin-Thompson V, Silver RC, Waitzkin H. When nurses double as interpreters: a study of Spanish-speaking patients in a US primary care setting. Soc Sci Med. 2001;52(9):1343–58.
36. Perez-Stable EJ. Language access and Latino health care disparities. Med Care. 2007; 45(11):1009–11.
37. Sheeran T, Rabinowitz T, Lotterman J, Reilly CF, Brown S, Donehower P, et al. Feasibility and impact of telemonitor-based depression care management for geriatric homecare patients. Telemed J E Health. 2011;17(8):620–6.
38. Vahia IV, Ng B, Camacho A, Cardenas V, Cherner M, Depp CA, et al. Telepsychiatry for neurocognitive testing in older rural Latino adults. Am J Geriatr Psychiatry. 2015;23(7):666–70.
39. Ament BH, Wolfs CA, Kempen GI, Ambergen T, Verhey FRJ, De Vugt ME. The benefit of a geriatric nurse practitioner in a multidisciplinary diagnostic service for people with cognitive disorders. BMC Res Notes. 2015;8:217.
40. Choi NG, Marti CN, Bruce ML, Hegel MT, Wilson NL, Kunik ME. Six-month post-intervention depression and disability outcomes of in-home telehealth problem-solving therapy for depressed, low-income homebound older adults. Depress Anxiety. 2014;31(8): 653–61.
41. Gellis ZD, Kenaley BL, Ten Have T. Integrated telehealth care for chronic illness and depression in geriatric home care patients: the Integrated Telehealth Education and Activation of Mood (I-TEAM) study. J Am Geriatr Soc. 2014;62(5):889–95.
42. Internet World Stats. Internet users in the world-distribution by world regions. 2011. http://www.internetworldstats.com/stats.htm. Accessed 30 Sept 2015.
43. Pedone C, Rossi FF, Cecere A, Costanzo L, Antonelli Incalzi R. Efficacy of a physician-led multiparametric telemonitoring system in very old adults with heart failure. J Am Geriatr Soc. 2015;63(6):1175–80.
44. Grant LA, Rockwood T, Stennes L. Testing telehealth using technology-enhanced nurse monitoring. J Gerontol Nurs. 2014;40(10):15–23.
45. Hu C, Kung S, Rummans TA, Clark MM, Lapid MI. Reducing caregiver stress with internet-based interventions: a systematic review of open-label and randomized controlled trials. J Am Med Inform Assoc. 2015;22(e1):e194–209.
46. Chi NC, Demiris G. A systematic review of telehealth tools and interventions to support family caregivers. J Telemed Telecare. 2015;21(1):37–44.

Suicide and Violence Prevention and Control: A Public Health Approach

25

Jason G. Roof, Glen L. Xiong, and Sidney R. Stacey

25.1 Background

Violence, whether directed toward others or toward oneself, is a multifaceted and complex issue for public health and prevention. While violence affects all ages, older populations are growing more rapidly than other populations and present unique issues related to violence and suicide. Between 2000 and 2010, the USA saw a 15 % population increase in individuals aged 65 and older. The only greater population increase involved individuals aged 45–54 years old at 31 % [1]. Supporting this trend of longer lives is a decrease in age-adjusted death rates for eight of the ten leading causes of death; however, one leading cause, suicide, has increased significantly in older populations [2]. This trend goes beyond the USA itself and the population aged 65 and older consistently presents itself as the demographic group with the highest suicide rate in most countries [3].

J.G. Roof, MD (✉)
Division of Psychiatry and the Law, Department of Psychiatry & Behavioral Sciences, University of California, Davis Medical Center, 2230 Stockton Blvd, 2nd Floor, Sacramento, CA 95817, USA
e-mail: jgroof@ucdavis.edu

G.L. Xiong, MD, CMD
Department of Psychiatry & Behavioral Sciences, University of California, Davis Medical Center, 2775 18th Street, Sacramento, CA 95818, USA
e-mail: gxiong@ucdavis.edu

S.R. Stacey, MHSc, FCCHL, FACHE
Department of Psychiatry & Behavioural Neurosciences, Faculty of Health Sciences, McMaster University, St. Joseph's Healthcare, West 5th Campus, 100 West 5th Street, Room B356, Hamilton L8N 3K7, ON, Canada
e-mail: sstacey@mcmaster.ca

A. Hategan et al. (eds.), *On-Call Geriatric Psychiatry: Handbook of Principles and Practice*, DOI 10.1007/978-3-319-30346-8_25

25.2 Suicide in Geriatric Populations

According to the World Health Organization, nearly 800,000 people die from suicide every year [4]. About three quarter of suicides occur in low- and middle-income countries. Although older age or geriatric age (defined herein as 65 years and older) is a well-known clinical risk factor for suicide, younger persons (ages 15–29) represent the highest risk age group, and suicide is the second leading cause of death in this age group. Suicide and attempted suicide have major societal and economic costs. In the USA, the estimated cost of suicide in 2005 was $34.6B [5] arising from 32,637 deaths including both direct health-care costs and inferred lost work productivity. Hospital and emergency room costs arising from self-harm were $6.4B. Effective public policy to promote suicide prevention and foster help seeking is challenging because of the complexity of integrating federal, state, and local initiatives. In a study of attempted suicide in persons 70 years and older in Sweden [6], key risk factors identified included being unmarried, living alone, low education level, history of psychiatric treatment, and previous suicide attempt. Interestingly, there was no association with major neurocognitive disorders (NCDs) (formerly dementia).

25.3 Violence Toward Others in Geriatric Populations

While younger patients tend to have higher rates of violence than older patients, aggression accounts for 15–40 % of community referrals for psychiatric services for older adults. Among these aggressive behaviors, 50–70 % of referrals were due to physical aggression [7]. Violence can be defined as abuse, threat, or assault toward others and may come in the form of verbal or physical aggression [7]. The causes of violence can be divided into (i) reactive, (ii) psychotically driven, and (iii) premeditated violence. Geriatric violence offenders can roughly be divided into three major categories: (1) persons with no psychiatric illness, (2) persons with psychiatric illness (including substance use disorders) other than NCD, and (3) persons with a major NCD.

Due to high prevalence of major NCDs, there are relatively more studies on patients with major NCDs than other chronic psychiatric illness. Verbal aggression tends to occur much more commonly than physical aggression. While verbal aggression commonly predates physical aggression, there is a lack of systematic studies to show whether early interventions at the verbal aggression stage would prevent physical aggression. It is clear that major NCD-related aggressive symptoms can be chronic [7]. In a small study of 52 geriatric psychiatry inpatients with major NCDs, nearly 10 % physically attacked others within 72 h of hospital admission [8]. Another long-term study found that 70 % of patients with mild Alzheimer's disease who exhibited aggression continued to do so after 2 years [9].

Although studies are scant, a history of aggression, personality traits (specifically antisocial traits), and medical conditions such as traumatic brain injuries (TBIs) and even hearing or vision loss have been associated with violence [7]. No particular psychiatric disorder has been found to be more predictive of violence in older patients compared to younger counterparts. However, among patients with major NCDs, delusional beliefs and misidentification are frequently associated with violence.

Assaults on family caregivers and nursing staff are particularly problematic, with the latter much better documented in the literature. While exceedingly rare, homicides committed by geriatric patients with major NCDs are disturbing and are a vexing concern for communities. In the UK, 73 % of nursing staff on geriatric inpatient wards were assaulted by geriatric patients with disorders including NCDs and TBIs [10]. In long-term care settings, a systematic review examined resident-to-resident physical aggression from 18 studies [11]. The review noted that perpetrators of aggressive behavior most frequently had a higher level of cognitive awareness and physical functionality as well as a history of aggressive behaviors. Victims are most likely female with cognitive impairment and with a history of wandering behavior. Aggressive episodes typically occurred in the afternoon in communal settings and were often triggered by communication issues, invasion of space, or were unprovoked [11].

In cases with legal implications, a lack of trial competency due to severe psychiatric illness may significantly affect a defendant's ability to understand trial proceedings and/or assist counsel in carrying out a defense. Patients with severe psychiatric illness, such as major NCDs, have a decreased likelihood of being able to reasonably participate in the preparation of their own defense. Forensic psychiatric evaluations may be required to determine competence to stand trial. Such evaluations may require a thorough psychiatric interview as well as neuropsychological tests and other medical workup. Due to both age and higher likelihood of comorbidity with systemic medical and neuropsychiatric illnesses, even for those without major NCDs, the restoration of competency for geriatric criminal offenders is likely to be more complicated and requires more treatment time. The delivery of clinical services to incarcerated geriatric patients is detailed in Chap. 22.

25.4 Public Health Approaches to Geriatric Suicide and Violence

Case Vignette: Depressed Delusion Mr. S's many decades of schizoaffective disorder characterized by intermittent episodes of partially remitted depression and paranoid delusions regarding being poisoned by a nearby manufacturing facility were being reevaluated during an outpatient psychiatric visit. A risk assessment was performed by his psychiatrist which revealed no reported suicidal thoughts, no homicidal thoughts, and no access to firearms. At the conclusion of the outpatient appointment, Mr. S softly remarked, "I don't know, maybe it's finally time that someone did something. Or maybe I've just reached the end of my long fight."

Public health approaches to geriatric suicide and violence are highly challenging but are increasingly receiving more general public awareness and political attention. While suicide and violence had been traditionally seen as societal issues, they are increasingly getting more attention at the individual level. Most of the initiatives have been to expand mental health services at the community level, so that patients can receive psychiatric treatment to improve their psychiatric symptoms to decrease the risk of suicide and violence. While there are few studies of intervention that have been shown to be effective to prevent violence against others, there is a growing evidence base for suicide prevention treatments. These include education of physicians on depression recognition and treatment and restricting patient access to lethal means such as firearms. Other promising methods include public education, screening, and media education.

Case Vignette: Displaced Depression

Mr. S's failing cognitive health resulted in his inability to function independently. He had become increasingly confused and unable to care for himself, while he was not actively taking any medications. His daughter, living several hundred miles away, arranged for him to live with her while she considered various care facilities nearby. Mr. S had always been private about his mental health treatment history and did not share that he had been treated for schizoaffective disorder with episodes of both depression and delusions. After living with him for several weeks, his daughter viewed a TV show program on depression and became concerned that her father might be depressed and could harm himself. She brought her father into a small community clinic to visit with a primary care physician (PCP). The PCP determined that there was evidence of a moderate stage, major NCD as well as some symptoms of depression, though could not determine where Mr. S might have received psychiatric treatment in the past. The PCP performed a basic risk assessment and determined that the daughter owned several hunting rifles and a revolver at home. The PCP also determined that Ms. S was unsafe to drive his car. The PCP, after his initial assessment, called his psychiatry backup on call, who advised him to assure that the weapons were safely secured and the driver license agency was contacted. The on-call psychiatrist advised the PCP to schedule a routine psychiatric appointment for further evaluation of NCD/depression/psychotic illness and to remind the patient's daughter to take him to the emergency department for any acute safety concerns or acute change in mental status. (See Chap. 10 for further details on assessment and on-call management of the chief psychiatric complaints.)

There are several challenges in designing public health suicide and violence prevention programs. Caine [5] noted a few of the challenges for suicide prevention, such as (i) an inability to discriminate relatively few true cases from large numbers of false-positive cases, (ii) a large number of false-negative cases that escape preventive detection, (iii) the inability of clinical services to reach patients who have suicidal intent, (iv) the paucity of knowledge about risk factors in diverse groups, and (v) the lack of coordinated strategies for suicide prevention among various local, regional, and national agencies and organizations. These same challenges would apply to violence prevention strategies. Discussions of firearm safety and public awareness of suicide/violence prevention, particularly in the USA, remain a topic for significant consideration and debate between medical professionals and policy makers [5].

In 2013, the American Association for Geriatric Psychiatry launched the Coalition on Mental Health and Violence Issues, calling for collaboration of mental health programs, federal and local government agencies, and the general public. In the USA, from 2005 to 2010, firearm injury accounted for 72 % of suicides among those aged 65 years and older compared to 51 % of all suicides [12]. In the Veterans Affairs health system, older men who died by suicide used a gun 79 % of the time. The Veterans Affairs system recommends clinicians to counsel family members about removing guns from patients with major NCDs [13].

25.5 Current Public Policy

Public health policy to reduce suicide among older adults requires early identification, suicide prevention training and education programs, stigma reduction, and health promotion strategies delivered at the local level that foster help seeking by reaching out to those who currently do not seek medical or psychological help [3]. Thomas Joiner's interpersonal theory of suicide [14] has been utilized by many suicide prevention agencies as an organizing framework to inform constructive public policy. Joiner stresses that three factors must be present for a suicide to be carried out: (1) thwarted belongingness, (2) perceived burdensomeness, and (3) acquired capability for suicide. Thwarted belongingness is a lack of meaningful connections to others and a strain or loss of previous solid relationships. Perceived burdensomeness occurs when the individual feels that they are a burden to the world and believe they not only do not make meaningful contributions to society but they are also a potential liability. These two factors combine to create the desire for suicide. Acquired capability for suicide is the third factor which involves the degree to which the individual is able to initiate the event. Repeated exposure to painful events and behaviors may desensitize a person to the formidable idea of suicide. Public policy needs to target early identification, health promotion and prevention, public education, and stigma reduction to foster enhanced levels of help seeking.

25.6 Policy Goals for the Future

Suicide prevention programs for the older adults must span a broad continuum to achieve the outcomes of reducing risk and preventing harm. Early detection initiatives with the help of family and community gatekeepers, treatment for high-risk patients, physician education, and increased outreach to older adults, such as periodic visits or telephone calls, are essential strategies for suicide prevention [3]. A practical guide for violence risk assessment in a clinical setting is available in Chap. 10. The decline in geriatric suicide rates in England and Wales was the result of several public health initiatives designed to promote better access to care and service [15]. Strategies included early identification and treatment of psychiatric illness and those at risk of suicide, adequate provision of comprehensive mental health services, and systematic follow-up of those who were recovering or had recovered from a psychiatric illness.

Innovative delivery models such as accountable care organizations [16] and collaborative models, which better integrate psychiatric care and primary care, are emerging strategies to foster better care for at-risk older adults. Policy goals must respond to the unique needs of the older adult and unite community organizations, mental health services, and resources to prevent death by suicide. Suicide prevention initiatives that promote early identification, reduce stigma, build resilience, and promote help seeking reflect the aim of preventing deaths and reducing the suffering of suicidal behaviors in the older adults.

Key Points

- Effective public policy to promote suicide prevention and foster help seeking is challenging, particularly in the USA because of the complexity of integrating federal, state, and local initiatives.
- Aggression accounts for 15–40 % of community referrals for psychiatric services for older adults, and 50–70 % of referrals are due to physical aggression.
- A history of aggression, personality traits (specifically antisocial traits), and medical conditions such as traumatic head injuries, and even hearing or vision loss, have been associated with violence.
- Public health policy to reduce suicide in the older adults requires early identification, suicide prevention training and education programs, stigma reduction, and health promotion strategies to foster enhanced levels of help seeking.

References

1. Howden L, Meyer J. Age and sex composition: 2010. Census.gov. 2011. http://www.census.gov/prod/cen2010/briefs/c2010br-03.pdf. Accessed 26 Nov 2015.
2. Xu J, Kochanek K. Products – data briefs – Number 168 – October 2014. Cdc.gov. 2014. http://www.cdc.gov/nchs/data/databriefs/db168.htm. Accessed 26 Nov 2015.
3. Lapierre S, Erlangsen A, Waern M, et al. A systematic review of elderly suicide prevention programs. Crisis. 2011;32(2):88–98.
4. Who.int. WHO | Suicide data. 2015. http://www.who.int/mental_health/prevention/suicide/suicideprevent/en/. Accessed 26 Nov 2015.
5. Caine ED. Forging an agenda for suicide prevention in the United States. Am J Public Health. 2013;103(5):822–4.
6. Wiktorsson S, Runeson B, Skoog I, Östling S, Waern M. Attempted suicide in the elderly: characteristics of suicide attempters 70 years and older and a general population comparison group. Am J Geriatr Psychiatry. 2010;18(1):57–67.
7. O'Callaghan C, Richman A, Majumdar B. Violence in older people with mental illness. Adv Psychiatr Treat. 2010;16(5):339–48.
8. Haller E, Binder RL, McNiel DE. Violence in geriatric patients with dementia. Bull Am Acad Psychiatry Law. 1989;17(2):183–8.
9. Eustace A, Coen R, Walsh C, et al. A longitudinal evaluation of behavioural and psychological symptoms of probable Alzheimer's disease. Int J Geriat Psychiatry. 2002;17(10):968–73.

10. Royal College of Psychiatrists' Centre for Quality Improvement. Healthcare Commission National Audit of Violence 2006–7 Final Report – Working Age Adult Services; 2008.
11. Ferrah N, Murphy B, Ibrahim J, et al. Resident-to-resident physical aggression leading to injury in nursing homes: a systematic review. Age Ageing. 2015;44(3):356–64.
12. Brauser D. Violence in elderly patients with dementia: overlooked? Medscape. 2014. http://www.medscape.org/viewarticle/827726. Accessed 26 Nov 2015.
13. United States. Department of Veterans Affairs (Corporate Author). Firearms & Dementia. Department of Veterans Affairs, Office of the Medical Inspector; 2012
14. Joiner TE. Why people die by suicide. Cambridge, MA: Harvard University Press; 2005.
15. Shah A. Does improvement in the treatment of those who attempt suicide contribute to a reduction in elderly suicide rates in England? IPG. 2009;21(04):768.
16. Shortell S, Addicott R, Walsh N, Ham C. Accountable care organizations in the United States and England: testing, evaluating and learning what works. 2014. http://www.kingsfund.org.uk/sites/files/kf/field/field_publication_file/accountable-care-organisations-united-states-england-shortell-mar14.pdf. Accessed 5 Dec 2015.

26 Aging with Neurodevelopmental Disorders: On-Call Assessment and Future Directions

Randi Hagerman, Andrew Ligsay, and Jeremy Goldberg

26.1 Background

There are many similarities neurobiologically between aging disorders and neurodevelopmental disorders. Many of the same proteins that are dysregulated in aging syndromes are also important for the development of the brain, and so the mechanisms of aging syndromes can also cause problems in neurodevelopment. Perhaps the most prominent example of this is the amyloid precursor protein (APP) which is an important protein for synapse formation in development, but also leads to amyloid plaques in Alzheimer's disease (AD). It is also located on chromosome 21, so it is overproduced in trisomy 21 leading to the early AD seen in Down syndrome.

The fragile X mental retardation 1 protein (FMRP) is another protein that is critical for development and aging. FMRP is a regulator of translation which controls hundreds of genes, many of which are important for synaptic plasticity and adult neurogenesis. FMRP controls the translation of approximately 30–50 % of the known genes that are mutated in autism spectrum disorders (ASD) [1, 2]. In the absence of FMRP because of a full mutation (>200 repeats in the *FMR1* gene on the bottom of the X chromosome leading to methylation and silencing of transcription), fragile X syndrome (FXS) occurs, which is the most common cause of inherited

R. Hagerman, MD (✉)
University of California MIND Institute, Sacramento, CA, USA

Department of Pediatrics, University of California Davis Medical Center,
2825 50th Street, Sacramento, CA 95817, USA
e-mail: rjhagerman@ucdavis.edu

A. Ligsay, MD
MIND Institute, University of California, Davis School of Medicine and MIND Institute,
Sacramento, CA 95817, USA

J. Goldberg, MD
Department of Psychiatry and Behavioural Neurosciences, McMaster University,
Hamilton, ON, Canada

A. Hategan et al. (eds.), *On-Call Geriatric Psychiatry: Handbook of Principles and Practice*, DOI 10.1007/978-3-319-30346-8_26

Table 26.1 Medical and psychiatric features associated with the fragile X premutation

Medical features	Psychiatric features
Fragile X-associated primary ovarian insufficiency (FXPOI) Fragile X-associated tremor/ataxia syndrome (FXTAS) Hypothyroidism, sleep apnea, hypertension, immune-mediated disorders, fibromyalgia, restless legs syndrome, seizures Autonomic dysfunction	Somatic symptom disorder Obsessive-compulsive disorder Interpersonal sensitivity Depressive disorders Social anxiety disorder Neurocognitive disorders Sleep disorders Attention problems/attention deficit hyperactivity disorder (ADHD) Social deficits Autism spectrum disorders (ASD)

Derived from Ref. [4]

intellectual disability and the most common known genetic cause of ASD. Therefore, any patient with ASD needs a fragile X DNA test as part of the medical workup. The fragile X premutation (55–200 CGG repeats in *FMR1*) is unmethylated and common in the general population, approximately 1 in 150–200 females and 1 in 400–450 males [3]. Most patients with the premutation have normal intellectual abilities, although ASD occurs in approximately 10 % of boys and anxiety and depression are seen in approximately 40–50 % of adults.

In aging, approximately 40 % of males and 16 % of females with the premutation develop a neurodegenerative disorder involving an intention tremor, cerebellar ataxia, neuropathy, and progressive memory and cognitive loss called the fragile X-associated tremor ataxia syndrome (FXTAS) [4] (see Table 26.1). The molecular underpinning of FXTAS is the opposite of FXS in that *FMR1* is overly active and produces between 2 and 8 times the normal level of the *FMR1* mRNA. This excess mRNA leads to an RNA gain-of-function toxicity where proteins that are essential for neuronal function are sequestered, such as DROSHA and DGCR8 [5]. DGCR8 stands for DiGeorge syndrome critical region 8 which is essential for the maturation of microRNAs, small pieces of RNA that regulate posttranslational processing of mRNAs. DGCR8 is deleted in the 22q deletion syndrome (22qDS), which is the most common genetic cause of schizophrenia and bipolar disorder in adulthood, but also causes neurodevelopmental disorders in childhood including attention deficit hyperactivity disorder (ADHD), anxiety, and ASD.

The pathophysiological interrelationships among neurodevelopmental disorders are remarkable, including the frequent occurrence of mitochondrial dysfunction, oxidative stress, production of reactive oxygen species (ROS), and vulnerability of neurons to toxins and early cell death [6]. For instance, mitochondrial dysfunction can lead to the slow movement of mitochondria in neuronal development, such that the connectivity of the CNS is impacted in many disorders including ASD and fragile X disorders [7, 8]. Gradual loss of mitochondrial function is part of the aging process leading to weakness, but it is accelerated in many aging disorders such as Parkinson's disease (PD) and AD. For many neurodevelopmental disorders (e.g., FXS, 22qDS), PD can be seen in aging at a higher frequency than the general population [9, 10].

26.2 Fragile X Spectrum Disorders

Case Vignette 1 of FXS and PD Mr. L was a 65-year-old male with FXS. His early development was marked by hyperactivity and social deficits leading to a diagnosis of ASD. He was language delayed and did not speak in sentences until 5 years old, although he was talkative throughout adolescence and adulthood. He had intermittent outburst behavior leading to the use of antipsychotics periodically in childhood and adulthood. He worked in an adult workshop for most of his adult life, but at age 55, he began to communicate less and gradually lost the ability to write his name. His movements gradually became slower, and he developed a shuffling gait in his late 50s. His mother, with whom he lived, died when he was 60, and he developed an episode of major depression. He had a gradual decline in his motor and cognitive function since age 60, and upon evaluation at age 65, he was unable to talk. The on-call evaluation of Mr. L demonstrated documentation of his fragile X full mutation of 450 CGG repeats. On communication with his caretakers, he has had significant depression for years that has not been treated. Because of his previous behavioral outbursts, he was on risperidone 5 mg a day which could have exacerbated his PD symptoms, so this medication was gradually tapered over a few weeks, and he was started on sertraline 50 mg daily to treat his depression. Thyroid function studies and vitamin deficiencies were evaluated; he was deficient in vitamin D, so this was supplemented at 5,000 IU per day. Mr. L was referred to neurology to treat his PD.

Case Vignette 2 of Fragile X Premutation Involvement Including Asperger Syndrome and FXTAS Mr. D was a 55-year-old male with a history of the fragile X premutation (with 72 CGG repeats in *FMR1*). His mother was a fragile X carrier, and she had a history of the fragile X-associated primary ovarian insufficiency (FXPOI) with menopause before age 40, years of fibromyalgia and migraines, and FXTAS with the development of tremor in her 70s followed by ataxia leading to the need for a wheelchair in her 80s and death from a cardiac arrhythmia and congestive heart failure at age 85. Mr. D was primarily raised by his mother since her depression, anxiety, and chronic pain symptoms led to a divorce of his parents when he was 10 years old. He did well in school, but he was always socially anxious and he had no friends. He was intensely interested in maps throughout childhood, and he became a cartographer in his adult work. He was diagnosed with Asperger syndrome in childhood because of his social deficits and intense interest areas that would dominate his conversations. He was married at age 40 because his wife felt that his social deficits were "sexy." Their daughter was a fragile X carrier but had normal development. At age 48 he developed memory problems that gradually worsened to executive function deficits. When he was evaluated at age 55, he had a slight intention tremor and significant ataxia and could not tandem walk. He had significant major neurocognitive disorder (NCD) (formerly dementia) on cognitive testing, and his MRI demonstrated white matter disease in the middle cerebellar peduncle (MCP sign; major FXTAS criteria for diagnosis; see Table 26.2) [4, 11], thin corpus callosum with white matter hyperintensity in the genu and splenium of

Table 26.2 Current diagnostic criteria for FXTAS

Examination and degree		
Molecular		
	Major	*FMR1* expansion in gray zone, premutation, or unmethylated full mutation range
Radiological		
	Major	MRI white matter lesions in middle cerebellar peduncle
	Minor	MRI white matter hyperintensities in the splenium of the corpus callosum
	Minor	MRI white matter lesions in cerebral white matter
	Minor	Moderate-to-severe generalized atrophy
Clinical		
	Major	Intention tremor
	Major	Gait ataxia
	Minor	Parkinsonism
	Minor	Moderate-to-severe short-term memory deficit
	Minor	Executive function deficit
	Minor	Neuropathy
Neuropathological		
	Major	FXTAS inclusions
Diagnostic category		
Presence of expanded CGG repeat (molecular)		
	Definite	Presence of one major radiological sign plus (i) one major clinical symptom or (ii) the presence of FXTAS inclusions
	Probable	Presence of one major radiological sign and one minor clinical symptom or two major clinical symptoms
	Possible	Presence of one major radiological sign and one major clinical symptom

Derived from Refs. [4, 11]

the corpus callosum (minor FXTAS criteria), and brain atrophy (minor FXTAS criteria). Treatment recommendations for him included donepezil 5 mg daily for his major NCD and FXTAS.

The on-call evaluation of aging patients with an intention tremor and cerebellar ataxia warrants fragile X DNA testing to assess if the premutation is present and an MRI looking for white matter hyperintensities (see Table 26.3) [12]. The premutation is common in the general population, and it can coexist with many aging disorders including AD, PD, multiple sclerosis, fibromyalgia, cardiac arrhythmias, congestive heart failure, hypothyroidism, and osteoporosis. The dysregulation of miRNAs because of DROSHA and DGCR8 sequestration also predisposes female carriers to immune regulation disorders, particularly hypothyroidism, fibromyalgia, and a central pain syndrome [13] that can include migraines, neuropathy, and back pain. Case 2 above had FXTAS, as did his mother, although his FXTAS initially presented with cognitive decline before motor symptoms, which is unusual. He may also have had AD in addition to FXTAS. Only the post-mortem study of brain pathology would clarify this. Those with FXTAS will have eosinophilic intranuclear

Table 26.3 Findings associated with cerebellar ataxia and/or action tremor in adults[a] that support testing for premutation alleles of *FMR1*

Associated feature	Additional comments	Independent indicator for *FMR1* testing[b]
Family members with intellectual impairment, autism, or autism spectrum disorder (ASD)	Fragile X syndrome is the leading monogenic cause of intellectual impairment and autism/ASD. FXTAS is common among older adults (>50 years) in fragile X families	Yes
Primary ovarian insufficiency (POI)	Premutation alleles of the *FMR1* gene constitute the leading monogenic cause of POI, often described in terms of early menopause/infertility (<40 years)	Yes
Hypothyroidism (women)	50 % of females with FXTAS, often associated with other evidence of immune dysfunction	No
Peripheral neuropathy	60 % of men and 53 % of women with FXTAS	No
Muscle pain/(fibromyalgia)	76 %/(43 %) among women with FXTAS	No
MRI hyperintensities within the middle cerebellar peduncles (MCP) or splenium of the corpus callosum	The MCP sign was one component of the original definition of FXTAS; involvement of the MCP and/or the splenium is highly characteristic of FXTAS	Yes
Family member with the premutation	At risk to be a carrier with no symptoms or any premutation-associated disorder	Yes

Derived from Ref. [12]

[a]Typical onset >50 years

[b]Features that would warrant testing for CGG-repeat expansions of *FMR1* irrespective of the presence of tremor or ataxia

inclusions that are tau and synuclein negative but positive for ubiquitin and the *FMR1* mRNA. In addition recent literature has demonstrated the presence of polyglycine protein (PolyG-FMRP) that occurs through RAN translation [14]. This means an aberrant protein that is translated from the *FMR1* mRNA with a non-AUG start site (RAN translation), such that misreading of the CGG produces a GCG or PolyG-FMRP that is toxic to the CNS [15]. In order to diagnose FXTAS, an MRI must be ordered, and the classic findings in FXTAS are the MCP sign as described above along with minor signs identified in Table 26.2 [4, 11].

26.3 Down Syndrome

Down syndrome (DS), also known as trisomy 21, is the most common genetic cause of significant intellectual disability (ID). It is due to the presence of all or part of a third copy of chromosome 21. In a small number of cases, some but not all of the cells are trisomy for chromosome 21; this is termed mosaicism.

Table 26.4 Common features and abnormalities in Down syndrome

Neurologic	Intellectual disability Early-onset Alzheimer's disease
Facial features	Flat facies and nasal bridge Upward slanting eyes with epicanthal folds at the inner corners
Hands and feet	Single palmar crease Deep groove between the first and second toes Lax ligaments
Ophthalmic	Congenital cataracts or glaucoma Refractory errors Strabismus Nystagmus
Otologic	Hearing loss
Cardiovascular	Septal defects Patent ductus arteriosus Tetralogy of Fallot Mitral valve disease
Endocrine	Thyroid disease Diabetes mellitus
Hematology/oncology	Polycythemia in newborns Acute myeloid leukemia Acute lymphoblastic leukemia

The phenotype for DS is characterized by a number of distinguishing features (see Table 26.4). Prevalence estimates for the rate of conception of DS fetuses have increased as the mean age of pregnant women has increased. However, the number of terminated pregnancies with DS has also increased, and so the prevalence of DS births has actually decreased from around 1/700 to about 1/900-1000.

The diagnosis of DS is made by chromosomal analysis. Prenatally, a blood test followed by cytogenetic diagnosis is offered to all pregnant women. In those diagnosed with DS, various guidelines for the medical management of these patients have been recommended [16, 17]. This includes a cardiac assessment with an echocardiogram after birth as about half of children with DS are born with congenital heart disease. Common cardiac lesions are atrioventricular septal defect, which occurs in 45 %; ventricular septal defect, which occurs in 35 %; isolated secundum atrial septal defect, which occurs in 8 %; persistent patent ductus arteriosus, which occurs in 7 %; and tetralogy of Fallot, which occurs in 4 % of DS infants. Symptoms of serious heart disease may be absent due to the tendency for children with DS to develop pulmonary vascular resistance. Furthermore, adolescents and young adults with no known intracardiac disease can develop mitral stenosis (46 %) and/or mitral regurgitation (17 %), and so a second cardiac assessment is recommended before children with DS reach puberty or young adulthood.

Assessment and treatment for hearing loss is another important aspect of the medical management of patients with DS, as between 38 and 78 % of patients with DS have a significant problem with hearing, which may be conductive, sensorineural, or mixed. Medical management for conductive hearing loss frequently includes treatment of otitis media and/or surgical interventions such as placement of pneumoeustachian tubes, tonsillectomy, and/or adenoidectomy. Subsequently, speech therapy, assisted communication, hearing aids, and/or cochlear implants is also used.

Ophthalmological assessments in DS should begin at birth or by no later than 6 months of age, in order to identify congenital cataracts or glaucoma. Ophthalmological disorders increase in frequency with age where the most frequent disorders identified are refractive errors (35–76 %), strabismus (27–57 %), and nystagmus (20 %). Ophthalmological assessments should therefore continue on a yearly basis throughout life.

Screening for thyroid disease typically occurs at birth, 6 months of age, and thereafter yearly with tests for thyroxine and thyroid-stimulating hormone. A number of other disorders including arthritis, atlantoaxial subluxation, diabetes mellitus, leukemia, obstructive sleep apnea, and seizure disorders occur more frequently among patients with DS; however, these disorders are not frequent enough to warrant routine monitoring.

Patients with DS are also more likely to have hematological aberrations, although most of these occur in childhood. These disorders include polycythemia in newborns, macrocytosis, transient myeloproliferative disorder, acute myeloid leukemia, and acute lymphoblastic leukemia. Obstructive sleep apnea is often noted in patients with DS, largely because of their mid-facial hypoplasia. However, surgical intervention does not always correct the problem, and conservative supplemental oxygen therapy under pressure is not easily tolerated. In the 8 % of patients with DS who develop seizures, the age of onset is bimodal (40 % occurring before 1 year and 40 % occurring in the third decade of life). In adults, partial, simple, or complex seizures may also develop.

Improvements in medical care for patients with DS have led to significant extensions of life span and enhanced quality of life for these patients. Consequently, up to the age of 35 years, mortality rates for these patients are comparable to those patients with ID from other causes [18]. However, after the age of 35, mortality rates double every 6 and a half years for people with DS as compared to 9.6 years for people with ID without DS.

Aging adults with DS are at increased risk for developing AD. The profile and sequence of cognitive impairments in these patients are similar to those seen with AD in the general population [18]. Memory processes are affected early in the course of DS-related, major NCD, while severe cognitive deterioration such as acquired apraxia and agnosia is reported in 28 % of patients with DS by the age of 30. In middle age, virtually all patients with DS have neuropathological changes consistent with AD including senile plaques and neurofibrillary tangles (NFT). However, not all of these patients will develop dementia. The earliest manifestation of major NCD in DS involves changes in personality, behavior, and socially deficient communication, which may be an early sign of frontal lobe dysfunction; this is a striking change from previously reasonably well-developed social capacities that are typically present in these patients.

The diagnosis of major NCD in DS can be challenging, given the background of intellectual and functional impairment; however, more reliable methods for the diagnosis of major NCD in DS include both informant-based and direct measures. Typically, the clinical signs of major NCD in DS are observed over the age of 50. In those patients suspected of AD, a comprehensive medical assessment should be done to detect any treatable disorders such as thyroid disease or depression.

US FDA-approved medications for treatment of AD in the general population have met with only mild-to-moderate success in the treatment of AD in DS. Therefore, other disease-modifying approaches are going to be critically important for the future therapeutics of AD in DS. Prevention may be the most promising approach to healthy aging for patients with DS, which may include both pharmacological (treating comorbid physical and psychiatric illness) and non-pharmacological interventions (such as diet, exercise, and fostering social interaction).

26.4 22q11.2 Deletion Syndrome (22qDS)

22qDS, also known as velocardiofacial or DiGeorge syndrome, is due to a hemizygous microdeletion on the long arm of chromosome 22. Its prevalence is estimated at 1 in 2000 to 1 in 6000 live births. Phenotypic features associated with 22qDS include abnormal facies, cleft palate, conotruncal cardiac anomalies, thymic aplasia and immune dysfunction, and hypocalcemia. A significant percentage of patients also have cognitive delay with patients typically scoring in the below average or borderline full scale IQ range. However, cognitive function also appears to decline with age [19].

Patients with 22qDS also have multiple psychiatric comorbidities. A recent study of 76 children with 22qDS showed a majority presented with elevated anxiety symptoms [20], which further substantiates previous reports of such an association. This is concerning because anxiety is associated with poor adaptive functioning and may interfere with cognitive potential as well [21]. Additionally, ADHD is notably present in 22qDS with the inattentive subtype being the most commonly diagnosed [22]. Major depressive disorder and, to a lesser degree, bipolar disorder are also linked with 22qDS. The prevalence of these problems also increases with age (15.75 % and 3.94 % by mature adulthood, respectively). Finally, there is an increased association with ASD with prevalence rates estimated between 6 and 19 % [23]. Despite these known comorbidities, there is very little published data identifying safety and efficacy of treatment trials targeting these symptoms.

Leading theories suggest a significant degree of dopaminergic dysregulation in 22qDS given its relationship with psychotic disorders and PD. Prevalence rates of schizophrenia spectrum disorders in 22qDS are estimated to be greater than 25 % [24], with the anxiety or depression being positive predictors for the development of psychotic disorders [25]. Case reports have suggested an association with early-onset PD [26], with a more recent study indicating the onset of motor symptoms to appear between 39 and 49 years old [10]. Because of the high prevalence of psychotic disorder in 22qDS, the use of antipsychotics could confound this diagnosis.

However, in many cases there was still a progressive decline in motor function despite the discontinuation of antipsychotic medications, yet a noticeable improvement with the use of antiparkinsonian medication (L-dopa).

26.5 Autism Spectrum Disorders

A recent paper documented on a large scale the rates of various psychiatric and physical comorbidities in adults diagnosed with an autism spectrum disorder (ASD) [27]. A majority of adults with ASD were found to have at least one additional psychiatric condition, with anxiety disorders (29 %) and depressive disorders (25 %) being the most common. There was also an increase in suicide attempts compared to the general population with an odds ratio of 5.05. However, the authors note that of the documented suicide attempts, many patients did not have an underlying diagnosis of depressive disorders suggesting that depressive disorders may be underdiagnosed in this population. Adults with ASD were also found to have a 22-fold increased rate of schizophrenia when compared to the general population. Many chronic systemic medical conditions (dyslipidemia, hypertension, diabetes, vitamin deficiencies, etc.) were more frequent as well.

Key Points

- Common medical problems, such as hypothyroidism and vitamin deficiencies, and common psychiatric illnesses, such as depressive and anxiety disorders, are also common in the aging of patients with neurodevelopmental problems as described here. These problems are straightforward to treat after an on-call evaluation.
- General lifestyle changes such as exercise; avoidance of toxins, such as alcohol or opioid abuse; and good nutrition including vitamins and antioxidants can also be helpful in aging to stimulate neurogenesis and avoid oxidative stress and ROS that can be detrimental to neurons.
- Currently many new targeted treatments are being studied for the neurodevelopmental disorders described here including GABA $\alpha 5$ inverse agonists for DS [28], GABA agonists and IGF1 analogue treatment for FXS [28, 29], and allopregnanolone treatment, a natural neurosteroid and GABA agonist that stimulates neurogenesis and repair of white matter disease, for FXTAS [30]. These treatments may not only alleviate the neurodevelopmental problems but also aide in aging problems perhaps for the general population also.

Acknowledgments This work was supported by NICHD grant # HD036071 and the MIND Institute Intellectual and Developmental Disabilities Research Center (U54 HD079125).

References

1. Darnell JC, Klann E. The translation of translational control by FMRP: therapeutic targets for FXS. Nat Neurosci. 2013;16(11):1530–6.
2. Iossifov I, Ronemus M, Levy D, Wang Z, Hakker I, Rosenbaum J, et al. De novo gene disruptions in children on the autistic spectrum. Neuron. 2012;74(2):285–99.
3. Tassone F, Iong KP, Tong TH, Lo J, Gane LW, Berry-Kravis E, et al. FMR1 CGG allele size and prevalence ascertained through newborn screening in the United States. Genome Med. 2012;4(12):100. doi:10.1186/gm401.
4. Hagerman R, Hagerman P. Advances in clinical and molecular understanding of the FMR1 premutation and fragile X-associated tremor/ataxia syndrome. Lancet Neurol. 2013;12(8): 786–98.
5. Sellier C, Freyermuth F, Tabet R, Tran T, He F, Ruffenach F, et al. Sequestration of DROSHA and DGCR8 by expanded CGG RNA repeats alters microRNA processing in fragile X-associated tremor/ataxia syndrome. Cell Rep. 2013;3(3):869–80.
6. Polussa J, Schneider A, Hagerman R. Molecular advances leading to treatment implications for fragile X premutation carriers. Brain Disord Ther. 2014;3. doi:10.4172/2168-975X.1000119.
7. Giulivi C, Zhang YF, Omanska-Klusek A, Ross-Inta C, Wong S, Hertz-Picciotto I, et al. Mitochondrial dysfunction in autism. JAMA. 2010;304(21):2389–96.
8. Kaplan ES, Cao Z, Hulsizer S, Tassone F, Berman RF, Hagerman PJ, et al. Early mitochondrial abnormalities in hippocampal neurons cultured from Fmr1 pre-mutation mouse model. J Neurochem. 2012;123(4):613–21.
9. Utari A, Adams E, Berry-Kravis E, Chavez A, Scaggs F, Ngotran L, et al. Aging in fragile X syndrome. J Neurodev Disord. 2010;2(2):70–6.
10. Butcher NJ, Kiehl TR, Hazrati LN, Chow EW, Rogaeva E, Lang AE, et al. Association between early-onset Parkinson disease and 22q11.2 deletion syndrome: identification of a novel genetic form of Parkinson disease and its clinical implications. JAMA Neurol. 2013;70(11):1359–66.
11. Leehey M, Hall D, Liu Y, Hagerman R. Clinical neurological phenotype of FXTAS. In: Tassone F, Hall D, editors. The fragile X-associated tremor ataxia syndrome (FXTAS). New York: Springer Science & Business Media, LLD; 2016.
12. Hagerman PJ, Hagerman RJ. Fragile X-associated tremor/ataxia syndrome. Ann N Y Acad Sci. 2015;1338:58–70.
13. Winarni TI, Chonchaiya W, Sumekar TA, Ashwood P, Morales GM, Tassone F, et al. Immune-mediated disorders among women carriers of fragile X premutation alleles. Am J Med Genet A. 2012;158A(10):2473–81.
14. Todd PK, Oh SY, Krans A, He F, Sellier C, Frazer M, et al. CGG repeat-associated translation mediates neurodegeneration in fragile X tremor ataxia syndrome. Neuron. 2013;78(3):440–55.
15. Buijsen RA, Sellier C, Severijnen LA, Oulad-Abdelghani M, Verhagen RF, Berman RF, et al. FMRpolyG-positive inclusions in CNS and non-CNS organs of a fragile X premutation carrier with fragile X-associated tremor/ataxia syndrome. Acta Neuropathol Commun. 2014;2:162.
16. Roizen NJ, Patterson D. Down's syndrome. Lancet. 2003;361(9365):1281–9.
17. Zigman WB. Atypical aging in down syndrome. Dev Disabil Res Rev. 2013;18(1):51–67.
18. Head E, Silverman W, Patterson D, Lott IT. Aging and down syndrome. Curr Gerontol Geriatr Res. 2012;2012:412536.
19. Green T, Gothelf D, Glaser B, Debbane M, Frisch A, Kotler M, et al. Psychiatric disorders and intellectual functioning throughout development in velocardiofacial (22q11.2 deletion) syndrome. J Am Acad Child Adolesc Psychiatry. 2009;48(11):1060–8.
20. Stephenson DD, Beaton EA, Weems CF, Angkustsiri K, Simon TJ. Identifying patterns of anxiety and depression in children with chromosome 22q11.2 deletion syndrome: comorbidity predicts behavioral difficulties and impaired functional communications. Behav Brain Res. 2015;276:190–8.
21. Angkustsiri K, Leckliter I, Tartaglia N, Beaton EA, Enriquez J, Simon TJ. An examination of the relationship of anxiety and intelligence to adaptive functioning in children with chromosome 22q11.2 deletion syndrome. J Dev Behav Pediatr. 2012;33(9):713–20.

22. Schneider M, Debbane M, Bassett AS, Chow EW, Fung WL, van den Bree M, et al. Psychiatric disorders from childhood to adulthood in 22q11.2 deletion syndrome: results from the International Consortium on Brain and Behavior in 22q11.2 Deletion Syndrome. Am J Psychiatry. 2014;171(6):627–39.
23. Richards C, Jones C, Groves L, Moss J, Oliver C. Prevalence of autism spectrum disorder phenomenology in genetic disorders: a systematic review and meta-analysis. Lancet Psychiatry. 2015;2(10):909–16.
24. Murphy KC, Jones LA, Owen MJ. High rates of schizophrenia in adults with velo-cardio-facial syndrome. Arch Gen Psychiatry. 1999;56(10):940–5.
25. Gothelf D. Velocardiofacial syndrome. Child Adolesc Psychiatr Clin N Am. 2007;16(3): 677–93.
26. Zaleski C, Bassett AS, Tam K, Shugar AL, Chow EW, McPherson E. The co-occurrence of early onset Parkinson disease and 22q11.2 deletion syndrome. Am J Med Genet A. 2009; 149A(3):525–8.
27. Croen LA, Zerbo O, Qian Y, Massolo ML, Rich S, Sidney S, et al. The health status of adults on the autism spectrum. Autism. 2015;19(7):814–23.
28. Hagerman RJ, Hendren RL, editors. Treatment of neurodevelopmental disorders. New York: Oxford University Press; 2014.
29. Lozano R, Hare EB, Hagerman RJ. Modulation of the GABAergic pathway for the treatment of fragile X syndrome. Neuropsychiatr Dis Treat. 2014;10:1769–79.
30. Irwin RW, Solinsky CM, Loya CM, Salituro FG, Rodgers KE, Bauer G, et al. Allopregnanolone preclinical acute pharmacokinetic and pharmacodynamic studies to predict tolerability and efficacy for Alzheimer's disease. PLoS One. 2015;10(6):e0128313. doi:10.1371/journal.pone.0128313.

Underprivileged Geriatric Patients: On-Call Intervention, Bridging, and Recovery

27

Mariam Abdurrahman and Ana Hategan

27.1 Background

The underprivileged geriatric population is a heterogeneous group including (i) the materially deprived (e.g., the homeless and the precariously housed, the impoverished but domiciled), (ii) the socially deprived (e.g., socially isolated seniors including elderly shut-ins, refugees, and disadvantaged immigrants with limited ability to navigate and utilize community support agencies), and (iii) the psychologically deprived (e.g., elderly recluses including extreme typologies captured in the Diogenes syndrome spectrum and/or those with severe and persistent psychiatric illness).

These underprivileged groups face significant systemic issues, many of which lie outside the healthcare system, but which can be addressed to variable degrees as part of medical encounters. Specifically, healthcare professionals are, in essence, gatekeepers to a variety of systems access points which should be used to provide practical assistance that extends beyond the traditional clinician-patient encounter. This may appear overreaching and somewhat daunting, but the reality is that the presenting medical complaint exists within a context of upstream health determinants, so that the effectiveness of on-call encounters depends on consideration of these factors and attempts to ameliorate such factors as much as is feasible.

Interventions for underprivileged geriatric patients are thus unique and challenging, but can be implemented using practical approaches listed in Table 27.1, particularly in the inpatient setting where the episode of care is longer and typically occurs in a multidisciplinary setting. On-call interventions with this heterogeneous

M. Abdurrahman, MD, MSc, Dip (GHEI) (✉)
Department of Psychiatry, St. Joseph's Health Centre, Toronto, ON, Canada
e-mail: mariam.abdurrahman@medportal.ca

A. Hategan, MD
Department of Psychiatry and Behavioural Neurosciences, Division of Geriatric Psychiatry, Michael G. DeGroote School of Medicine, Faculty of Health Sciences, McMaster University, Hamilton, ON, Canada

A. Hategan et al. (eds.), *On-Call Geriatric Psychiatry: Handbook of Principles and Practice*, DOI 10.1007/978-3-319-30346-8_27

Table 27.1 Practical interventions in the management of underprivileged geriatric patients [1, 3, 4]

Item	Issue	Recommendation
Access to primary care	Lack of primary care physician (PCP) Frequent acute care service usage due to lack of PCP	Confirm health coverage, facilitate renewal as needed Make referral to accepting PCPs Provide information about mobile primary care clinics, mobile dentistry, and street- and shelter-based health clinics Provide information on local public health programs and services including dental and vaccination clinics
Bridging	Patient no longer requires acute admission but requires supportive environment to facilitate adherence with post-discharge recommendations	Identify respite care settings, e.g., medical shelter beds Liaise with community care services to provide medical support (wound care, medications, escort to medical appointments in post-discharge period) Day program referral to bridge until placement occurs
Housing	Homeless, precarious housing Housing inappropriate for functional needs	Liaise with community housing agencies for long-term shelters catering to older adults Social work referral for affordable housing unit Occupational therapy or home care nurse assessment for adaptive housing needs and level of independence
Immigration health needs	Complex presentation due to language barrier, lack of medical documentation, stigma	Identify and use cultural brokers if available Provide information about local agencies offering programs and services to recent immigrants Linkage with culturally relevant community services
Discharge planning	Patient with low level of health literacy, cognitive deficits, or communication deficits Continuity of care Complex psychosocial needs	Use transitional care facilitators including shelter-based patient navigators if available Provide patient a copy of discharge record and pocket cards listing most recent laboratory results and current medications Obtain case management to take effect at discharge Utilization of discharge principles described in Chap. 9

Table 27.1 (continued)

Item	Issue	Recommendation
Medication	Expense	Apply for old age drug card or disability drug
	Medication adherence	Blister packing, home support worker
	Polypharmacy	Medication reconciliation and simplification, identify high-risk medications and consider alternatives if possible
Preventive healthcare Infectious disease risk management	Vaccine preventable diseases: hepatitis B, influenza, pneumococcal and meningococcal vaccines TB screening	Administration as per national standards and guidelines
Sanitation	Infestation, e.g., bedbugs Functional barriers to cleaning Hoarding	Advocate for landlord to treat patient's unit Home care worker if patient qualifies Home care assistance with cleaning with patient consent Liaise with local health department to facilitate decongestion if health hazard exists
Service delivery model	Traditional primary care model incongruent with patient needs	Outreach case management model to assist patients with service navigation and facilitate communication between healthcare and social service professionals, thus improving patient engagement and follow-up

population will vary depending on the particular vulnerable group and the location of presentation. This chapter will largely focus on the materially deprived group of geriatric patients, particularly the aging homeless who now constitute almost a third of the homeless population in keeping with recent demographic shifts [1–4]. Aging homeless persons are recurrent users of acute care services [1–7] and are thus encountered often in on-call situations.

27.2 The Emergency Department Setting

Case Vignette: A complex patient of no-fixed address Mr. E was a 58-year-old man of no fixed address. He presented to the emergency department (ED) with recurrent falls that had been worsening over the preceding month. He had a history of schizoaffective disorder, alcohol abuse, and diabetes mellitus but was not followed for any of these conditions and did not take any medications. His presentation was notable for his aged appearance, postural instability, tremor, heavily stained and worn clothing, and the odor of urine which emanated heavily.

He was well known to the ED, with numerous episodic visits for nonurgent concerns. He was subsequently admitted to the general medical ward with an admitting diagnosis of "social admission" and then transferred to the psychiatric ward for treatment optimization for his schizoaffective disorder.

During the course of Mr. E's psychiatric admission, he was medically detoxified, but his gait symptoms appeared to be unchanged and he frequently complained of headaches, so computed tomography of head was conducted. He was then diagnosed with normal pressure hydrocephalus, which was missed on prior ED visits due to the impression that his postural instability, tremor, and general presentation were associated with alcohol abuse. Following surgical intervention and involvement of allied health professionals on the psychiatric ward, Mr. E was discharged to a respite facility for bridging in collaboration with a community support agency until accommodation became available in a supported independent living facility. He was discharged on a depot antipsychotic to facilitate adherence.

His admission was also instrumental in the renewal of his health insurance enrollment and application for disability benefits which instrumentally provided him with a pharmacy benefit card. Mr. E was still pre-contemplative with respect to his alcohol use but agreed to join a harm reduction program as he wanted assistance with moderating but not discontinuing his alcohol use. The ED and the supportive living agency completed an ED care plan with Mr. E, who agreed to use the agency's clinic for nonurgent health concerns.

The case vignette above reflects the recent but growing phenomenon of the graying of the homeless population, with reported high utilization of the ED [1–3, 5–7]. Relative to the conventionally defined geriatric age of 65 years and older, homeless persons age at a faster rate than their domiciled counterparts and are considered to be physiologically "aged" above the age of 50 [3, 8], with elevated prevalence rates of geriatric syndromes [1] as demonstrated in the case vignette. This accelerated aging is thought to stem from psychological and metabolic stressors associated with the harsh life of the streets [8]. Further discussion of geriatric syndromes in the aging homeless will emphasize the importance of screening underprivileged patients like the patient in the vignette.

The aged homeless population is vulnerable to a number of geriatric syndromes including functional impairment, cognitive impairment, depression, falls, frailty, sensory impairment, and urinary incontinence, at rates exceeding their age-matched domiciled counterparts as well as the general geriatric population [1–3, 5]. In fact, rates of these syndromes surpass the rates in non-homeless older adults 20 years older than homeless adults in the 50–64-year-old age group [1]. These geriatric syndromes are potentially amenable to amelioration but need to be detected; thus, screening is a key intervention in healthcare encounters with the aging homeless.

A number of abbreviated variations of geriatric screening instruments can be used efficiently in the fast-paced environment of the ED. The Mini-Cog, MoCA, and similar tools could be applied to identify those with major neurocognitive disorders as this is a red flag that contradicts discharge back to the streets or shelters where they are at high risk of victimization, further deterioration, and adverse events, particularly as they are unlikely to be able to adhere to medications, follow-up appointments, and aftercare on discharge [1, 4].

Those with a positive cognitive screen or with frank cognitive impairment unrelated to substance intoxication should trigger disposition to an appropriate setting. The presence of social workers in the ED to facilitate the process may potentially allow the application of more extensive screening tools such as the Identification of Seniors at Risk (ISAR) screening tool which was developed to improve the recognition of older ED patients at risk for adverse outcomes [9, 10]. The ISAR tool examines social, physical, and mental risk factors, medical history, and the use of medical services, medications, and alcohol, with the most specific and sensitive items related to sensory impairment, medications, and depression. The ISAR screener also serves as a predictor of return visits to the ED within 30 days [10–12]. Predictors of return include depressive symptoms, frailty, history of heart disease, history of diabetes mellitus, poor self-reported health, poor baseline functional status, having ever been married, not drinking alcohol, a recent ED visit, lack of support, age 85 years or older, and living alone [11, 12].

Falls present another geriatric syndrome commonly seen in geriatric ED patients. A number of hospitals utilize a fall risk assessment tool to identify high-risk patients. While numerous such tools exist, the challenge is in identifying one that can be seamlessly used in the ED. Patients with a single geriatric syndrome likely have more than one syndrome and should thus trigger evaluation for additional geriatric syndromes. Most of the syndromes mentioned above have screening tests that can be administered in less than 5 min [2] and should thus be incorporated into encounters with aging homeless patients.

Beyond treating the immediate chief complaint, practical interventions in such encounters requires consideration of housing status which is often overlooked [7] but is essential to post-discharge prognosis, particularly the likelihood of presenting to the ED again. Homeless persons consistently report that they are not asked about their housing status in the course of a hospital visit although this is a key determinant in their ability to follow through on post-discharge treatment and follow-up. Patients discharged to homeless shelters often report being resigned to poor coordination and poor transitions in care between the hospital and shelter [7]. Additionally, this expectation and reality of suboptimal transition exacerbates delays in seeking care, which contributes to end-stage disease presentations and the increased mortality rates seen among the homeless persons [1–3]. The essential role of handover during transitions is discussed in further detail in Chap. 9.

Access to non-acute health services by homeless adults is usually limited by difficulty in navigating health and social service systems and limited self-efficacy in competing for health and social services in the traditional institutional settings [13, 14]. As such a number of homeless older adults utilize the ED for routine care as they also have difficulty accessing and/or following up with scheduled primary care appointments. Another barrier lies in the lack of valid identification and current health insurance (as in Canada's publicly funded universal health insurance system) or lack of enrollment for health insurance coverage in the US medical system that commonly occurs among homeless persons. An ED visit for nonurgent care presents an opportunity to provide linkage with case management agencies, public programs, and community health centers that can provide unscheduled primary care visits and assist with completing applications for medical insurance coverage and other social benefits. The ED social worker is in a position to initiate such links, as a number of aging homeless may not know about social benefits they are entitled to and how to access them.

ED visits labeled with a chief complaint of "social visit" should not be trivialized, as homeless patients frequently have underlying chronic medical conditions that should be addressed as part of the visit, in addition to linking patients with community support agencies. The case vignette is not an uncommon occurrence, with missed diagnoses and missed opportunities to intervene and bridge patients earlier in their course of acute care usage thus preventing further deterioration and use of limited acute care service resources.

In the case of socially deprived groups such as refugees and disadvantaged immigrants, cultural considerations are an important factor in identifying how best to provide acceptable bridging, intervention, and recovery-oriented supportive care. Cultural factors may limit or skew expressions of psychiatric illness, thus contributing to missed opportunities for on-call intervention. Shame and stigma may limit patients' willingness to accept bridging services, particularly if perceived to be outside the bounds of "treatment." Those new to the country face challenges in navigating community programs and services that are well versed in assisting those with psychiatric illness and may thus present to the ED with nonurgent concerns. Part of the healthcare encounter will need to include education and redirection to more appropriate care and service settings. The use of case management is again advantageous when available as it facilitates advocacy for the underprivileged patient.

The psychologically deprived group perhaps presents the most challenging group of underprivileged geriatric patients. In particular, elderly recluses and uncommon extremes such as Diogenes syndrome require very careful attempts at intervention [15]. They rarely present voluntarily and typically come to attention because of concerned neighbors, family members, or public authorities such as the fire, police, or other municipal departments. Although research on this group is limited, an outreach model of bridging, intervention, and supportive care is perhaps the best way to negotiate access on an ongoing basis as they are highly unlikely to utilize acute care services and are similarly unlikely to attend follow-up.

27.3 The Inpatient Setting

The inpatient admission provides a wider window for initiating more comprehensive interventions much as illustrated in the case vignette. Similarly, many of the practical interventions suggested in Table 27.1 are likely best accomplished in the inpatient setting as part of the treatment plan. On admission, the multidisciplinary team should evaluate not only the chief complaint and comorbidities, but the outpatient context in which these conditions occur so as to optimize discharge planning.

Screening tools are again invaluable in identifying and stratifying patient risks. Extensive screening tools such as the comprehensive geriatric assessment (CGA) [16] or equivalent should ideally be applied to all geriatric patients on admission to identify high-risk patients and implement interventions aimed at risk management while also reducing the likelihood of return visits and readmission. The CGA covers four major domains: (i) a 7-item somatic domain (which notably includes mobility and stability, medication, nutrition, continence, skin, pain and allergies), (ii) a 5-item psychological domain, (iii) a 6-item functional domain, and (iv) a 3-item social domain [16]. For psychiatric wards with an underpowered multidisciplinary team, it is important to consider consulting other services such as geriatric medicine to assist with a more comprehensive assessment of vulnerable patients.

Beyond management of the admitting diagnosis, discharge planning is perhaps the single most important element during the course of admission. As with the ED, consideration of domicile status is essential as this is a key factor in the likelihood of failed discharge. Other essential aspects of discharge planning include assessment of access to primary care and referral to a primary care physician for those lacking one. For the highest risk patients and the most marginalized patients, where possible, facilitation of case management is essential to post-discharge care and treatment adherence, particularly in those with chronic systemic medical and psychiatric illnesses [1, 3, 4] (see Table 27.1).

Medication reconciliation constitutes another key element of discharge planning (see Chap. 9) in order to optimize the likelihood of adherence and follow-up. Linkage with a community health center with multidisciplinary staffing including pharmacy counseling, social workers, and nutrition educators presents an ideal primary care setting if available. Discharge planning should also consider the risk of readmission, flagging those at high risk in order to triage post-discharge follow-up and select an appropriate setting for outpatient care coordination, particularly for patients that lack a primary care physician. Essential items to consider in the readmission risk assessment are illustrated in Fig. 27.1 [10–12, 17].

In summary, the underprivileged geriatric population comprises of a heterogeneous group, each with unique health vulnerabilities that require recognition in order to tailor and optimize on-call interventions, bridging, and recovery. Furthermore, recognizing the underprivileged population is important as healthcare encounters with them uniquely require clinicians to look beyond the chief complaint lens and consider other factors driving the presentation. Consideration of health factors upstream of the chief complaint, notably determinants of health like housing and social supports, is required in order to deliver more informed interventions to this diverse vulnerable population.

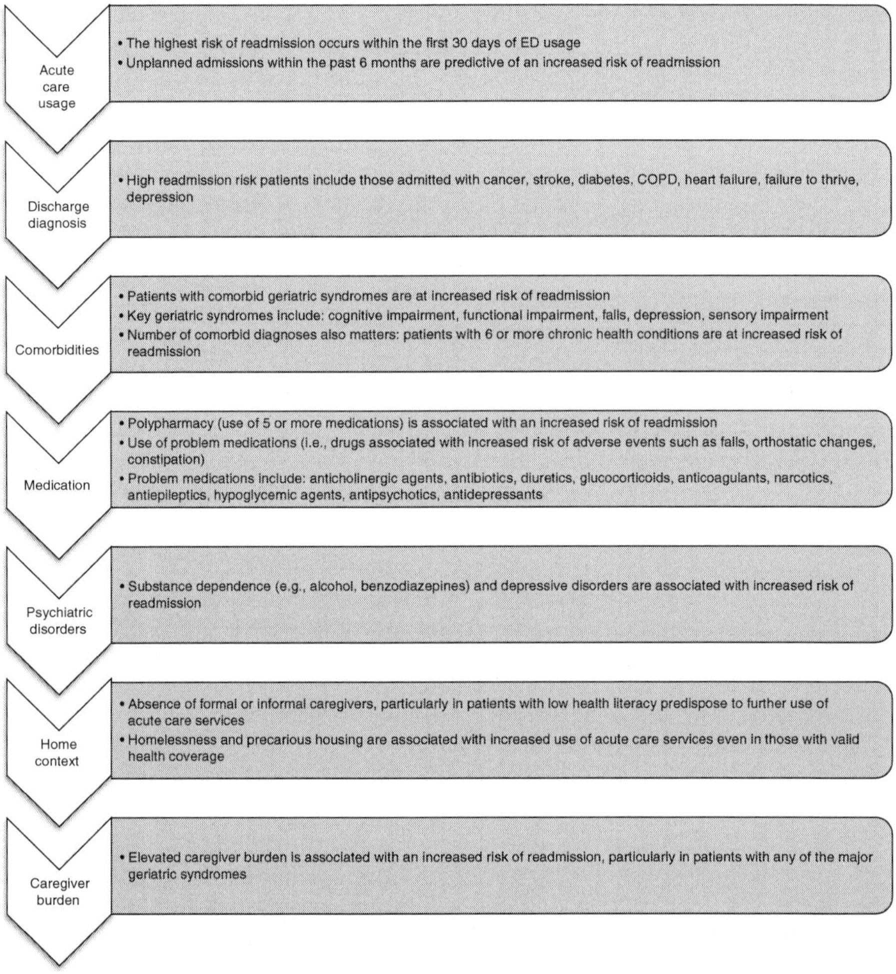

Fig. 27.1 Factors contributing to readmission of underprivileged geriatric patients [10–12, 17]

Key Points

- Underprivileged geriatric patients include a diverse spectrum of individuals.
- Underprivileged groups face significant systemic issues that require shifting the healthcare lens beyond the traditional chief complaint lens.
- ED encounters with underprivileged patients should require a high index of suspicion to apply screening tools in identifying the highest risk patients.
- The homeless age faster than their domiciled counterparts and should be viewed as being aged with more complex health issues once beyond the age of 50.

- Geriatric syndromes are present at higher rates among the aging homeless than their domiciled counterparts and the general geriatric population.
- Geriatric syndromes common among the homeless include cognitive and functional impairment, frailty, falls, depression, sensory impairment, and urinary incontinence.
- Inpatient encounters should optimize the use of a multidisciplinary team in attending to the systemic issues facing underprivileged patients.
- Discharge planning should include consideration of housing status and discharge location as factors determining adherence to follow-up plans.
- Evaluation of the risk of readmission is an essential element of discharge planning.
- Recognition of underprivileged populations is essential in tailoring and optimizing on-call interventions, bridging, and recovery.

References

1. Kushel M. Older homeless adults: can we do more? J Gen Intern Med. 2013;27(1):5–6.
2. Brown RT, Kiely DK, Bharel M, Grande LJ, Mitchell SL. Use of acute care services among older homeless adults. JAMA Intern Med. 2013;173:1831–4.
3. Hahn JA, Kushel MB, Bangsberg DR, Riley E, Moss AR. The aging of the homeless population: fourteen-year trends in San Francisco. J Gen Intern Med. 2006;21(7):775–8.
4. Sermons MW, Henry M. Demographics of homelessness series: The rising elderly population. Homeless Research Institute: National Alliance to End Homelessness. 2010. http://www.endhomelessness.org/page/-/files/2698_file_Aging_Report.pdf. Accessed 10 Aug 2015.
5. Brown RT, Kiely DK, Bharel M, Micthell SL. Geriatric syndromes in older homeless adults. J Gen Intern Med. 2012;27:16–22.
6. Brown RT, Kimes RV, Guzman D, Kushel M. Health care access and utilization in older versus younger homeless adults. J Health Care Poor Underserved. 2010;21(3):1060–70.
7. Greysen SR, Allen R, Lucas GI, Wang EA, Rosenthal MS. Understanding transitions in care from hospital to homeless shelter: a mixed-methods, community-based participatory approach. J Gen Intern Med. 2012;27(11):1484–91.
8. Epel ES. Psychological and metabolic stress: a recipe for accelerated cellular aging? Hormones. 2009;8(1):7–22.
9. McCusker J, Bellavance F, Cardin S, Trépanier S, Verdon J, Ardman O. Detection of older people at increased risk of adverse health outcomes after an emergency visit: the ISAR screening tool. J Am Geriatr Soc. 1999;47:1229–37.
10. Wilder S. Geriatric emergency medicine. 2012. Available http://newfrontiers.americangeriatrics.org/chapters/pdf/rasp_3.pdf. Accessed 14 Aug 2015.
11. McCusker J, Cardin S, Bellavance F, Belzile E. Return to the emergency department among elders: patterns and predictors. Acad Emerg Med. 2000;7:249–59.
12. McCusker J, Bellavance F, Cardin S, Belzile E, Verdon J. Prediction of hospital utilization among elderly patients during the 6 months after an emergency department visit. Ann Emerg Med. 2000;36:438–45.
13. Garibaldi B, Conde-Martel A, O'Toole TP. Self-reported comorbidities, perceived needs, and sources for usual care for older and younger homeless adults. J Gen Intern Med. 2005; 20(8):726–30.

14. Nakonezny PA, Ojeda M. Health services utilization between older and younger homeless adults. Gerontologist. 2005;45:249–54.
15. Waserman J, Hategan A, Bourgeois JA. Harnessing neuroplasticity in Diogenes syndrome: a proposed mechanism to explain clinical improvement. Gen Hosp Psychiatry. 2014;36(6):761.e3–5.
16. Buurman BM, Parlevliet JL, van Deelen BA, de Haan RJ, de Rooij SE. A randomised clinical trial on a comprehensive geriatric assessment and intensive home follow-up after hospital discharge: the Transitional Care Bridge. BMC Health Serv Res. 2010;10:296.
17. South Carolina Hospital Association. Best practice report project BOOST: better outcomes for older adults through safe transitions. 2012. http://www.scha.org/files/documents/bpr_project_boost_better_outcomes_for_older_adults_through_safe_transitions.pdf. Accessed 20 Sept 2015.

On-Call Teaching and Education 28

Sheila Harms and Karen Saperson

28.1 Background

While psychiatry residents may have on-call experiences in a variety of settings such as inpatient units or chronic care facilities, the emergency department (ED) is likely the most common setting for postgraduate residents in psychiatry to encounter a spectrum of psychiatric problems marked by patient heterogeneity, acuity, and crisis. For this reason, the authors focused on the ED as a setting where supervisors and postgraduate residents in psychiatry were most likely to encounter geriatric patients and related psychiatric presentations. It is important to note that most psychiatry supervisors in the ED setting do not have specialized training in geriatric psychiatry; however, it will require requisite knowledge and skills within geriatric psychiatry to provide adequate care for this patient population. Although the practice of supervision is commonplace for most general psychiatrists, formal training in teaching and supervisory skills remains uncommon [1]. When considering care for geriatric patients with psychiatric problems in the ED, the role of the supervising psychiatrist differs from other settings because of the associated acuity, systemic medical comorbidity, and the increased time required for managing complex problems. The emergency room can therefore be a daunting place for both teaching and learning specific to the geriatric psychiatry patient. The supervising psychiatrist

S. Harms, MD (✉)
Department of Psychiatry and Behavioural Neurosciences, Faculty of Health Sciences, Michael G. Degroote School of Medicine, McMaster University, McMaster University Medical Centre, Hamilton Health Sciences Corporation
1200 Main St. West, Hamilton, ON L8S 4K1, Canada
e-mail: harmssh@hhsc.ca

K. Saperson, MBChB
Department of Psychiatry and Behavioural Neurosciences, Division of Geriatric Psychiatry, Faculty of Health Sciences, Michael G. Degroote School of Medicine, McMaster University, St. Joseph's Healthcare, W5th Campus, 100 W5th Street, Hamilton, ON L8N 3K7, Canada

A. Hategan et al. (eds.), *On-Call Geriatric Psychiatry: Handbook of Principles and Practice*, DOI 10.1007/978-3-319-30346-8_28

may alleviate challenges within the ED environment by recognizing the supervisor competencies necessary to optimize learning for trainees in this setting.

In answering the question "what makes a good clinical teacher in medicine?," Sutkin and colleagues [2] identified "cognitive" and "noncognitive" characteristics of effective medical teachers/supervisors in a systematic literature review. While the ability to demonstrate clinical competence (i.e., technical skills and clinical reasoning) and to impart knowledge were labeled as cognitive characteristics, skills necessary for excellence in teaching and supervision were frequently designated as noncognitive abilities. The latter included the ability to establish a positive relationship with a resident, create a supportive learning environment, demonstrate excellence in communication skills, display enthusiasm in a way that motivates the resident and finally, exhibits self-awareness leading to reflection and improvement about one's teaching abilities. Scheepers and colleagues [3] noted that extraverted physicians are consistently rated as better supervisors. While these innate personality traits are helpful in the educational milieu, the authors also found that providing a motivating learning climate, clearly communicating learning goals as well as providing constructive feedback is also important for an educator to consider.

Case Vignette You supervised a third-year resident on call. During the shift, the resident had been asked to assess a 79-year-old male from a local assisted living facility, who presented in the ED with:

- A recent history of confusion, paranoid delusions, and aggressive behavior
- Marked impairment in functioning (i.e., not eating, refusing to bathe) and judgment
- Previously diagnosed hypertension and diabetes mellitus

On examination, the resident described the patient as markedly agitated and malodorous. He flinched when approached by hospital staff, and the resident noticed bruises on his scalp, right wrist, and flank. The resident asked you to attend the ED in person to assist with the clinical complexity.

After arriving in the ED and directly observing the resident, you made the following observations:

- The resident was eager to learn but struggled to elicit a complete history. Additionally, the resident described lack of clarity about privacy legislation and permitted "circle of care" for the purpose of information gathering.
- The resident demonstrated a lack of familiarity with the recommended workup for delirium.
- The resident articulated concerns about how to approach the issue of possible elder abuse.
- The resident requested support in responding to ED pressures to determine a rapid disposition for the patient.
- The resident struggled with the challenge of managing this complex situation as a priority with several other patients waiting for assessment.

Applying the literature to the case scenario suggests that creating an inspiring learning atmosphere, which motivated the resident to be intellectually curious about potential learning opportunities, is one of the first critical tasks for the supervisor. This can be done through role modeling one's own curiosity about the case and engaging the resident in clarifying a few pertinent learning questions for consideration while on shift. Given the described challenges articulated by the resident as well as the inherent complexity associated with the clinical vignette, it is important to acknowledge the probable apprehension on the part of the resident in tackling this particular learning challenge, at the same time recognizing the other responsibilities for the resident in the ED. This form of rapport building is also noted to be an important strategy in establishing the supervisor-resident relationship. In addition to these noncognitive abilities, taking the opportunity to ask directed questions which allow the resident to grapple with some clinical issues related to diagnostics (i.e., possible delirium and related differential diagnosis) and management is also essential in this vignette.

The movement toward competency-based medical education (CBME) in North America has led to scholarly discussions about the "competencies" required of medical educators. Srinivasan and colleagues [4] developed a framework to support such teaching standards using the Accreditation Council for Graduate Medical Education (ACGME) criteria and the CanMEDS roles as defined by the Royal College of Physicians and Surgeons of Canada [5]. They identified six core competencies as appropriate for all medical supervisors/educators: content knowledge specific to the medical discipline, resident centeredness, skills in the domain of communication and interpersonal relatedness, role modeling and professionalism, practice-based reflection, and system-based practice.

An important component of the psychiatrist's role as a supervisor is to not only teach and model the art and science of psychiatry but also provide the resident with meaningful feedback for ongoing educational development while role modeling the provision of excellent clinical care [6]. Specific applications to the current case scenario suggest an opportunity for the supervisor to role model a firm, respectful and fair approach with ED colleagues in insisting on sufficient time to interview the patient and caregivers, as well as the completion of an adequate medical workup prior to disposition decisions. The psychiatry supervisor can then take the opportunity to specifically highlight the various physician roles associated with the case including advocating for patient-centered care as well as insisting on appropriate investigations required to work through a reasonable differential diagnosis for delirium; a condition which carries significant mortality and morbidity if not adequately managed. This may require consultation from and collaboration with internal medicine colleagues prior to transferring the patient. The supervisor may also take the opportunity to note elements of the case that would necessitate urgency as it pertains to priority setting within the ED environment. In our case, this would include a requirement to skillfully and sensitively probe the issue of elder abuse (also see Chaps. 13 and 14) and to address potential ageism in colleagues who may see elderly confused individuals as "less deserving" of acute care resources (also see Chap. 5).

28.2 Context Is Everything: Supervision in the Emergency Department

The notion of *context specificity* is recognized as a salient learning influence in medicine. Residents who demonstrate clinical skills and problem-solving abilities in one setting may or may not perform similarly in other educational milieus [7]. In geriatric psychiatry, residents may obtain clinical mastery in the community where assessments occur over several hours often in collaboration with interprofessional colleagues, but struggle to apply these skills within the ED where, comparatively, time and human resource constraints are common. The very nature of the ED creates a unique educational environment marked by large patient volumes and diverse clinical presentations with variable acuity. Brief patient encounters with frequent interruptions and high turnover rates in often overcrowded spaces separate the ED from other practice settings. This, along with divergent opinions about the establishment of a patient's medical stability prior to psychiatric referral, sets the stage for a challenging teaching, learning, and working environment.

In order to adequately support residents, psychiatry supervisors must be aware that geriatric patients presenting to the ED have unique clinical and service needs. Colenda and colleagues [8] note that the ED is often the gateway to access mental health services for geriatric patients. Common emergency room presentations for older adults necessitating psychiatric evaluations include dementia-related bizarre or aggressive behaviors, delirium, psychosis, depression, substance use disorders (including withdrawal states), neuropsychiatric symptoms secondary to general medical conditions, and psychosocial difficulties such as caregiver burnout, isolation, neglect, or elder abuse. It is imperative that the psychiatry supervisor appreciates the many barriers that exist in delivering effective psychiatric emergency services for geriatric patients. Commonly, there is a lack of coordination between primary care providers and community-based psychiatry services making it difficult for the older adult to obtain effective services in the community [9]. Once in the ED, it is not uncommon for the geriatric patient to have difficulty articulating a "chief complaint." An example is the geriatric depressed patient who presents with a chief complaint of constipation, demonstrating rumination and preoccupation with bowel function, resulting in depressive symptoms being missed (also referred to as "depression without sadness"). Supervisors need to be vigilant for negative attitudes toward older individuals and in particular adverse stereotypes toward older adults with mental illness [10, 11].

Geriatric psychiatry supervisors must be familiar with the literature that suggests geriatric patients are less likely to receive an adequate medical workup in the ED, therefore possibly leading to ineffective treatment [12]. Long periods of time are often required to obtain an adequate psychiatric history from a geriatric patient, which includes collateral information from reliable resources such as other family members or caregivers. Supervisors must encourage residents to slow the interview pace with a geriatric patient to ensure an adequate and fulsome understanding of concerns, something which is often counterintuitive to the tempo within a busy ED setting. Other issues constraining the psychiatric interview with the geriatric patient may be related to sensory loss (i.e., hearing, vision), language spoken, and lack of privacy, decisional capacity for informed consent, as well as concomitant physical discomfort or pain. Attending to these aspects of care can make a substantial difference in the interview experience for the patient but may require extra work in a setting that feels rushed or overextended at times. The net effect for both psychiatry residents and supervisors alike in the emergency department can be an overwhelming sense of chaos, if not adequately prepared. However, unique learning opportunities are available if the supervisor understands what knowledge, skills, and attitudes are required of the resident in the ED.

Milestones as defined by the Accreditation Council for Graduate Medical Education (ACGME) are behaviorally anchored, observable clinical skills, behaviors, or outcomes for medical trainees within a supervised residency or fellowship program [13]. Milestones are used to determine "competency" and provide meaningful feedback on the trainee's performance across the training spectrum. The milestones are graded and therefore reflect a continuum of skill acquisition throughout the training spectrum, from the novice postgraduate trainee to the independently practicing physician. Similarly, the Royal College of Physicians and Surgeons of Canada have developed an educational paradigm referred to as "Competence by Design" (CBD), which articulates a learning progression throughout postgraduate training [14] and into consultancy, consisting of developmental milestones which are considered to be the "building blocks" of "entrustable professional activities" (EPAs) that constitute the work of a competent psychiatrist. Within CBD, competencies for seven essential physician roles are developed for each specific discipline. These roles include medical expert, communicator, scholar, advocate, manager/leader, collaborator, and professional and are referred to as the "CanMEDS roles." Specific competencies for geriatric psychiatry are in various stages of development across Canada and the USA; however, at the time of publication, no specific milestones and EPAs had been formally developed for residents training in geriatric psychiatry. Bourgeois and colleagues [15] argue that the current educational arena embracing competency-based education provides a unique opportunity for residents to focus on scholarship within their learning experience where scholarship extends beyond the idea of research. In the authors' opinions, scholarship is defined broadly as discovery, integration, application, and teaching [16].

The supervising physician in the case scenario must be aware of competencies at various levels of training and use graded expectations as an objective benchmark for the resident's learning. Specifically, the supervisor's presence in the ED and ability to observe the resident in real-time engenders an opportunity for rich, specific feedback about the resident's strengths and struggles. Respectfully and authentically engaging the resident in a self-reflective exercise to better identify specific areas of content deficit is essential in determining a realistic, resident-focused education plan. Using milestones as achievement anchors, the supervisor can assist the resident in determining specific learning goals that map directly onto current skills and abilities. Once the learning foci are explored and agreed upon (e.g., evaluation of capacity for the purpose of sharing medical information), an effective strategy for the supervisor would be to ask the resident to engage in a learning prescription about these concepts, follow-up with the supervisor a few days after the call-shift to discuss what the resident learned and how the learning could be integrated and applied in other cases. The resident could then be encouraged to consolidate this learning through teaching residents in more junior years.

28.3 Specific Teaching Strategies in the Emergency Department

Molinaar and colleagues [17] have developed a teaching framework that highlights specific educational requirements for supervisors. These authors suggested that educators in the emergency room must have an understanding of how educational experiences for residents in the emergency setting are different compared to other organized educational experiences embedded into other core learning activities. For psychiatry supervisors, it is essential to appreciate what educational opportunities related to geriatric psychiatry patients are inherent within the ED so that appropriate teaching strategies and techniques can be applied. Table 28.1 summarizes some "teaching on the fly" strategies that may be utilized in a busy setting such as the ED in order to enhance resident experiences [5, 17–21].

Table 28.1 Teaching strategies in the emergency department [5, 17–21]

Teaching strategies	Brief description
1-min preceptor method	1. *Get a commitment:* ask the resident a direct question and have them verbally commit to an answer Example: "What treatment options would be appropriate for this patient?" 2. *Probe for supporting evidence*: ask the resident to provide clinical reasoning or cite studies to support their answer 3. *Give feedback*: reinforce what the resident did well and discuss areas for further learning 4. *Teach a general principle:* explain how the information learned can be generalized to other situations 5. *Conclusion:* ask the residents about additional questions or clarifications [17, 18]
SNAPPS (summarize, narrow, analyze, probe, plan, and select)	In the resident-centered framework, the resident is first asked to summarize the history and physical findings of a clinical case and then narrow the differential diagnosis through clinical reasoning. The resident then probes the supervisor with questions or clarifications to assist with the development of a management plan. Finally, the resident selects areas for ongoing learning and research so as to improve any areas of performance that the supervisor felt to need attention [19]
"Aunt Minnie"	In this teaching model, the supervisor focuses on assisting the resident develop rapid pattern recognition. In other words, if the resident sees a person who looks like your Aunt Minnie – she probably is your Aunt Minnie. Using this framework, the resident completes a history and physical independently and then presents a short summary to the supervisor with a differential diagnosis and preferred diagnosis. The supervisor then independently sees the patient and develops a management plan. The supervisor and resident then discuss the case, while the supervisor highlights teaching points. This model can be particularly efficient in the emergency room setting [20]

Table 28.1 (continued)

Teaching strategies	Brief description
The teachable moment	Within each clinical exchange, there are many moments worth highlighting, making them relevant to a resident's needs. In this teaching framework, the supervisor intentionally emphasizes a specific and salient learning point, otherwise referred to as the "brief clinical pearl" for the resident. Using direct observation, the supervisor can promote the "teachable moment" whereby he/she provides feedback about a particular observed skill [5]
Ask-tell-ask	In this "feedback sandwich" model, the supervisor indicates to the resident that he/she will be providing feedback. Prior to doing so, the supervisor asks the resident to evaluate his/her performance (i.e., how do you think you did?). Following this, the supervisor provides both positive and corrective feedback based on his/her observations, comments on the resident's self-assessment, and suggests a learning plan moving forward. The supervisor ends by asking the resident about his/her understanding of the educational plan and identified strategies for improvement [21]

Key Points

- Supervisors must create a stimulating learning environment to engage postgraduate residents. This involves taking the time to inspire intellectual curiosity for the resident as it relates to geriatric psychiatry.
- For a multitude of reasons, older adults are less likely to receive an adequate medical workup in the ED, possibly leading to ineffective treatment. This clinical challenge needs to be highlighted for residents in the ED and role modeled where appropriate.
- Longer periods of time are often required to obtain an adequate psychiatric history from a geriatric patient, often necessitating multiple sources to corroborate an accurate picture. Encourage residents to take this time to complete a thorough ED assessment.
- Medical complexity is the norm in geriatric patients, requiring a broad differential diagnosis in the face of behavioral presentations for older adults. Residents must be challenged to problem solve through numerous etiologies and request help from other disciplines where relevant.
- Residents must be aware of the impact of sensory impairments and concomitant physical discomfort/pain on the assessment process of emotional and behavioral disturbance in geriatric psychiatric syndromes.
- Psychiatry supervisors must familiarize themselves with current information about developmental milestones in order to provide appropriate "stage of training" and behaviorally anchored feedback to residents.
- Knowledge of evidence-informed educational frameworks and teaching tips will be an asset to psychiatry supervisors in the ED.

Acknowledgment The authors would like to acknowledge Dr. Shadi Aminololama-Shakeri for editorial contributions in the writing of this chapter.

References

1. Hatem CJ, Lown BA, Newman LR. The academic health center coming of age: helping faculty become better teachers and agents of educational change. Acad Med. 2006;81:941–4.
2. Sutkin G, Wagner E, Harris I, Schiffer R. What makes a good clinical teacher in medicine? A review of the literature. Clin Ed. 2008;83:452–66.
3. Scheepers RA, Lombarts KMJMH, van Aken MAG, Heineman MJ, Arah OA. Personality traits affect teaching performance of attending physicians: results of a multi-centre observational study. PLoS One. 2014;9(5):e98107. doi:10.1371/journal.pone.0098107.
4. Srinivasan M, Li ST, Meyers FJ, Pratt DD, Collins JB, Braddock C, et al. "Teaching as a Competency": competencies for medical educators. Acad Med. 2011;86(10):1211–20.
5. Competence by design -http://www.royalcollege.ca/portal/page/portal/rc/resources/cbme/resources. Accessed 26 Aug 2015.
6. Birnbaumer DM. Every physician is a teacher: bedside teaching in the Emergency Department. Seattle: American College of Emergency Physicians' Scientific Assembly; 2007.
7. Eva KW. On the generality of specificity. Med Ed. 2003;37(7):587–8.
8. Colenda CC, Greenwald BS, Crossett JH, Husain MM, Kennedy GJ. Barriers to effective psychiatric emergency services for elderly persons. Psychiatr Serv. 1997;48(3):321–5.
9. Beland F, Lemay A, Philibert L, Maheux B, Gravel G. Elderly patients' use of hospital-based emergency services. Med Care. 1991;29(5):408–18.
10. Greenstein RA, Ness DE. Psychiatric emergencies in the elderly. Emerg Med Clin North Am. 1990;8(2):429–41.
11. Kennedy GJ, Lowinger R. Psychogeriatric emergencies. Clinics Ger Med. 1993;9:641–53.
12. Waxman HM, Carner EA, Dubin W, Klein M. Geriatric psychiatry in the emergency department; characteristics of geriatric and non-geriatric admissions. J Am Geriatr Soc. 1982; 30:427–32.
13. The psychiatry milestone project – http://www.acgme.org/acgmeweb/Portals/0/PDFs/Milestones/PsychiatryMilestones.pdf. July 2015. Accessed 26 Aug 2015.
14. Neher JO, Gordon KC, Meyer B, Stevens N. A five-step "microskills" model of clinical teaching. JABFP. 1992;5(4):419–24.
15. Bourgeois J, Hategan A, Azzam A. Competency-based medical education and scholarship: creating an active academic culture during residency. Perspect Med Educ. 2015;4(5):254–8. doi:10.1007/s40037-015-0218-4.
16. Glassicm CE. Boyer's expanded definitions of scholarship, the standards for assessing scholarship and the elusiveness of the scholarship of teaching. Acad Med. 2007;75:877–80.
17. Molinaar WM, Zanting A, van Beukelen P, de Grave W, Baane JA, Bustraan JA, et al. A framework of teaching competencies across the medical education continuum. Med Teacher. 2015;31:390–6.
18. Walsh A. The one-minute preceptor. Five microskills method. 2004. http://fhs.mcmaster.ca/facdev/documents/oneminutepreceptor.pdf. Accessed 26 Aug 2015.
19. Wolpaw TM, Wolpaw DR, Papp KK. SNAPPS: a resident-centred model for outpatient education. Acad Med. 2003;78:893–8.
20. Irby DM, Wilkerson L. Teaching when time is limited. BMJ. 2005;336:384–7.
21. Konopasek L, Mutnick A, Encadela J. Beyond the feedback sandwich: fun tools for improving feedback skills. 2014. http://restech.ccnmtl.columbia.edu/mod4/Mod4_Feedback.ppt. Accessed 4 Aug 2015.

Index

A. Hategan et al. (eds.), *On-Call Geriatric Psychiatry: Handbook of Principles and Practice,* DOI 10.1007/978-3-319-30346-8

B

Q

R

S